Cardiac Catheterization and Angiocardiography

Cardiac Catheterization and Angiocardiography

DAVID VEREL M.A., M.D., F.R.C.P.
Consultant Cardiologist to Sheffield Area Health Authority (Teaching)
Lecturer in Cardiology in the University of Sheffield
Sometime Beit Memorial Research Fellow

RONALD G. GRAINGER M.D., F.R.C.P., D.M.R.D., F.R.C.R., F.A.C.R.(Hon.)
Northern General Hospital, Sheffield 5
Consultant Radiologist to Sheffield Area Health Authority (Teaching)
Clinical Teacher in Radiodiagnosis in the University of Sheffield
Visiting Professor, Radiology Department, Stanford University, Palo Alto, California, U.S.A.

With a chapter on echocardiography by

D. R. NAIK M.B., Ch.B., D.M.R.D., F.R.C.R.
Consultant Radiologist to Sheffield Area Health Authority (Teaching)
Clinical Teacher in Radiodiagnosis in the University of Sheffield

Foreword by
SIR JOHN McMICHAEL M.D., F.R.C.P., F.R.S.

Sometime Director, Postgraduate Medical Federation, London
Sometime Professor of Medicine, Royal Postgraduate Medical School, London

THIRD EDITION

CHURCHILL LIVINGSTONE
EDINBURGH LONDON AND NEW YORK 1978

CHURCHILL LIVINGSTONE
Medical Division of Longman Group Limited

Distributed in the United States of America by
Longman Inc., 19 West 44th Street, New York,
N.Y. 10036 and by associated companies,
branches and representatives throughout
the world.

© Longman Group Limited 1978

First Edition 1969
Second Edition 1973
Third Edition 1978

ISBN 0 443 01374 8

Library of Congress Cataloging in Publication Data
Verel, David.
  Cardiac catheterization and angiocardiography.

  Bibliography
  Includes index.
  1. Cardiac catheterization. 2. Angiocardiography.
I. Grainger, Ronald Graham, joint author.
II. Title. [DNLM: 1. Angiocardiography.
2. Heart catheterization. 3. Heart catheterization-
Instrumentation.   WG141 V491c]
RC683.5.C25V47   1976   616.1′2′07572   76–28433

Printed in Great Britain by
T. & A. Constable Ltd., Edinburgh

Foreword

Dr Verel and Dr Grainger are rendering a valuable service in outlining the place of cardiac catheterization and angiographic methods in the modern study of cardiac problems. Without this vast increase in precision of diagnostic techniques, the miracles of modern cardiac surgery would be impracticable. In commending their book, it may be salutary to recall some of the early history of the development of these valuable procedures and the generally conservative attitudes with which they were at first received.

The story goes back to 1929 when Dr Werner Forssmann was a resident in the Augusta Victoria Hospital at Eberswald, near Berlin. In those days, anaesthetic deaths were not uncommon and he had had the experience of seeing intrapericardial haemorrhage result from the heroic intracardiac injections of adrenalin normally used in such emergencies. He conceived the idea that it would be safer to inject adrenalin through a catheter passed via an arm vein into the heart. To prove its safety he asked a fellow resident to undertake this procedure on his own person. The catheter was passed as far as the axilla when Forssmann's associate took fright but Forssmann himself with the catheter in position walked to the radiological department and, with a radiographer holding a mirror in front of the screen, completed the procedure and took pictures of the catheter in his own right atrium. He felt nothing and no harm resulted. Naturally excited by the possibilities, he later made several further efforts including the injection of concentrated sodium iodide to obtain rather faint angiograms of the right heart and pulmonary vessels. He catheterized his own heart nine times in all and after this, was unable to do any more as he had used up all his available superficial veins. He contacted Professor Sauerbruch, then the leading surgeon in Berlin, to see whether any use could be made of the catheterization procedure in diagnosis or management in a cardiac surgical clinic. Sauerbruch's reaction was that 'he ran a clinic not a circus'! Orthodoxy banished Forssmann from the university world. In 1949 when I visited Germany on behalf of the British Council, I asked 'Where was Forssmann?' His name had been forgotten but Professor Spang of Heidelberg located him in practice in a small town in the Rhine valley. I was able two years later to enlist Forssmann's help in recording the story of catheterization in a teaching film made by I.C.I. and a few years later Forssmann justifiably shared a Nobel Prize with Cournand and Richards.

Forssmann's work, however, was not neglected in other countries. Jimenez-Diaz in Spain realized the possibility of using this technique to get right heart samples for the measurement of cardiac output. He recorded one such attempt but did not follow the matter up. In Portugal, De Carvalho and colleagues used the technique to obtain angiograms of the root vessels of the lung, clarifying much confusion in the interpretation of the branching shadows in the lung roots. Ameuille and others in Paris made similar pictures but all these procedures involved 'quick in and quick out' intracardiac injections. By the time of the outbreak of war in 1939, however, there were on record no less than about 110 occasions on which intracardiac catheterization had been done without trouble to the patient or any recognizable harm.

The war then demanded effort by investigators on the nature of wound shock and a great deal of the investigative endeavour would naturally fall on civilian hospital teams. At the Bellevue Hospital, New York, civilian accident cases came under the investigative supervision of Dr D. W. Richards and Dr André Cournand. They asked their hospital board's permission to study such gravely injured patients by intracardiac catheterization and permission was given. In 1941 Cournand and Ranges published their paper in the Proceedings of the Society for Experimental Biology and Medicine.

I had been intrigued by the possibility of measuring the cardiac output which started with my student contact with Meakins and Whitteridge Davies in Edinburgh. They had made many efforts to obtain the gaseous composition of right heart blood by various indirect rebreathing techniques and the results sometimes seemed surprising, such as a fairly normal cardiac output in the presence of cardiac valvular disease. Such findings led to widespread doubts about the validity of these methods! I had been working (1930–33) on portal congestion and the regulation of portal venous pressure in Aberdeen and in University College Hospital Medical School, London. My interest in the regulation of venous pressure led me to consider making a study of the general congestive phenomena of cardiac failure. In 1932 Grollman had published his book on cardiac output based on the use of the acetylene method for its estimation. I talked to Samson Wright about this and he invited me to come to his department at the Middlesex, a short walk from University College, where he put Grollman's apparatus at my disposal. There were considerable technical difficulties in getting good results with the acetylene method owing to analytical inaccuracies from the high solubility of acetylene in the carbon dioxide absorbent. Realizing the difficulty, Samson Wright suggested that we eliminate this by using a very small volume of caustic soda in a manometric Van Slyke apparatus which would at least reduce and standardize the amount of acetylene which disappeared in solution. This involved the construction of a special Van Slyke gas chamber with a trap at the bottom for ejection of the gas absorbent mixtures. A small glass blower near Queen Square made it for me very cheaply and I took it with me when I returned to the Physiology Department in Edinburgh. The method worked out splendidly. My first paper on cardiac output was rejected for Clinical Science as Thomas Lewis at that time thought that 'the readers of Clinical Science had little interest in the cardiac output'!

In 1935 Professor T. R. Harrison published his book on *Failure of the Circulation*. In this book he took into account all published reports of the measurement of cardiac output in heart disease and, accepting the finding that the cardiac output might not be unduly depressed even in heart failure, he evolved the concept that heart failure was a 'dyskinetic syndrome', output being maintained at the expense of venous congestion. I found this an exciting and challenging concept and as I was now given charge of beds in Professor Ritchie's wards in the Edinburgh Royal Infirmary, I extended my cardiac output studies in heart failure with resulting confirmation of the validity of many of Harrison's views.

When I returned to London in 1939, I was able to continue with the acetylene technique. Although the method was practicable and indeed sufficiently accurate to give results of great interest, it was cumbersome and took the better part of a day to work out and cross-check a single estimation. With my colleague Sharpey-Schafer at Hammersmith, we were indeed trying to make use of the acetylene method for the estimation of cardiac output changes following venesection in blood donors, but the results were too difficult to obtain to give any adequate sequence of cardiac output changes following blood loss.

When we read Cournand and Ranges's paper in 1941, new possibilities suddenly appeared. We realized that Cournand had shown that it was possible to put the catheter into the right atrium and *leave it in situ* for periods of an hour or so, during which sequential observations could be made. It took a little while to persuade our radiological colleagues to cooperate in cardiac catheterization but we began work in the autumn of 1942. The first patient studied was a young man with asthma who became extremely cyanotic in the attacks and whose cyanosis was far in excess of what might be expected from our lung function tests at that time. He proved to have an atrial septal defect through which he was developing a right to left shunt during his attacks. We also began to study patients in heart failure, and to document the consequences of digitalis administration. The improvements in circulatory states which followed our efforts led some of the patients in subsequent hospital admissions to complain of the delay in putting the 'tubes' into their arms!

Our growing experience was convincing us of the wide range of applicability of the new technique. We wished to extend our experience with normal subjects acting as blood donors and I went to see Sir Edward Mellanby, then Secretary of the Medical Research Council. We wanted to get the blessing of the Wound Shock Committee on a request for volunteers. Mellanby's reaction was that no Committee could give its approval of such an unorthodox procedure and that the responsibility must lie with ourselves. He would have no objection, however, to a personal approach from ourselves to the Friends Ambulance Unit and this was made. The first volunteer for cardiac output determination during a venesection indeed bore the name of Cadbury. In order to get the maximum information from these volunteers, we had now obtained the cooperation of Professor Henry Barcroft and Dr O. G. Edholm, who were in a position to make peripheral blood flow studies simultaneously with measurement of the total circulation. I well remember the excitement of observing for the first time the intense vasodilatation of the forearm vessels during a post-haemorrhagic faint. While the war continued with its inevitable increase in the hazards to life, volunteers were not difficult to persuade as they had the feeling that they were contributing to the war effort by helping in these researches.

In December 1943 Sharpey-Schafer and I made our communication to the Physiological Society at University College Hospital Medical School. Sir Thomas Lewis was in the chair. He described our opening paper as 'startling' and at the lunch-table he shook his head hinting that we should abandon the procedure. Sir Henry Dale also at the table, however, took a different view and said that the total record of experience which we had assembled (394 cases) seemed to establish the practicability and safety of the technique and that it was too valuable to be dropped. His powerful and influential support was indeed a great encouragement.

It was already becoming clear that the diagnostic possibilities of the method were enormous as well as the value of the technique in the study of pharmacological and therapeutic effects. We were at that time timidly limiting ourselves to right atrial catheterization and simple saline manometry. The results obtained were precise as far as they went but we went wrong in our interpretation of digitalis action as we failed to realize that a reduction of right atrial pressure could result from improved ventricular function *irrespective* of cardiac output change. Our early approach was, perhaps understandably, too conservative and we did not get round to making optical records of changes in intraventricular pressure through the cardiac cycle until 1948. Indeed, we had hesitated to record from the right ventricle because of possible risks and in any case we thought that optical recording from a long catheter might be misleading and inaccurate. Furthermore, the habit of economy was ingrained in the penury of wartime academic life. We had no special laboratory, no radiological equipment of our own, and most of our apparatus was home made. By 1948 Cournand and his colleagues in New York had gone well beyond what we had achieved with our simpler and more limited techniques. The development of surgery for congenital heart disease by Blalock and Taussig in Johns Hopkins had also opened a new chapter. The method of catheterization made modern cardiac surgery possible and the subsequent development of cardio-angiography soon arrived. It now became fashionable and justifiable to demand increasingly costly apparatus. Special radiological laboratories were fitted out as the procedures became obligatory for precision of diagnosis and safety for the patients.

I am grateful for the opportunity to put a little of the early struggles on record. The modern application of these techniques is splendidly outlined in this book which I can heartily commend.

1969   JOHN MCMICHAEL

Preface to the Third Edition

It is a measure of the rapid advances is the field of cardiovascular investigation that extensions and much rewriting should be needed so soon after the last edition. A new section on echocardiography has been written by Dr D. R. Naik; the sections on calculated data and coronary arteriography have been considerably extended and the chapter on radiographic equipment completely rewritten to include information on the latest equipment.

We have resisted the suggestions of some reviewers to expand this book into a textbook of cardiovascular disease. We hope it remains a primer, an introductory manual to be read critically as a guide to a difficult craft. The atlas should be treated as a picture book showing, in the main, common conditions, and limited by the impossibility of showing cine film.

Throughout the text of the manual it has been our policy to select illustrations which are of average quality obtained at routine cardiac catheterisation. This inevitably means that features such as alternating current interference with the electrocardiogram will appear as they will frequently do in most catheter laboratories. Similarly, many pressure tracings are of less than perfect quality because on many occasions such tracings have to be accepted as the best obtainable under the conditions of work. The illustrations in the atlas section have all been obtained at routine diagnostic cardiac catheterization. The angiographic radiographs were all taken on a bi-plane Schönander AOT changer and have been selected from a very large number of patients studied in the last 15 years. The basis of their selection is their relative high quality, suitability for reproduction as illustrations and because of the wide range of conditions which they illustrate.

While many conditions mentioned in the text are illustrated in the atlas, both text and atlas are intended to complement each other and may be studied separately.

The text has been thoroughly revised throughout, the atlas extended, and the bibliography has been enlarged. The comments of reviewers of this manual have been of real value in preparing this edition.

D.V.
R.G.G.

1978

Preface to the Second Edition

In this second edition the text has been completely revised and several chapters have been re-arranged and extended. Recently introduced equipment and procedures have been included, and a new chapter on coronary arteriography has been added.

The Atlas section of the book has been considerably extended by the addition of many new angiocardiograms, and the section has been re-arranged and numbered so that illustrations of the same patient are now included under the same Figure numbers (e.g. Fig. 57 A, B, C, D).

As in the first edition, the emphasis is on attempting to provide a rational explanation of the technical methods employed in the current practices of cardiac catheterization and angiocardiography. It is hoped that the second edition will continue to provide a practical manual both for the cardiologist and the radiologist.

D.V.
R.G.G.

Sheffield, 1973

Preface to the First Edition

Cardiac catheterization has been used for the diagnosis of disease of the heart for nearly a quarter of a century. During this time the techniques have remained basically three: the visualization of the heart chambers, the identification of shunts and the measurement of pressure in the heart chambers and blood vessels. Advances in technique have included an increasing refinement of apparatus and a multiplication of the methods available for the demonstration of the three parameters measured. Cardiac surgery has been established as a result of the diagnostic precision achieved by cardiac catheterization: the results of cardiac surgery have, *pari passu,* justified the development of cardiac catheterization.

The increasingly complex instrumentation available for cardiac catheterization has been accompanied by a corresponding increase in the complexity of the investigations themselves. Most noteworthy in this respect has been the development of selective angiocardiography and its incorporation as part of the catheterization along with oximetry, pressure measurement, and other techniques. This has brought together what were, as recently as ten years ago, separate investigations. The postgraduate entering the field of cardiac catheterization is therefore faced by a complex discipline which makes use of a wide range of different techniques.

We have found that, despite wide reading, postgraduate students have difficulty in making an appropriate choice of method during cardiac catheterization. There appears to be no simple manual which presents the available techniques as parts of a single integrated investigation. In general, cardiologists have more experience of venous catheterization, whilst radiologists have developed a considerable experience of arterial puncture and catheterization. Because of this, a tendency has developed in many departments for cardiologists to undertake right heart catheterization and angiography, while radiologists practise retrograde left heart catheterization and angiography. Our department has tended to adopt a similar pattern of work, but there is no sharp division. Indeed, it is our belief that both the cardiologist and the radiologist who undertake cardiac catheterization should be competent in catheter approaches to both sides of the heart. In writing this book we have tried to present an introductory account of a single craft which makes use of many widely different techniques. We hope that it will provide the trainee cardiologist with a sufficient background knowledge of the radiological aspects of angiocardiography, and inform the radiologist of the basic concepts of haemodynamics and modern investigation techniques so that both may become competent and versatile in adopting an integrated approach to cardiac catheterization and angiocardiography. We have included only a few references: a full bibliography will be found in Zimmerman's series of monographs.

Inevitably, an account of this kind is coloured by our own experience and practice. We have both, however, watched catheterizations performed in many other centres at home and overseas. Our own practice has therefore been modified by that of others, and in writing this book we have tried to take some account of preferences other than our own.

The techniques of cardiological diagnosis discussed in this handbook are entirely dependent on the coordinated efforts of many people. In particular, we wish to record our thanks to Dr R. E. Nagle, Dr N. H. Stentiford and other registrars who have undertaken many catheterizations, to our cardiological technicians, our radiographers and our nursing staff. We owe a real debt to the thousands of patients whom we have investigated. Without their fortitude and confidence we would have accomplished little.

The illustrations of the text and of the atlas are the work of the Photographic Departments of the Sheffield Area Health Authority (Teaching). We are particularly grateful for the excellent service which they have so willingly provided, and for the admirable blocks made by our publishers.

Several secretaries have typed our manuscripts, and to these also, our thanks are proffered.

We are honoured to include a foreword by Professor Sir John McMichael, F.R.S.

D.V.
R.G.G.

Sheffield, 1969

Contents

1. Methods of Recording

Recording characteristics

In the course of investigating the cardiovascular system it may be necessary to record a wide variety of phenomena. Events as different as the respiratory cycle and the heart sounds may have to appear upon the same record. Satisfactory work is only possible if there is some understanding both of the characteristics of the phenomena being recorded and of the apparatus in use. Since all observations depend ultimately upon some recording system for their expression, it is desirable to begin a work of this type with a general consideration of the available recording techniques. Certain properties are common to all recording systems and must be understood by those working with them. We shall consider: (1) frequency and frequency response; (2) amplitude of response; (3) linearity of response and (4) damping and overswing.

Frequency is a term usually applied to a phenomenon that is repeated in a regular cycle. Thus, one may speak of respiration having a frequency of 16 or 50 cycles per minute, depending on its rate. Similarly the heart rate may have a frequency of 70 or 250 per minute depending on circumstances, while the heart sounds may have frequencies of several thousand cycles per second (c.p.s., or Hz for 'hertz'). A 'cycle' implies that the phenomenon repeats itself. One complete waveform from start to finish constitutes a cycle (Fig. 1.1). When the event is

non-repetitive, for example the rise in skin temperature that follows peripheral nerve block, the term 'cycle' is not appropriate, but the recurrent rise and fall in finger tip temperature that follows immersion in ice water (what Lewis termed 'hunting') can fairly be called a cycle although its 'period' (the time for a complete cycle) is several minutes.

The frequency response of a recorder is the maximum frequency that can be recorded faithfully. This may be low, as in the float recorders used in limb plethysmography or spirometry, which may become inaccurate at rates over about 25 cycles per minute (c.p.m.), particularly if the excursion made by the instrument is large. Alternatively the frequency response may be high, as in the cathode ray oscilloscope, which can follow precisely anything likely to be encountered in cardiovascular work. In considering the purchase of equipment, the nature of the work to be recorded must be carefully related to the frequency response of the apparatus (Fig. 1.2).

The amplitude of the response is a fundamental property in any recorder. It ranges in complexity from the length of the wooden spill attached to a float recorder to make the excursion on a smoke drum equal approximately (say) 1 cm rise for each 5 ml increase in volume, to the electronics needed to provide a range of responses in an oscilloscope enabling any voltage from 1000 to 1 V to give a deflection of precisely the same degree in the electron beam. In considering equipment, the cost and amplitude of response are usually closely linked, high sensitivity and high cost going together. Here the likely use of apparatus is again of prime importance. There is no point in spending large sums of money on sensitive equipment if it is only to monitor the electrocardiogram in postoperative cases. Equally, if a direct writing recorder is in use, it is not going to produce the high sensitivity necessary for a precise analysis of the wave form of an intracardiac pressure tracing. The pros and cons of various recording systems are considered later.

Linearity of response is now found in most recording systems available commercially. By 'linearity' is implied a constant excursion for a given change over the whole range of the recorder movement. The usual fault in recording systems is a progressive lessening in the movement produced by a given change as the recording rises above the base line. For example, in a recorder which is tracing blood pressure, it may be that a change from 0 to

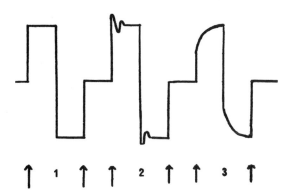

FIG. 1.1 Diagrammatic representation of a square wave oscillation. 1. Critically damped. 2. Underdamped showing overswing. 3. Overdamped showing loss of the square wave form. In each case a complete cycle has been represented as a positive deflection followed by an equal negative one. An example of a square wave with a wholly positive deflection is shown in Fig. 1.4.

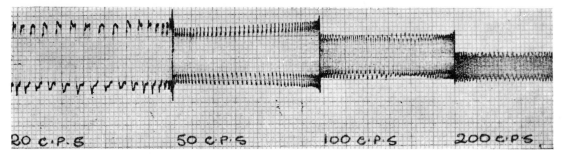

FIG. 1.2 The effect of increasing the frequency beyond the capacity of a recorder. The instrument was a standard direct writing electrocardiograph of Continental make. A square wave is recorded at 20, 50, 100 and 200 Hz (c.p.s.), the voltage being constant. Even at 50 Hz the recorder shows a falling off in the amplitude of the response, with a progressively poorer performance as the frequency is increased. Clearly the phonocardiograph attachment sold with this instrument can give only a crude indication of the sounds occurring in the cardiac cycle.

10 mmHg causes a rise of 1 cm while a change from 100 to 110 mmHg causes a rise of only 0·6 cm. Clearly a recording system of this kind presents great difficulties if it is used for anything more than a qualitative record.

Damping is a term which is applied to any reduction in the frequency or amplitude of a phenomenon caused by the characteristics of the recording system. Such a reduction may be deliberate or accidental, and it is necessary to distinguish clearly between them. Undesirable damping may occur in a simple float recorder if the needle bearings, about which the float rotates, are too tightly screwed up. Similarly, in the recording of intracardiac pressures by electronic transducer, damping will occur if the recording system contains an air bubble, or if blood or X-ray contrast medium fills the catheter instead of the less viscous saline or dextrose solution, or if the hot stylus is adjusted to press too hard on the heat sensitive paper of a direct writing recorder (Fig. 1.3). Whatever the cause, the effect is a reduction in the amplitude of the recording and of the frequency response of the system.

Damping is deliberately introduced into recording systems for a variety of reasons. That most commonly found is concerned with 'over-swing' (Figs. 1.1 and 1.4). This use of damping is similar to that employed in the springing of a motor car. Here the frequency of the springs of the car is such that if no damping were applied the passengers would soon be bounced into travel sickness. The car dampers apply a graduated friction which smooths the natural oscillations imparted to the springs by the irregularities in the road surface. Examples of this type of damping are built into recording systems to prevent the inertia of the system causing oscillations—

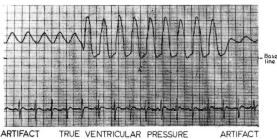

ARTIFACT   TRUE VENTRICULAR PRESSURE   ARTIFACT

FIG. 1.3 A pressure tracing showing the artefact which may be produced by damping. Throughout this tracing the catheter tip lay within the ventricle. Initially, a small air bubble was present in the catheter. The removal of this produced a normal ventricular tracing and at the end of a period of recording, the tap between the pressure head and the catheter was turned off. The pressure head was sufficiently sensitive to record a pressure tracing despite the rather loose tap obstructing the fluid column. Similar damping might be due to blood clot in the catheter or contrast medium of high viscosity.

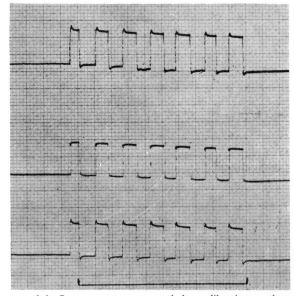

FIG. 1.4 Square waves generated by calibrating a three channel electrocardiograph. The centre channel is slightly overdamped, the other two slightly underdamped. Recorded at 50 mm/s.

for example, most galvanometers are just sufficiently damped by some mechanical device to make them swing steadily to an indicated reading and then stop. Such damping is precisely calculated to reduce the overswing to a desired degree without affecting the amplitude of the response, and is termed '*critical damping*'. Without it the recorder swings beyond the end point and then reaches its final deflection after a series of diminishing oscillations. Too much damping reduces the frequency response, obliterating fine detail, and reduces the amplitude of the response progressively as the damping increases until an oscillation such as the electrocardiogram (E.C.G.) is converted to a straight line. Damping of this degree is used in pressure recorders for obtaining mean pressure recordings. The degree of damping is usually ascertained by recording a so-called 'square wave'. This may be a change in pressure, volume, electrical potential or voltage, depending on the recorder, but whatever the quantity changed, it has the characteristics shown in Figure 1.1, i.e. the transition from one value to another is achieved as nearly instantaneously as possible.

Deliberate damping may be employed for a rather different reason in the recording of pressure during cardiac catheterization. The pressure transducers used in this work are necessarily extremely sensitive with a high frequency response. They will, therefore, record not only the pressure waves occurring in the heart and vessels but also pressure changes of higher frequency originating in the liquid filled catheters which connect the pressure sensitive device to the site from which the record is being made. These high frequency pressure oscillations are similar to the vibrations in an organ pipe which is resonating, or in a length of central heating pipe which is struck by a hammer. They are generated by the movement imparted to the catheter by the beating heart and their frequency is a function of the bore of the catheter, having lower frequencies in wider bore catheters. They may occur throughout the pressure cycle or be generated only at certain times in the cycle, as, for instance, at the onset of the systole when the movement of the heart is particularly likely to tap the side or end of the catheter (Fig. 1.5). Undesirable oscillations of this kind may be removed by suitable damping. The mechanism for achieving this is built into the amplifiers in most apparatus and acts by reducing the frequency response. In some centres critical damping is applied to each catheter by introducing a suitable length of capillary tubing between the catheter and the pressure transducer. This latter technique is not easy and carries the hazard that any oscillation occurring in the tracing which has the frequency that is being damped out will be eliminated—in other words the damping process cannot distinguish between pressure changes generated in the heart and those generated in the catheter if they are of the same frequency. In general it is safest to record a length of un-

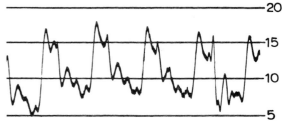

FIG. 1.5 A very badly distorted pulmonary artery tracing. This normal pulmonary artery pressure (15/5) is grossly distorted by harmonic pressure waves in the catheter tubing. The basic pressure change due to the heart action is overlayed by a coarse oscillation having a frequency of about 0·2 s.

damped tracing followed by a tracing with as much damping as is needed to clarify the record. When the artefact is large, it may be impossible to eliminate it without applying so much damping that the amplitude of the recording is reduced and the tracing thereby falsified.

Finally, there is the *natural resonant frequency* inherent in any fluid-filled system. This property is used in the organ pipe which is tuned to the frequency of the reed at its base so that the sound is amplified. In the cardiac catheter system, resonance is a complex function of the length of the catheter, its bore, the elasticity of its walls, the shape of the chamber in the transducer and the nature of pressure-sensitive element of the transducer. The ideal system should have a flat response to frequencies above those encountered in the heart beat. Scruggs *et al.* (1975) in a study of the properties of catheters and transducers found that the best recording characteristics are found in short, wide-bore catheters with stiff walls such as the U.S.C.I. trans-septal Brockenborough catheter. The longer, thin-walled polyethelene catheters had the least satisfactory characteristics. The semiconductor transducer which has a minute pressure displacement gave a better performance than the straingauge transducer which has an oscillating metal diaphragm.

Types of recorder
Recorders used in cardiovascular work are, with very few exceptions, designed to measure changes in voltage, or by a mechanical system to appreciate displacement or volume change. It can be surprisingly difficult to record a large mechanical movement with a small electrical one as anyone who has tried to get the output from a venous occlusion plethysmograph on the same record as an electrocardiogram and a pressure tracing can testify. In most recording systems some compromise also has to be reached between the frequency response of the recording (this is usually limited by the mass of the recording stylus), the frequencies of the parameters being measured, and the cost of the apparatus. Other considerations may

also play a part—for example the amount of processing needed to render a recording available, or the need for having records in a permanent, durable form suitable for incorporation in hospital notes. In deciding on methods, delineating the scope of an investigation, and assessing the value of results, a thorough knowledge of the potentials and limitations of the various recording systems available is essential.

Brodie bellows

In its original form the Brodie bellows consisted of a small bladder which lay between a fixed lower platform and a hinged upper plate to which a stylus was attached. The stylus inscribed a smoke drum. Volume changes were imparted to the bladder which moved the hinged plate. The record produced by this simple system is not linear, but a more sophisticated version of the same thing does give a linear record over a considerable part of its range, and is easily made from plastic sheet and either celluloid or perspex. It is a sensitive recorder which has little inertia and can be made in any size from about 1·5 cm diameter up to over 30 cm diameter (Fig. 1.6). It has many advantages over the float recorder.

Float recorder

This exists in many forms, two being common. In one, a hinged open box traps air in a water bath, and a stylus

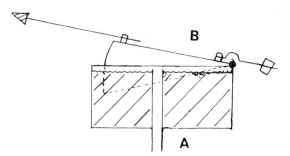

FIG. 1.7 A float recorder. In this instrument a thin brass float with an open lower surface traps air over a water-filled tank (A). The pointer is counterbalanced and the inertia of the float considerable. The sensitivity depends on the area of the water surface trapped and on the pointer length. Increasing the length of the pointer makes the instrument more sensitive and the record more nearly linear but also increases inertia and so increases the tendency for the water in the reservoir to oscillate, thus offsetting by counteroscillation the gain in sensitivity. Rapid movements are damped out by this water movement.

moves up and down to record changes in volume (Fig. 1.7). The bell recorder (Fig. 1.8) has the advantage of being precisely linear over the whole of its range. It is usually employed for this reason for spirometers. The float recorder is not precisely linear, but the error is negligible over much of its range, and when used at right angles to the recording paper can usually be arranged to stop recordings when it reaches a significantly alinear part of its range, by the simple device of having a pen length so short that the point leaves the paper. In arranging this type of recorder there is again a compromise: the longer the stylus the more nearly linear the record and the greater the inertia of the recording system. The bell recorder is obviously less sensitive than the float.

The main disadvantage of these recorders is their failure to record accurately when the excursion demanded of them is either rapid or large. This comes about because the water which acts in both types as a seal can move up and down in the opposite phase to the recorders themselves. This means that in rapid deep breathing, for example, as the bell of a spirometer is forced up by expiration there is a simultaneous movement of the water in the bell going downwards, with a complementary upwards movement of the water outside the bell. Bernstein and Mendel (1951) have proposed a partial solution to this dilemma: a very light bell of wide diameter, but this is attaining a more accurate record by sacrificing sensitivity, for a wider bell will have a smaller excursion per unit of volume.

Bubble recorder

The inertia of the preceding recorders is considerable, and they are incapable of making faithful records of rapidly changing events. Where considerable changes in

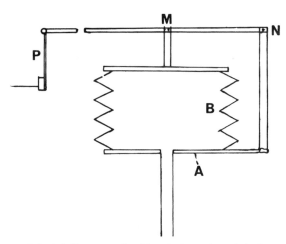

FIG. 1.6 A bellows recorder. The platform, A, and the levers are made of perspex or celluloid. M and N are light joints made with hypodermic needle tubing pinned through the plastic. The pen (P) is made from a celluloid tube and sheet with a stainless steel tubing stylus. The bucket reservoir of the pen holds a drop or two of ink. In this type of recorder the linearity of the record depends on the relations between P, M and N, and the sensitivity on the length of M to P (as well as the area of the bellows, B). Increasing the distance M–P makes the recording more sensitive as well as more nearly linear. The light weight of the moving parts makes this a relatively sensitive recorder.

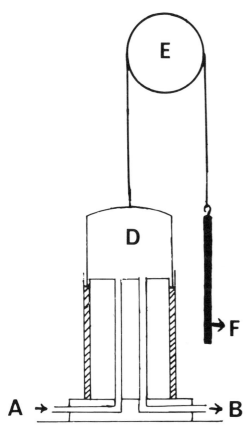

FIG. 1.8 A bell recorder. The tube (A) leads air into the bell (D) in which air is trapped over a water seal which is shown hatched. Air leaves the bell by tube (B). A counter-weight and pointer (F) balance the bell by means of a pulley (E). This apparatus gives a linear record over its whole range. The sensitivity is a function of the area of the bell and so of its diameter. Large oscillations of low frequencies are well recorded but rapid or small movements are damped by movements of the water which is forced down inside the bell and up outside when the bell is blown rapidly up, and vice versa.

volume or displacement are concerned. it is surprisingly difficult to devise a recording system that is of low inertia and that is genuinely recording the change observed, and not some function such as pressure change or rate of change of pressure which is dependent on the phenomenon under observation. For example, the device sold with most multichannel E.C.G. recorders for arteriometry is a piezo-electric crystal. Placed over an artery or other pulsation, it will produce what appears to be a convincing record of movement. Comparison with a recorder which is truly recording displacement, however, reveals that the the record is distorted, and is really a record of the *rate of change* of position. Small displacements can be accurately followed by suitable devices, e.g. those used by Mounsey (1962) and by Nagle (1967),

but large volume changes are difficult to record in detail. The bubble recorder is sometimes a convenient answer to this problem. It consists of a suitable length of glass tubing which is wet inside with a detergent solution. A bubble is formed in the tube which is connected by wide bore tubing to the apparatus whose pulsation is to be recorded. The recording tube is arranged along the slit of a photographic recorder and the bubble illuminated so that its shadow falls on the recorder paper.

Galvanometers

The great majority of data recorded in cardiovascular work is recorded by galvanometers of some sort or another. For the purposes of this discussion they may conveniently be divided into three groups—direct writing, ink jet and photographic.

Direct writing instruments consist of a stylus attached to a magnet which oscillates in a magnetic field. The changes recorded are made to affect the field and so the position of the magnet. Suitable damping is built in to the apparatus to prevent overswing, and most instruments are linear in their response. The record is inscribed either by a hot wire on heat sensitive paper or by a capillary tube touching the paper which draws an ink line by capillary attraction. The advantages of this type of recording are that it is immediately available for inspection, is reasonably permanent, and is easily copied. The main disadvantages are the poor frequency response and its limited capacity for recording detail at high sensitivity. These recorders cannot exceed a frequency of about 90 Hz (Fig. 1.2), and attempts to record at high sensitivity are often limited by the limited excursion of the recording arm. It is also impossible to superimpose simultaneous recordings. Despite these limitations they remain the most frequently employed recorders, being used universally for routine electrocardiography and many other purposes. They have the same limitations as the previously described mechanical recorders—a large movement needs a long and heavy lever.

Ink jets are a partial answer to the poor frequency response of the direct writer. In those instruments the stylus tip does not quite touch the paper and the ink either runs out by siphonage or is blown out under pressure. The stylus writes in an arc (as does the ink direct writer) which makes the records difficult to quantitate if the area described by the writer is important. The line traced is rather thick. Some instruments have an exasperating habit of going dry at inconvenient moments, and some have an equally disastrous capacity for making puddles of recording ink on records. Frequency responses as high as 500 Hz are claimed for the more sophisticated instruments. With the latest instruments the tracings can be superimposed.

Photographic recording dispenses with the inertia of the recording stylus and the drag of friction on recording paper. Small mirrors are mounted on the coils of the galvanometers and are used to reflect light which shines through a suitable slit. The light may impinge on bromide paper which provides an excellent black on white record, but which requires development and fixing like any bromide photographic print. Alternatively, immediate recording paper using an ultraviolet light source is available. The records obtained with the latter system are adequate, but have rather poor contrast, making reproduction difficult. This is important as the records may fade if exposed to light. On the whole, the increased complication of bromide paper recording, despite its delays and risks of spoiled records is preferable in the authors' view to the present direct photographic recording systems. Frequencies up to 1000 Hz can be recorded with suitable galvanometers, making this the only system really suited to the production of permanent phonocardiograms of high quality, and the nature of the light beam makes it possible to use the full width of the recording paper for any parameter measured. It is also possible to increase the sensitivity so that only part of a tracing takes up the full width of the record, making detailed analysis of parts of tracings possible. This type of recording is essential for most units undertaking research, but is time consuming in circumstances where much routine work is done. A satisfactory compromise where circumstances allow is achieved by providing both direct writing for routine work and photographic recording for research.

Oscilloscopes

These provide the most sensitive records available, having practically no limit to their frequency response and being capable of tremendous amplification. Their main limitation is the problem of providing permanent records of the tracings described by the electron beam on the oscilloscope tube. Photography, either with a conventional camera or a polaroid instrument is useful, e.g. for recording vector cardiograms, but the use of oscilloscopes is largely in *monitoring* changes to avoid the continuous recording of phenomena of little permanent interest. The most up to date instruments can be supplied so that the record seen on the oscilloscope is precisely that to be recorded on the photographic paper. On others with independent amplification in the oscilloscopes, the records may differ in a misleading fashion, e.g. an adequate oscilloscope movement may be present when the amplification on the recording paper is far too small. Mention of vector cardiography is a reminder of the use of the oscilloscope as a tool for integrating data. By applying data to the X axis and Y axis of the oscilloscope simultaneously, it is possible to record the resultant of two factors, e.g. the vector cardiogram. Similarly a continuous pressure–flow record can be made to show changes in resistance.

Tape recording

This provides a convenient method of storing large quantities of data. The commonly available types used for sound recording are not suitable for the low frequencies of the E.C.G. and pressure records, but need frequency modulation circuits which at present make them expensive. The main disadvantage is the mass of data that can be collected. Continuous records of the E.C.G. over several days are easily collected, but not easily analysed, even by a very sophisticated computer. In the field of radiology of the heart, however, the storage of image-intensifier records on videotape has become standard practice, and created a revolution in technique.

Another new technique which permits the storage and retrieval of large amounts of data for oscilloscope display and complex calculation is storage on discs. With modern instruments on line, analysis and calculation can be made during catheterization by connecting the recorders directly to the computer.

Computer recording

This is used in this context as a somewhat unsatisfactory name for a promising development in this field of technology. Just as the oscilloscope permits the integration of two variables, so it is possible to use electronic circuits to partially process data before recording them. An obvious example is found in the recording of 'mean' pressure where the application of a long time constant to the recorder results in the obliteration of pressure oscillation so that the record is reduced to a straight line at the mean position. A more advanced example is found in the electronic integration of the area under a curve such as is used in the estimation of cardiac output by dye dilution. Great advances are occurring in this field, as mentioned above.

Preservation of records

The preservation of biological records is a matter of very great importance. It is rarely possible to reproduce precisely the conditions under which some phenomenon has occurred. Each record has, therefore, a unique value. Records may be rendered useless in a variety of ways. They may be lost, destroyed by fire or water, or rendered unintelligible by the failure to record in sufficient detail the conditions under which they were made. Certain types of recording paper (particularly the heat sensitive paper used for much cardiological work) are sensitive to heat, to damp and to pressure and if mounted in hospital notes may be defaced by the pressure of writing on pages overlying the record.

A satisfactory system must permit ready access to results with precautions to avoid loss. This may be achieved by the retention of all original records in files within the department and the provision of copies for the hospital records. Adequate indexing and cross indexing are essential. The bulk of these records are electro-cardiograms, phonocardiograms and the tracings taken at cardiac catheterizations and cardiac operations. They consist either of photographic recordings made on bromide paper or recordings made with heated stylus on heat sensitive paper. A first essential in preserving the records is an efficient copying machine. With modern copying machines it is possible to produce a positive copy of a recording for a few pence. Photocopies of original recordings on heat sensitive paper are of excellent quality, those of phonocardiographs made on bromide paper are adequate for a rough reference but do not provide suitable copies for the interpretation of fine detail unless the original recording is of unusually good quality. Accordingly, the processing of the two types of records should be somewhat different.

Original photographic records, after developing and drying, are cut into suitable lengths, backed with dry mounting paper and mounted permanently on cards the size of hospital notes. Each record is mounted in dupli-cate, one set of records is placed in a binder in the hospital notes together with a suitably annotated report; the other record is filed in a manilla envelope in the department. *Heat-sensitive records* are first mounted on card using a suitable adhesive ('cowgum' is currently used) and, in the case of pressure recordings, the edge of every record is clearly marked with the calibration at the time of mounting. A failure to take this precaution may result in records being quite worthless when, after a year or two, they are found to have no indication of the pressure range used during recording. The records are then photocopied and the copies are issued for the hospital notes and also to other parties who may have a need for them. The originals and several spare copies are filed in manilla envelopes in the department. The re-mainder of the tracings which are not used for mounting are rolled up and stored in boxes for a period of some years, at the end of which time they are destroyed.

Indexing

For all recording activities a comprehensive day book is kept in which, under the appropriate investigations, are entered the patient's name, age, diagnosis and other relevant data. On discharge from hospital, the index diagnosis is entered in three separate indexing systems. A record is kept in the hospital indexing system, a second diagnostic index in which all diagnoses are entered is kept within the department and a third index-ing system is maintained on punch-cards. In this way it is possible to proceed from the index diagnosis to the patient or from the patient to the diagnosis, and similarly, if an analysis is required of the departmental work done, it can be assembled in a matter of an hour or two from the daybooks which are available.

Mounted records are best filed chronologically using a numerical system. A card with each patient's name is kept and the number of the relevant record with a note of its content and any unusual points of interest is filed alphabetically on an index. Filing records alphabetically sooner or later gets unworkable as the number of records grows. Both these and the patients' case notes are kept in the departmental filing system within easy reach of the staff working in the department. In a similar fashion, copies of all summaries relating to patients are filed apart from the notes so that in the event of notes being lost it is usually possible to assemble the bulk of the data from sources within the department.

The responsibility of keeping daybooks and filing records may be divided. Each technician making a particular recording should be responsible for filling up the daybook, cutting the record, mounting it and making sure that it is filed correctly. He may also be responsible for the typing necessary to label the finished reports as a typist will not be familiar with the recording. Photo-copying is done either by the technicians making the record or more easily by a less skilled assistant. Filing of case notes within the department, together with typing and filing of summaries, may be the responsibility of the secretarial staff or, if the work justifies it, a filing clerk may be employed solely for this job. Cardiological data and diagnoses are particularly suited to storage on the recently developed discs. Eventually most units of any size are likely to use these instead of conventional notes.

References

BEILIN, L. & MOUNSEY, J. P. D. (1962). The left ventricular impulse in hypertensive heart disease. *Br. Heart J.* **24,** 409.

BERNSTEIN, L. & MENDEL, D. (1951) The accuracy of spiro-graphic recording at high respiratory rates. *Thorax,* **6,** 297.

NAGLE, D. E. & TAMARA, F. A. (1967) The left parasternal impulse in pulmonary stenosis and atrial septal defect. *Br. Heart J.* **29,** 735.

SCRUGGS, V., PIETRAS, R. J. & ROSEN, K. M. (1975). Fre-quency response of fluid filled catheter-micromanometer systems used for measurement of ventricular pressure. *Am. Heart J.* **89,** 619.

2. Methods of Measuring Pressure

It is not easy to measure pressures at cardiac catheterization. The chamber in which the pressure changes are occurring is connected to the recorder by a column of liquid which may be as long as 150 cm and as narrow as 0·5 mm. If such a system is connected to a standard laboratory mercury manometer, the mercury float will rise to a pressure which is an accurate measurement of the mean pressure in the chamber in which the catheter lies. The mercury recorder, however, will show no oscillation of any kind as the inertia of the recording system is too great. Accurate records of the pressure changes in such a chamber can only be made if the volume displaced in the recording head (or transducer) is extremely small. The most sensitive gauges at present available are nearly all variations on a manometer devised by Hamilton. This consists of a closed brass tube, the end of which is formed by a flexible metal diaphragm about 3 mm across on which is mounted a small mirror. Alterations in pressure inside the brass tube flex the diaphragm at the end and so oscillate the mirror. A simple light beam is arranged to fall on the mirror and be reflected on a photographic plate. The modern derivatives of this apparatus make use of various tricks to record the oscillations of a metal diaphragm. These include capacitance where the diaphragm forms one plate of a condenser with a coil and condenser in series; strain gauges; or a light beam system similar to that of Hamilton, in which the light falls on a photoelectric cell. Any device which converts a pressure change to an electrical one is called a transducer. Whatever the method used, the measure of sensitivity is the displacement in terms of volume produced by a measured change in pressure. This is most conveniently expressed in cubic millimetres displacement per 100 mmHg change in pressure. A reasonably sensitive gauge produces a change of 0·04 mm^3 per 100 mmHg rise in pressure and a very sensitive one 0·01 mm^3 per 100 mmHg. Even greater sensitivity may be achieved with transducers in which the sensitive element is a semiconductor.

The other factor of prime importance in such a system is the frequency response. Here it is as well to consider the recording system. If a direct writing system is in use with a maximum frequency response of 100 Hz, there is not much point having a pressure sensing head capable of responding to 1000 Hz, since the sensitivity in this respect would be completely lost in the recording side. Most gauge heads on the market have an adequate frequency response for all ordinary pressure measurements and this aspect of their function can usually safely be neglected. The sensitivity in terms of volume change, however, is of fundamental importance since an insensitive gauge quickly diminishes the possibilities in a unit. Even as simple an exercise as recording pressure accurately down a No. 5F catheter may be rendered quite impossible by an insensitive gauge head which is entirely adequate, and indeed may be preferable, for use with the wider bore catheter. It follows that in any unit where small babies are investigated it is essential to insist on the most sensitive possible transducer.

Associated with the problems of recording pressure is the necessity for keeping the cardiac catheter clear of clotted blood. In some centres it is customary to run a slow infusion continuously down the catheter. This is not without danger. However carefully arranged, air may enter the system and be blown through the catheter; pressure feed is necessary since the intra-cardiac pressures may exceed those of any ordinary gravity system and so transfuse blood into the catheter. Particularly in small babies, a considerable load of fluid may enter the patient during a prolonged procedure. It is safer and entirely satisfactory to use no continuous infusion during cardiac catheterization. The catheter is connected directly to the pressure head and when necessary a small quantity of 5 per cent dextrose solution containing 5000 units of Heparin per litre is injected down the catheter. Saline should not be used since it may be responsible for increasing the cardiac failure in some small infants.

Damping has been mentioned in the section dealing with recording systems. It is a common source of confusion in the recording of pressures through cardiac catheters. The frequency of oscillation in pressure records ranges from about 1 per second to as much as 20 or 30 Hz. The beginner should examine the effect on a pressure tracing of flicking the cardiac catheter with his finger. This should induce a violent and rapid oscillation whose frequency is related to the size of the catheter, being lower with long large bore catheters. It is a vibration not dissimilar to that produced in a musical instrument and is subject to the same harmonics and overtones. The high frequencies encountered in the fine bore catheters usually have no significant effect upon the recording, but with the larger catheters (6F upwards) mechanical movements may produce undesirable oscillations which are superimposed on the natural pressure change (Fig. 1.5). These are frequently seen in recordings from pulmonary artery and are not infrequent in recordings from other sites. They are rarely seen in recordings made by direct needle puncture of a blood vessel. Their elimination is a matter of great difficulty. 'Critical' damping can be achieved by the inter-position of a small length of fine bore tubing adjusted to eliminate the oscillations of the catheter. This will have the inevitable effect of eliminating any naturally occurring oscillation of the same period and as the artefacts due to catheter oscillation are mostly seen with large catheters they are, therefore, of relatively low frequency. It is, therefore, precisely in the case where elimination of abnormal record is most desirable that the elimination carries the risk of obliterating an important (low frequency) detail in the trace. Provision for damping the record is built into most recorders. It is an electrical device which reduces the rapidity of the frequency response. In most recorders it is stated that it does not affect the amplitude of the pressure response, but careful checking against a variety of pressure records is desirable before such a statement can be accepted. In any case where damping is applied, the degree of damping used should be noted on the record and a length of undamped tracing recorded.

Damping of undesirable character may arise from a number of causes. It has already been noted that the volume changes inside the recording heads are extremely small. The presence of an air bubble, the presence of blood or contrast medium in the recording tube and the presence of a lax length of plastic tubing in the system are all sufficient to damp down the record and render it valueless. Examples of different forms of damping are shown in Figure 1.3.

A further point of some importance is that in a liquid-filled system, the zero point is related to the position of the recording head. This is of great importance when the patient is catheterized on a tilting table. It is usual to take the mid-axillary point as zero and place the pressure head at this level, but some centres prefer a fixed distance related to the angle of Louis and in others a fixed distance above the table top is used. Again the beginner is recommended to try the effect on the pressure record of raising and lowering the transducer (pressure head). If the recording system is filled with fluid it will be found that an elevation in the pressure head produces a negative pressure while lowering it produces an increasingly positive pressure (Fig. 2.1).

Typical normal atrial pressures are shown in Figures 2.2 and 2.3. The pressure changes consist essentially of two waves termed the A wave, coinciding with contraction of the atrium, and the V wave, which occurs during the filling of the right atrium in ventricular systole. The fall in the pressure succeeding the A wave is termed the X descent, and that after the V wave the Y descent. The X descent is usually interrupted by a small rise in pressure termed the C wave. This coincides with the beginning of ventricular systole and is due to the bulging of the mitral or the tricuspid valve into the atrial cavity. Normal right atrial pressure is usually 5/0 mmHg. Normal left atrial pressure is somewhat higher, perhaps 10/2 mmHg. An increase in the A wave is found in conditions in which ventricular filling is more difficult than

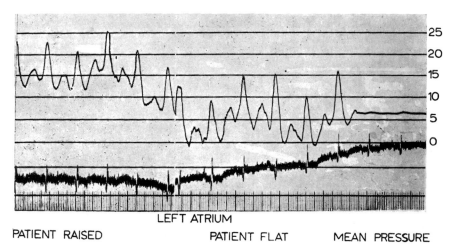

LEFT ATRIUM

PATIENT RAISED   PATIENT FLAT   MEAN PRESSURE

FIG. 2.1 The effect of changing the inclination of the X-ray table when the pressure head and heart are at different levels. At the left of the record the patient was tilted at 20 degrees, head up, the pressure head being placed about level with the midthigh. The pressure recorded is 25/12. The table was then tilted horizontal thus reducing the hydrostatic difference between the level of the heart and pressure head. A true pressure of 15/0 is now recorded with a mean pressure of 6 mmHg. The record has been shortened by excising a length recorded during tilting. Catheter in left atrium.

B

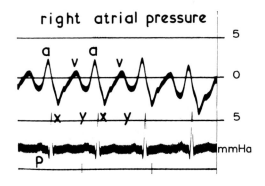

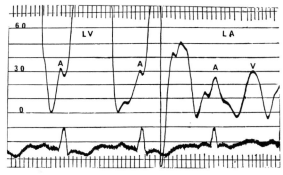

FIG. 2.4   An A wave in the left ventricle and atrium in aortic stenosis. The same case as that illustrating aortic stenosis in Fig. 2.10. Comparison of these tracings illustrates the flexibility of photographic recording. Despite the large V wave there was no mitral incompetence in this case.

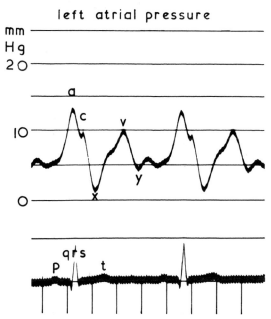

Atrial fibrillation modifies this tracing as the A wave is absent. The result is a somewhat featureless and variable tracing, in which the V wave is the most prominent feature (Fig. 2.7).

The typical tracing from the ventricle is reminiscent of a square wave (Fig. 2.8). A low pressure phase of ventricular filling occurs in diastole, not infrequently terminating in a rise in pressure, easily recognizable as the A wave of the atrium (Fig. 2.4). This is followed by a sharp rise to systolic pressure, the opening of the pulmonary or aortic valve, a phase of ejection and subsequent fall in pressure coinciding with the onset of diastole. In a normal ventricle the systolic phase has often a bifid appearance. This is usually absent in a ventricle in which the outlet is stenosed. Systolic pressure in the right ventricle is usually under 30 mmHg and pressures as low as 12 mmHg may be encountered in normal subjects.

Arterial pressure has a more complex form (Fig. 2.8). Ventricular systole produces a sharp rise following the opening of the outlet valve from the ventricle and a rounded tracing which falls more or less gradually towards diastolic pressure. This fall is interrupted by a distinct dicrotic notch more or less coinciding with the closure of the outlet valves of the ventricles. Stenosis of the aortic or pulmonary valves results in a slower rise in

FIGS. 2.2 and 2.3   Normal right atrial and left atrial pressures recorded by cardiac catheterization. In this case there was no obvious C wave in the right atrium, but a very clear C wave in the left atrium. In this patient with insignificant mitral stenosis the pressures are normal. Notice that the A wave follows the P wave of the E.C.G. occurring about 0·1 s later.

usual, for example, in stenosis of the outflow from the ventricle, in pulmonary or aortic valve stenosis, in ventricular hypertrophy due to hypertension in the pulmonary or systemic systems, or in stenosis of the mitral or tricuspid valve (Fig. 2.4). Incompetence of the mitral or tricuspid valve will result in a large V wave in the appropriate atrium if it is considerable in degree (Fig. 2.5). A raised diastolic pressure in the atrium is found in any of these disorders if they are sufficiently severe. A high right atrial pressure with deep X and Y descents is typical of constrictive pericarditis, but may occur in severe right heart failure of any cause (Fig. 2.6).

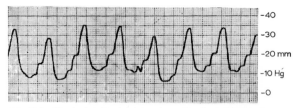

FIG. 2.5   Typical left atrial tracing of mitral incompetence. There is a large V wave. The Y descent is rapid and the X descent absent. Note the high ventricular filling pressure (atrial diastolic) of 10 mmHg.

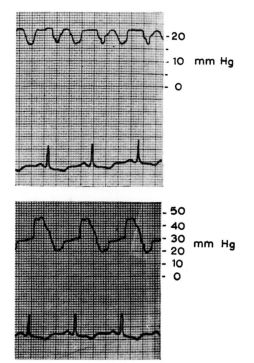

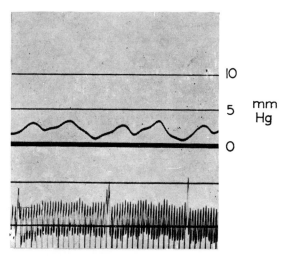

FIG. 2.7 Right atrial tracing from a patient with atrial fibrillation. At first sight there appears to be both an A and a V wave. The wave form in atrial fibrillation is variable, only the V wave being a constant feature. Note the A.C. interference from the X-ray generators distorting the E.C.G. record.

FIG. 2.6 Typical tracing of constrictive pericarditis. The upper trace shows the pressure in the right atrium with a high filling pressure of 17 mmHg, to which the atrial contraction contributes little on most beats. The X and Y descents are steep. The lower tracing (at half the sensitivity) shows the very brief Y descent at the end of right ventricular systole followed by the sharp plateau as the constricted heart sharply fills. The abrupt tensioning of the heart is associated with vibrations which are usually loud enough to be audible with the stethoscope.

systolic pressure, and often a more featureless fall in pressure—the anacrotic pulse. Incompetence of these valves may produce a fall in diastolic pressure in the aorta or pulmonary artery, but has to be considerable in degree before its effects are obvious. In many cases with mixed aortic stenosis and incompetence, a curious double peak is found in the arterial pulse. This is termed the pulsus bisferiens.

Pressure gradients can give information of the greatest importance. They are found most frequently at the site of valves. When the inlet valve of a ventricle is narrowed, there is a rise in the pressure of the chamber proximal to the valve during ventricular diastole (Fig. 2.9). Similarly, when there is a stenosis at the site of an outflow valve, there is a rise in the systolic pressure proximal to the valve with a loss of the normal contour of the ventricular tracing (Fig. 2.10). Complex narrowings may be detected by careful pressure measurement, for example, the presence of pulmonary valve stenosis with infundibular stenosis proximal to the valve will be detected and similarly subvalvar stenosis may be identified by pressure

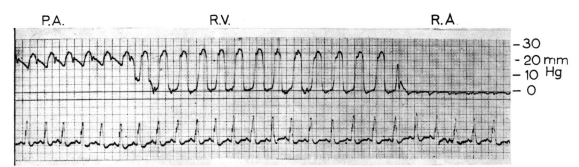

FIG. 2.8 Withdrawal tracing from pulmonary artery to right atrium in a normal subject using a direct writing recorder. There are no extrasystoles. The single abnormal beats recorded at the transition from pulmonary artery to ventricle and from ventricle to atrium are artefacts due to the angiographic catheter which has a series of side holes at the tip. For these single beats, these holes are astride the valves. Note that the normal end diastolic pressure in the ventricle is not the nadir, but that the pressure is beginning to rise indicating an increasing resistance to filling.

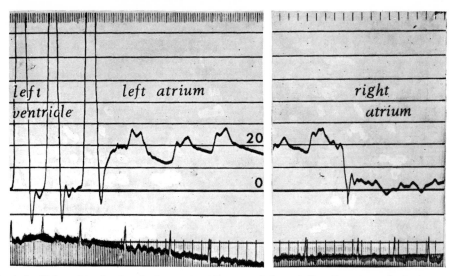

FIG. 2.9   A typical withdrawal tracing in mitral stenosis with atrial fibrillation. The recorder is a photographic one permitting great magnification of the tracing. On the left the diastolic part of the ventricular pressure record shows oscillations generated in the catheter. The left atrial diastolic pressure is about 15 mmHg above the ventricular diastolic,

and the end diastolic pressure is the lowest atrial pressure recorded. On the right the catheter is drawn back through the atrial septum into the right atrium where the pressure is normal. Transseptal catheterization using the Ross needle and Seldinger wire.

measurement. The commonly encountered pressure gradients are illustrated diagrammatically in Figure 2.11.

Occasionally measurements of pressure can be misleading. There may exist in the presence of large left to right shunts a marked fall in systolic pressure at the site of the pulmonary valve, and yet at surgery no pulmonary valve stenosis may be apparent. The cause of this change in pressure can frequently be predicted from the com-

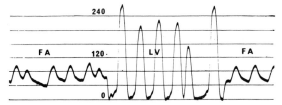

FIG. 2.10   Simultaneous measurement of the pressure in the left ventricle and femoral artery in a patient with aortic stenosis. The ventricular pressure is measured by a catheter passed through the atrial septum by the Ross needle and Seldinger wire. The femoral artery pressure is measured by needle puncture. A single pressure head is connected to both sites using a 3-way tap. The tap is turned from one position to the other providing an immediate comparison without any risk of error due to differences in the responses of two pressure heads. In this case the femoral pressure is 100/60, the ventricular pressure 220/0 indicating a significant stenosis. The normal ventricular diastolic pressure indicates that there is little difficulty in filling the ventricle as yet. The atrial trace from this case (Fig. 2.4) however shows a prominent A wave showing that the atrium is working harder than usual to fill the ventricle—i.e. the thickening of the ventricular wall is beginning to make the impedance rise.

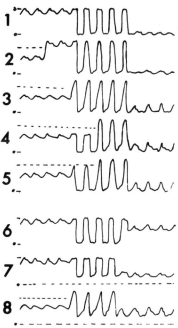

FIG. 2.11   Diagrammatic representation of characteristic pressure tracings. The normal systolic and zero pressures are indicated on the left. 1. Normal. 2. Stenosis beyond aortic or pulmonary valves—supravalvar stenosis, coarctation or pulmonary artery stenosis. 3. Pulmonary or aortic valve stenosis. 4. Infundibular stenosis, normal aortic or pulmonary valve. 5. Infundibular and valve stenosis. 6. Mitral or tricuspid stenosis. 7. Heart failure. 8. Aortic or pulmonary valve stenosis with thickening of the ventricular wall leading to an increased ventricular filling pressure (reduced ventricular compliance).

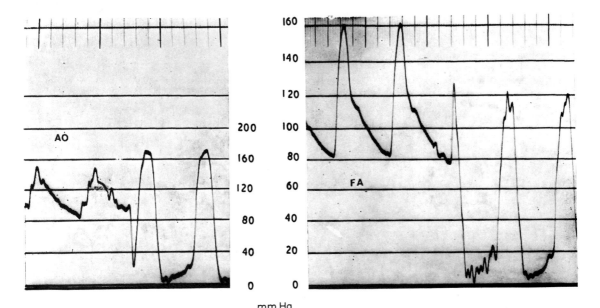

mm.Hg

FIG. 2.12 A curious anomaly occasionally encountered in recording pressure, usually, as in this case, in mixed aortic valve disease. On the left the aortic pressure is recorded by an aortographic catheter passed from the femoral artery to a position close to the aortic valve in the ascending aorta. The aortic pressure is about 140/80, the ventricular pressure 170/0. In the same patient the pressure in the femoral artery recorded by needle puncture some time earlier during the Seldinger procedure for aortography was 160/80 with a simultaneously recorded ventricular pressure of 120/0. The ventricular pressure is recorded in both cases by a Brockenborough catheter passed to the left ventricle through the atrial septum, and in both cases the traces are continuous, the catheters being connected to the same 3-way tap. A number of explanations have been advanced to account for the paradoxical rise in systolic pressure as the length of the aorta is traversed. It is rarely as marked as that shown here.

bination of a marked left to right shunt together with a fall from raised right ventricular pressure to a pulmonary artery pressure which is within normal limits. In true pulmonary stenosis the pulmonary artery pressure is usually much below normal limits. Angiocardiography will usually confirm the nature of the outlet obstruction in doubtful cases.

An occasional cause of confusion is the physiological change in the character of the pulse wave in the aorta. In Figure 2.12 the femoral artery pressure recorded by needle puncture shows a systolic pressure greater than that in the left ventricle. When the aortic pressure is recorded close to the aortic valve this phenomenon is abolished and a small gradient is revealed.

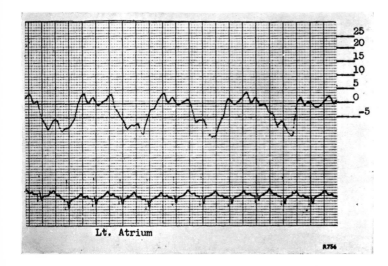

FIG. 2.13 Left atrial pressure recorded in a two month old infant investigated for failure to thrive. A ventricular septal defect and patent ductus were present. A marked negative pressure associated with inspiration is superimposed on the pressure changes due to the heart action. The catheter was passed to the left atrium through the foramen ovale.

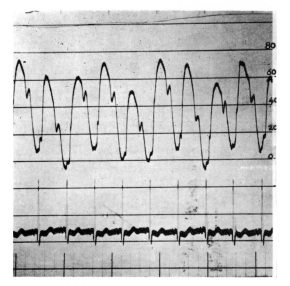

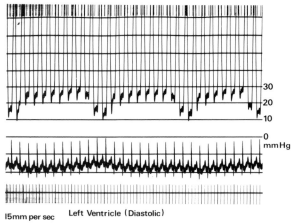

I5mm per sec   Left Ventricle (Diastolic)

FIG. 2.14b   Record of left ventricular diastolic pressure during snoring. The patient, in left ventricular failure following myocardial infarction, fell asleep during catheterization. No pre-medication, local anaesthesia.

FIG. 2.14a   Tracing from right ventricle of an infant with pulmonary congestion due to patent ductus arteriosus. The appearance of ventricular alternans is due to respiratory changes in intrathoracic pressure. This is evident from inspection of the ventricular diastolic pressure which approximately mirrors the systolic variations.

Marked changes in intrathoracic pressure may occur in some dyspnoeic patients. These changes are most commonly seen in recordings of atrial pressure when they are superimposed on the intracardiac pressure changes (Fig. 2.13). In ventricular recordings, a superficial resemblance to pulsus alternans may be produced (Figs. 2.14a, 14b).

The effect of exercise and of pressor drugs may be of assistance in assessing organic and functional ventricular outflow obstruction. In Figure 2.15 the effect of simple leg raising on the gradient across an aortic valve is shown.

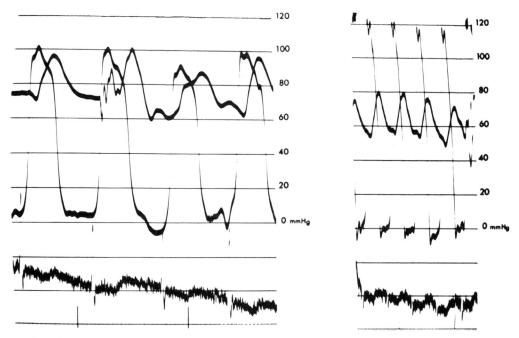

FIG. 2.15   Effect of exercise on aortic valve gradient on an 11-year-old boy. The tracing on the left taken before exercise shows no aortic valve gradient. That on the right, recorded during straight leg raising, shows an increased systolic pressure in the ventricle and a fall in aortic pressure. Aortic pressure recorded by P.E. 160 catheter, left ventricular pressure recorded by F.7 Brockenborough trans-septal catheter in left ventricle. Local anaesthetic only.

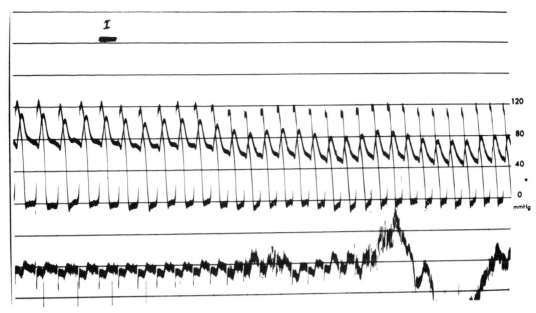

FIG. 2.16   Effect of 1·0 mg of isoprenaline (1) injected into aorta on left ventricular and aortic pressure. Same patient as 2.15.

The patient was an 11-year-old boy. Exercise has increased the height of ventricular systole and reduced the aortic pressure. In the same patient the intravenous injection of a small quantity of isoprenaline causes a fall in aortic pressure without any rise in ventricular pressure (Fig. 2.16). This reaction is likely to be an example of the vasodilator action of isoprenaline which appears to be fairly commonly seen if small doses of about 0·2 mg per kg are injected. With larger doses the ventricular pressure increases. The effect upon the arterial pressure of both exercise and pressor drugs in aortic stenosis is somewhat unpredictable. In many patients the ventricular pressure rises and the valve gradient increases. In some patients

with a considerable gradient at rest (e.g. 100 mmHg) exercise causes no change in the pressures measured in the left ventricle and aorta. The reason for this has not been elucidated in our patients who have been risky subjects for investigation.

The development of a considerable gradient due to increased ventricular pressure after injection of adrenergic drugs in a patient who has no gradient at rest is characteristic of functional outflow obstruction (e.g. H.O.C.M., see Fig. 2.17). However, a similar response may be seen occasionally in fixed outflow obstructions (e.g. valve stenosis, supravalve stenosis, subvalvar diaphragm). It is therefore necessary to confirm the

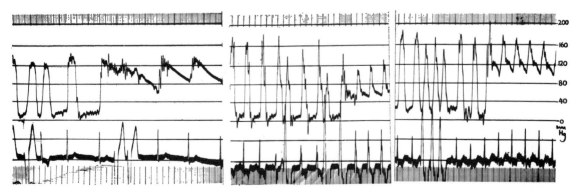

FIG. 2.17   Effect of isoprenaline given intravenously in a patient with hypertrophic obstructive cardiomyopathy (H.O.C.M.). Left—control withdrawal trace from left ventricle to aorta shows no gradient. Centre—gradient after injection of 0·3 mg isoprenaline. Right—repeat injection of 0·3 mg isopranaline after the intravenous administration of practolol shows no gradient. Beta adrenergic blockade has prevented the effect. Catheterization by Dr G. A. Batson.

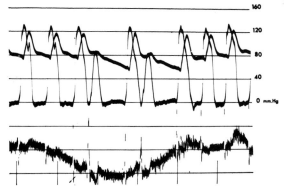

FIG. 2.18 Effect of extrasystoles on pulse pressure. Extrasystoles stimulated by rotating the Brockenborough catheter in the left ventricle. Note the normal response, the longer filling resulting in a larger pulse pressure than normal. Same patient as Figs. 2.15 and 2.16.

diagnosis of functional obstruction by angiocardiography (Fig. 2.18) and by the demonstration of a paradoxical response to extrasystoles as described below (Fig. 2.19).

Confirmatory evidence suggesting functional outflow obstruction may be obtained by stimulating ventricular extrasystoles while monitoring ventricular and arterial pressure simultaneously. In a normal response the increased stroke volume of the heart which follows an extrasystole causes an increase in aortic valve pressure (Fig. 2.18). In functional outflow obstruction the ventricular systolic pressure of the heart is increased but the arterial pulse pressure is diminished (Fig. 2.19). Note, however, the anomalous tracing in Figure 18.6.

Destruction of the aortic valve by acute bacterial endocarditis can result in a haemodynamic situation of the utmost gravity. In free aortic incompetence of this degree the aortic diastolic pressure can be transmitted to the left atrium causing acute pulmonary oedema and

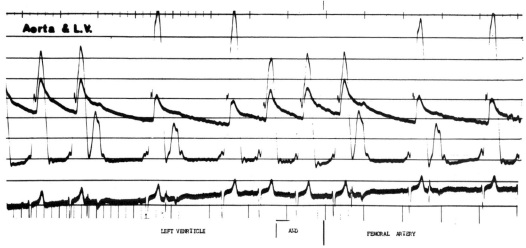

FIG. 2.19 Typical left ventricular and aortic pressure trace from a patient with functional ventricular outflow obstruction, in this case H.O.C.M. Note that the increase in the ventricular pressure after an extrasystole is accompanied by a fall in pulse pressure.

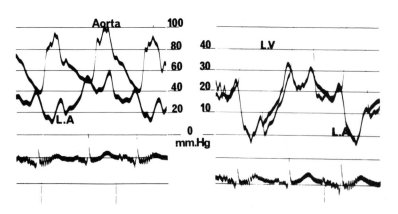

FIG. 2.20 Recording of aortic, left ventricular and left atrial pressures in a patient with acute bacterial endocarditis of the aortic valve due to *staphylococcus aureus*. Free aortic incompetence results in the equalization of all three pressures at the nadir of the aortic diastolic pressure.

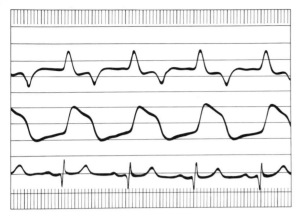

FIG. 2.21 Differential pressure measurement. Tracing, showing from below upwards, the electrocardiogram, the right ventricular pressure measured with an intracardiac manometer (0–40 mmHg), and top, the differential or rate of pressure change (dp/dt).

premature closure of the mitral valve. Only emergency aortic valve replacement can save the patient (Fig. 2.20).

Differential pressure measurement. The rate with which the ventricle contracts is a useful measure of its functional state. Accurate measurements of this can only be made with an intracardiac manometer. In this device, the transducer is placed at the end of the catheter so that it is introduced into the chamber from which the presssure is being recorded. The output from this manometer is passed through a differentiating circuit which then records the rate with which the pressure changes inside the chamber concerned. This measurement together with an assessment of ventricular contraction obtained by angiocardiography or by echocardiography is of value in determining the state of ventricular function both before and after surgery (Fig. 2.21).

References

BRAUNWALD, E. & ROSS, J., Jr. (1963). Ventricular end-diastolic pressure. *Am. J. Med.* **34,** 147.

BROCKENBOROUGH, E. C., BRAUNWALD, E. & MORROW, A. G. (1961). A hemodynamic technic for the detection of sub-aortic stenosis. *Circulation,* **23,** 189.

FOWLER, N. O., MANNIN, E. P. & NOBLE, W. (1957). Difficulties in the interpretation of right heart catheterization data. *Am. Heart J.* **53,** 343.

NIXON, P. F. G. & WOOLER, G. (1963). Phases of diastole in various syndromes of mitral valve disease. *Br. Heart J.* **25,** 393.

WELLS, B. G. (1958). The diagnosis of mitral incompetence from left atrial pressure waves. *Br. Heart J.* **20,** 321.

Cardiovascular Fluid Dynamics, edited by Bergel, D. H.; Academic Press (1972), may be consulted by those seeking a comprehensive account of techniques of measurement.

3. Shunt Detection and Other Methods of Investigation

Methods of measuring oxygen saturation in blood have been devised specifically for cardiac catheterization. The traditional methods of estimation by gas analysis (van Slyke, Haldane and others) require at least 5 ml for accurate duplicate estimates and are extremely time-consuming. To get a fair measurement of oxygen saturation 20 minutes per sample is needed and this throws an intolerable load on the staff of the majority of cardiovascular units. One method of gas analysis suitable for catheter work is the microsyringe method of Roughton and Sholander (1943). This permits multiple estimates on small samples, but again has the disadvantage that duplicate measurements require something like 20 min per sample. The methods specifically adopted for cardiac work are mostly based on absorptiometry. A light beam is passed either through a solution of blood and the percentage oxygenation assessed by the colour absorbed by the haemoglobin, or the blood is placed in a suitable cuvette and light reflected from its surface. In either case two wave lengths are used. One is a reference which changes little with changes in oxygen saturation and the other is greatly affected by the degree of saturation of the blood. Where the light passes through the solution the technique is termed absorptiometry. Where a reflected beam of light is used the instrument is usually called a haemoreflector. In choosing between techniques it is desirable to consider a number of factors. The absorptiometric technique can be applied to any high quality absorptiometer and is, therefore, obtainable with standard laboratory equipment. It is not affected by the addition of coloured tracer substances to the circulation. Measurements made with it are extremely accurate and a relatively junior technician can produce consistent results with the instrument. Against this, the solutions have usually to be haemolized and the blood is, therefore, not available for return to the patient or for other measurements.

The haemoreflector in our hands has not proved as reliable as absorptiometry. When in use it has been our practice to check at least three samples against an independent method in each run of investigations. With some models it is possible to return the blood to the patient and to make an indefinite number of estimations. In this type of apparatus, however, cleaning the cuvette is a matter of great difficulty and its use is a possible source of reactions in the patient. It is possible that direct methods of measuring oxygen in blood using polarographic probes or glass fibre catheters will eventually allow the measurement of oxygen saturation within the patient without the removal of samples.

Recently developed instruments are capable of measuring partial pressure of gases in solution. These provide another rapid method of oxygen analysis of small samples of blood. They are not as easy to use as the absorptiometry instruments, but if they are in regular use for blood P_{CO_2} and pH measurements, the additional use for P_{O_2} presents little difficulty.

The saturation of samples is conveniently recorded on a diagram such as that shown in Figure 3.1.

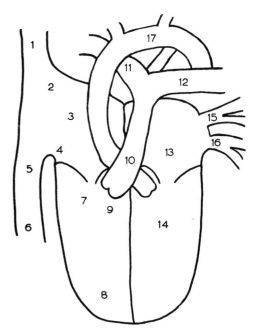

FIG. 3.1   A diagram used to record the oxygen saturations of blood samples taken from the heart. 1. Superior vena cava. 2. High right atrium. 3. Mid right atrium. 4. Low right atrium. 5. High inferior vena cava. 6. Low inferior vena cava. 7. Inflow of right ventricle. 8. Apex of right ventricle. 9. Outflow of right ventricle. 10. Main pulmonary artery. 11. Right pulmonary artery. 12. Left pulmonary artery. 13. Left atrium. 14. Left ventricle. 15. Right pulmonary vein. 16. Left pulmonary vein. 17. Aorta. A diagram of this type is of use in the rapid appreciation of the results of oximetry.

Shunt detection by Oximetry
Oxygen saturation

The simplest way of detecting a shunt is to identify the presence of blood coming through a defect from the other side of the heart by *oximetry*. However, this apparently satisfactory technique is not without its difficulties. There is considerable variation in oxygen saturation in a normal heart chamber from one part to another, in particular in the different parts of the right atrium where the two venae cavae, the coronary sinus and the vena azygos may all contribute blood of different saturations. Not infrequently, patients with hot hands and hot feet have blood returning from the periphery at over 85 per cent and even as high as 90 per cent saturation. This high saturation makes the results of oximetry uncertain (p. 154).

It may be difficult on screening to be reasonably certain whether a catheter lying in the upper part of the inferior cava is at the level of the entrance of the hepatic veins or not. Many of the statements that the inferior vena caval blood is more desaturated than that descending from the head and neck in the superior vena cava may be based on a misapprehension of this kind. It is easy to place a catheter in the inferior vena cava, draw it back until it appears to lie just below the right atrium and take a sample to be labelled 'inferior vena cava', when, in fact, the catheter is lying at the lowest extremity of the right atrium, opposite the coronary sinus. This is because the liver viewed on the X-ray table often lies in front of the lower part of the right atrium. Samples taken from this position may have a very low oxygen saturation as coronary sinus blood is usually very desaturated. In fact, blood from the inferior vena cava is usually better oxygenated than that coming from the superior vena cava. Difficulties of this kind make an independent method for detecting shunts of great value. Cardioangiography is, in some ways, the most useful of these, but the detection of an injected tracer substance has many advantages. It can be a great deal cheaper than cardioangiography and may be capable of detecting very much smaller shunts. A considerable number of methods has been developed and we shall deal here in detail with only three. These are: the injection of coloured dye, the injection of ascorbic acid, and the injection or inhalation of radioactive substances.

Tracer techniques

The use of tracer techniques has diminished since the first edition of this book was published insofar as the identification of intracardiac shunts is concerned. Increasing confidence in the use of angiocardiography by cine, 100 mm and full-sized film techniques has, to a very large extent, replaced them.

In this section the use of tracer techniques to further the diagnosis of heart disease is considered. Their use for the measurement of cardiac output is dealt with elsewhere. An increasing number of substances is in use for the identification of cardiac lesions by tracer techniques. Essentially all methods consist of the introduction of some substance into the circulation and its identification at one or more sites. It is possible to measure either the time at which it appears at a selected point, or the concentration achieved in the circulation, or both these factors. In some techniques both concentration and appearance time are measured. In other techniques, however, the change in the concentration of the indicator is the essential measurement, while in some techniques the appearance time is the critical factor.

Dye dilution. Perhaps the most widely used technique is *dye dilution* and as this makes use of both appearance time and concentration, description of this method will permit a ready understanding of all methods. In its most usual form the dye, which may be blue or green, is injected into the circulation through a catheter, placed on the right side of the heart, and its appearance in the arterial circulation is measured by a suitable photoelectric device attached to the ear lobe of a patient. Cardiogreen (1 to 2 ml) is the most widely used dye for this purpose. In a normal subject, injection into the right atrium, ventricle or pulmonary artery is followed after an interval of usually five to eight seconds by a deflection in the recorder attached to the ear which has a characteristic double hump shape (Fig. 3.2). The initial deflection recording the appearance of the dye in the circulation at the ear, is followed by its disappearance, the second deflection being a recirculation of incompletely mixed dye. It is not usual to see further deflections as mixing is substantially complete at the end of the second circuit. The tracing does not return to the original baseline as the plasma is coloured by the injection. This characteristic curve is distorted in the presence of lesions in the heart. It is convenient to consider them in two groups—the changes that may be seen in patients in whom there are no shunts and the changes resulting from the presence of shunts.

In the heart in which no shunts are present the dye curve may be distorted by the presence of either substantial leaks at valves or by gross dilatation of the chambers between the site of injection and the appearance point (Figs. 3.3 and 3.4). Both of these act in much the same way by broadening the normal curve. It may be a matter of considerable difficulty to be certain that the curves are not normal when minor changes are present and the technique is not suitable for the detection of minor degrees of incompetence except in the most experienced hands. In general the closer to the valve concerned that the injection is made, the more certain the results; for example, when mitral incompetence is under investigation the dye injection is most usefully made through a Ross needle into the left atrium. Injection into the pul-

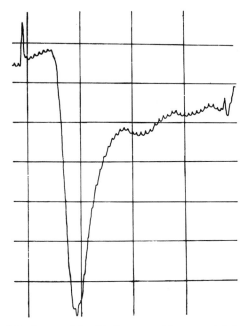

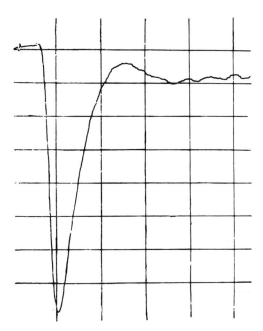

FIG. 3.2   A normal dye dilution curve. The upward deflection at the left of the tracing is the point of injection of 0·5 ml. Coomassie blue into the right atrium. The large downward deflection due to the appearance of the dye at the ear follows 7 seconds later. The tracing shows considerable pulsation which was not abolished by adjusting the apparatus, and the recirculation deflection was small. Arterial pulsation is more easily reduced in later types of apparatus. The interval between the vertical graph lines is 10 seconds.

FIG. 3.3   Injection of dye into the right pulmonary artery in Ebstein's anomaly. The curve is normal as the circulation from this point to the ear is normal.

monary artery in such cases can produce a rather misleading curve.

The value of tracer techniques in identifying intracardiac shunts depends to some extent on the other resources of the diagnostic department. In circumstances in which diagnostic work is done without easy access to selective

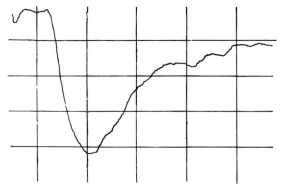

FIG. 3.4   Injection of dye into the right atrium in the same case of Ebstein's anomaly as in Fig. 3.3. The same volume of dye produces a much lower, broader curve due to the mixing into the large volume of blood in the atrium, and the slower clearing from it.

angiocardiography in the course of a routine cardiac catheterization and in which the results of oxygen analysis from samples are not immediately available, tracer techniques can provide information of the greatest possible value by indicating, with reasonable certainty, the site of intra-cardiac shunts. They thus make possible a much more intelligent appreciation of the situation during catheterization than would otherwise be feasible. On the other hand, where immediate oxygen analysis is possible the information obtained from tracer techniques is less critical because it is usually possible to assess the type of significant shunts immediately from oxygen analysis or from selective angiocardiography performed in the course of the catheterization.

The abnormal curves found in the course of conventional dye studies made from the right side of the heart are fundamentally two. In patients with a left to right shunt in the heart, injection of dye is followed by a normal interval during which the dye traverses the lungs and reaches the ear lobe oximeter. The recirculation curve is, however, to a varying degree abnormal as some dye passes from the left heart to the right side, then through the lungs and back to the ear. Examples are shown in Figures 3.4 and 3.6. In a large shunt there is a slow fall towards the final concentration of dye. In a small shunt, a rapid fall is followed by a flattening out of the curve.

In patients with a right to left shunt there is a more dramatic change. If the dye is injected proximal in the circulation to the site of the shunt, a quantity will escape

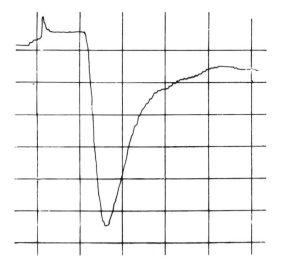

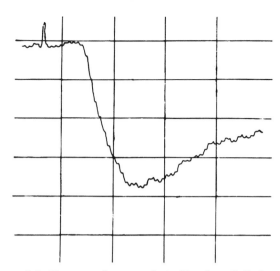

FIG. 3.5 Dye curve recorded by ear oximeter in a patient with a small shunt through an atrial septal defect. The injection of dye into the pulmonary artery is signalled 9 seconds before the appearance at the ear. The return of the recorder towards the base line is more gradual than normal and there is no recirculation peak. Compare this curve with a normal one (Fig. 3.2) and the curve recorded in the presence of a large shunt. Clearly, in cases with only small shunts, interpretation can be difficult.

FIG. 3.6 Dye curve from a patient with a large L–R shunt through an atrial septal defect. Injection into the right atrium is followed 8 s later by a deflection due to the dye reaching the ear. Thereafter there is a gradual return towards the baseline, only part of which is shown. Large shunts of this kind are usually clinically obvious, and are readily demonstrated by oximetry, tracer techniques or angiocardiography.

to the left side of the heart through the defect, and pass immediately to the ear. The appearance time is therefore greatly shortened and in most cases the increasing concentration of dye shows a double contour (Fig. 3.7) due to the initial right to left shunt followed by the main concentration of dye coming through from the lung. Clearly if dye is injected into the left side of the heart in a normal subject, or into a right ventricle which largely empties into the aorta, a short circulation time with no hump on the upstroke will be found. In the presence of a large intracardiac shunt the fall off in concentration will be slow. Similarly in a heart in which there is a right to left shunt, if dye is injected beyond the site of the shunt, there will be a normal transit time through the lung followed by a slow fall off produced by the intracardiac shunting.

Further developments of the tracer techniques have moved in two directions. The first is towards methods devised for injecting tracer substances into the arterial side of the circulation in order that the site of a left to right shunt can be identified. The second is towards a simple test intended to indicate the presence of an intracardiac shunt without defining precisely its site. This has value in outpatient screening in possible cases of congenital heart disease.

Two simple methods of introducing tracer methods to the left side of the heart are available. The first is the inhalation of an identifiable substance which passes from

the alveoli to the blood in the lung. The use of hydrogen and radioactive xenon for this purpose will be described. The other technique is the injection of ascorbic acid into the right side of the heart and its subsequent identification

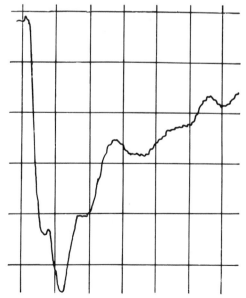

FIG. 3.7 A rather unconvincing example of L–R shunting in Fallot's tetralogy. The early appearance following injection into the right ventricle is followed by a further rise in concentration. This curve was probably complicated by rather slow clearance of dye from the ventricle.

when it comes to reach the left side of the heart and pass through a defect back to the right side again.

Hydrogen

The use of *hydrogen* depends upon its property of generating a potential when it comes into contact with platinum black. A standard cardiac catheter is modified by the provision of a platinum ring at the tip connected to an electrode at the hub of the catheter. This platinum is converted to platinum black by an appropriate process and with suitable amplification a record can be obtained of the arrival of the hydrogen at the tip of the catheter. The technique is comparatively simple once the catheter and amplifying system are prepared. The amplifier normally used for electrocardiography has a suitable sensitivity for this purpose. Hydrogen is obtained in cylinders and is kept outside the catheter room. A small rubber bag with a capacity of perhaps 500 ml is connected to a standard anaesthetic mask. The patient is catheterized with the electrode catheter and its position confirmed by pressure measurement and blood sampling. The mask is placed over the patient's face. He is in-

structed to take a single deep breath and the time of this breath is marked on the recorder. When the hydrogen encounters the electrode, a sharp deflection occurs and the time between the breath and the deflection is noted. A typical series of results is shown in Figure 3.8. This illustrates well both the sensitivity and the limitations of the technique in our hands. In this patient a small-ventricular septal defect was not shown with the standard oximetry. A series of samples was taken from a number of places in the right ventricle and hydrogen curves recorded. At one site only, a sharp deflection occurred early in response to hydrogen. However, the blood sample taken at this site also showed a sharp rise in oxygen saturation and testing with hydrogen in the main pulmonary artery failed to produce any convincing deflection. It has been our experience with this technique that it will readily demonstrate left to right shunting and will indicate the site of a shunt with great accuracy. However, if oxygen estimation is made by a precise method, the hydrogen technique does not seem to us to have a superiority over the combination of blood sampling and cardioangiography sufficient to merit the routine use of a time-consuming and somewhat cumbrous technique.

Radioactive gas technique

Similar objections apply to *radioactive gas technique* with the added difficulty of the blood sampling needed to identify the radioactivity and the risk of contamination with the radioactive gas which necessitates careful exhaust ventilation over the patient.

Ascorbic acid technique

The *ascorbic acid techniqye* depends on the generation of a potential when ascorbic acid impinges on platinum which is rendered sensitive by a small current. It is capable of detecting shunts in either direction if a platinum electrode catheter is used in conjunction with a platinum catheter inserted into an artery. A solution of ascorbic acid is injected through the catheter and this generates a deflection at the platinum ring on the catheter tip. The time at which the arterial system is reached is recorded by the indwelling arterial electrode and the return to the starting point by a further deflection from the electrode on the injection catheter. When the injection is made proximal to a right to left shunt, an early arterial appearance is recorded. If the starting point for the injection is distal to the site of a left to right shunt then deflection is recorded early on the right side by the shunted blood, for example, if ascorbic acid is injected into the right ventricle in a patient with an atrial septal defect, the injection causes an initial deflection. This is followed by a second early deflection due to ascorbic acid passing through the atrial septal defect to reach the right ventricle. If, however, the electrode on the catheter lies in the right

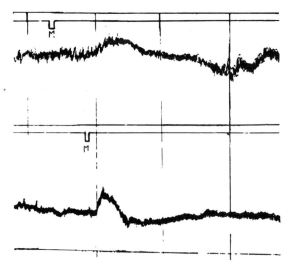

FIG. 3.8   Tracing of two hydrogen curves from the same ventricle. Hydrogen was inhaled at M in both. The upper curve shows a deflection after 7 s and was recorded with the platinum black electrode at the apex of the ventricle. There is no indication of a shunt. The lower curve shows a more obvious deflection 2 s after inhalation, indicating a shunt. In this case the electrode lay close to the septum in the stream of arterial blood coming through a surgically insignificant defect. The quantity of blood shunted was not enough to cause a significant rise in the oxygen saturation in the pulmonary artery, and the platinum electrode showed no early deflection at this site. The amplification needed for this technique results in the platinum electrode recording the intracardiac electrocardiogram as well as deflection due to the hydrogen. The large oscillations of the electrocardiogram obscure the deflections due to hydrogen, and have been omitted in these tracings.

heart proximal to the site of a left to right shunt, a normal circulation time to the right side of the heart is recorded.

This technique using ascorbic acid is at present the most generally useful of the tracer techniques available for the detection of intracardiac shunts. It has the advantage of permitting identification of both left to right and right to left shunting. It employs a non-toxic, indeed physiological, tracer; repeated injections do not produce undesirable cumulative effects and the apparatus is comparatively simple. Circuits have been described which are safe and a number of refinements are possible, for example, electrode catheters bearing two electrodes are available, so that simultaneous recording can be made from two sites at the right side of the heart as well as from the arterial circulation.

The main limitation of the tracer techniques described is their inability to distinguish between shunting and valve incompetence. This is of particular interest in the right ventricle where blood may enter either through a defect in the ventricular septum or through an incompetent pulmonary valve. Tracer techniques will not distinguish clearly between pulmonary valve incompetence due to a hypertensive patent ductus without ventricular septal defect, and the coexistence of a ventricular septal defects with patent ductus. Similarly in the atrium the tracer technique may suggest the presence of a ventricular septal defect where, in fact, a low atrial septal defect is present. However, they are of great value in many situations, for example, they will show clearly the presence of high atrial septal defects of the sinus venosus type and it is possible to document precisely the site at which arterial blood is entering the atrium in a way which can be very difficult on the basis of oxygen sample analysis.

Methods of screening outpatients to detect intracardiac shunting have been devised; for the most part they depend upon some form of external assessment of intracardiac build up of a detectable substance, usually an isotope. A collimated counter may be positioned over the heart, an injection of isotope labelled protein given. The form of the resulting curve is somewhat similar to that seen in the dye dilution technique. Where intracardiac shunting occurs, there is loss of the characteristic rise and fall in concentration seen in a patient with intact septa. These techniques are of value where large shunts are present, but they are subject to the considerable limitation that small shunts may be difficult to identify. They cannot, of course, distinguish between the patient in whom a small shunt is present because of a small defect, and the patient in whom shunting is reduced by increased resistance in the pulmonary circulation.

Scintillation gamma scanning

The scintillation gamma-scan camera is now able to provide, by computer analysis, comprehensive data on heart function without formal catheterization. Following injection of a suitable tracer such as ^{99m}Tc into the superior vena cava, the instrument can calculate blood volume, cardiac output, stroke volume, left ventricular ejection fraction, end-diastolic volume and quantitate shunts (Weber *et al.*, 1972). In its simpler form without the computer it can identify shunts and areas of diminished blood supply to the myocardium (Ennis *et al.*, 1975; Alazraki *et al.*, 1972; Flaherty *et al.*, 1967).

Intracardiac phonocardiography

The sounds generated inside the heart chambers may be recorded by a suitable sensing device mounted on the end of a catheter. The technique may have a place in routine diagnostic work, although its use has so far been mainly directed to the elucidation of physiological problems. An example of diagnostic application is the detection of systolic murmurs within the ventricular cavity in cases of ventricular septal defect. In pulmonary stenosis the murmur is usually only found beyond the pulmonary valve. The detection of a systolic murmur proximal to the valve by intracardiac phonocardiography may be the only way of demonstrating the presence of a small ventricular septal defect associated with pulmonary valve stenosis in certain cases in which the small size of the defect, together with the small gradient between the ventricles, renders other methods of identifying its presence ineffective.

Intracardiac electrocardiography

An electrocardiogram is readily obtained from the cavity of the heart and great vessels by means of a platinum tipped electrode of the type used for the ascorbic acid tracer technique. The tracings obtained from the great vessels, ventricles, atria and coronary sinus are different and readily identified (Fig. 3.9). They may, therefore, supplement the pressure tracing as a means of determining the site of the catheter tip, and are occasionally of considerable diagnostic value. For example, in cases of infundibular pulmonary stenosis without valve stenosis, the pressure tracing may be equivocal, but the site of the valve may be clearly shown on the intracardiac electrocardiogram and its separation from the site of the pressure gradient confirmed. It is claimed that a similar diagnostic precision is achieved in cases of Ebstein's anomaly, where the intracardiac electrocardiogram in the ventricular part of the right atrium is said to give ventricular electrocardiographic complexes while the pressure record is atrial. In several cases investigated by this way by the author the results were unconvincing the diagnosis being established angiocardiographically.

Adequate intracardiac electrocardiograms may be recorded by angiographic catheters if these are filled with a suitable conductor such as bicarbonate solution. This

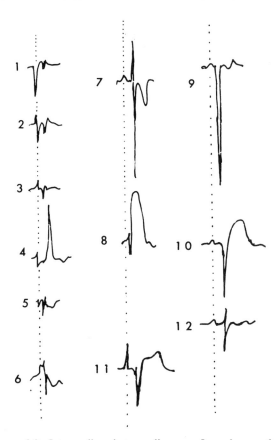

FIG. 3.9   Intracardiac electrocardiograms. In each case the dotted vertical line indicates the atrial complex. 1. High right atrium. 2. Mid right atrium. 3. Low right atrium. 4. Right atrial appendage. 5. Left atrial cavity. 6. Left atrial wall. 7. Right ventricle cavity. 8. Right ventricle wall. 9. Left ventricle cavity. 10. Left ventricle wall. 11. Coronary sinus. 12. Great vessel.

technique provides a simple and safe check before angiocardiography in the ventricle. If the catheter tip touches the wall of the ventricle there is a considerable risk that the contrast medium may be forced into or even through the ventricular wall causing so-called 'stripping' of the muscle. The ventricular wall and the ventricular cavity, however, have easily differentiated electrocardiographic patterns. We therefore record the intracardiac E.C.G. routinely before any selective angiocardiogram into a ventricle if there is any doubt that the tip of the catheter is not lying free in the cavity of the ventricle. If the tracing indicates that the tip is lying against the heart wall, a further manipulation is made to get it into a more favourable site. No intramural injections have occurred when this has been done (Figs. 3.10 and 3.11).

Anyone interested in this technique should read the excellent accounts by Watson (1962) and Stentiford (1968).

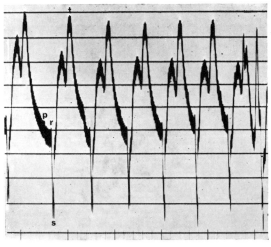

FIG. 3.10   Intracardiac electrocardiogram recorded through an angiographic catheter filled with 5 per cent sodium bicarbonate. Note the gross elevation of the S–T segments. Angiocardiography is contraindicated as the catheter tip is touching the wall of the ventricle.

The usefulness of the intracardiac electrocardiogram (I.C.E.C.G.) in float catheterization can hardly be exaggerated. It is often difficult to be sure from the pressure tracing whether the tip of a float catheter has passed from the right ventricle to the pulmonary artery since the damping of the record in many cases results in a tracing which approximates to a mean pressure. Furthermore, when float catheterization is undertaken without radiological screening, it may be uncertain even whether

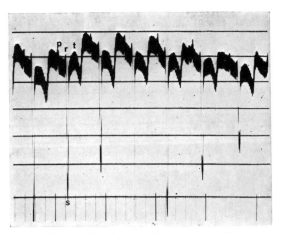

FIG. 3.11   Intracardiac electrocardiogram recorded in the same patient as that shown in Fig. 3.10. The catheter has been repositioned and now shows a cavity potential with normal S–T segments. The catheter tip lies in the ventricular cavity, confirmed by a hand injection of contrast medium viewed by fluoroscopy. Angiocardiography is not likely to cause local damage to the ventricle.

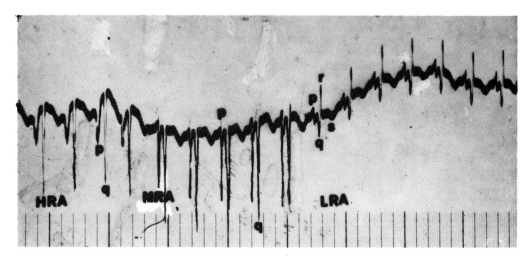

FIG. 3.12 Intracardiac electrocardiogram recorded from the right atrium. Note the progressive change in the form of the P wave and QRS as the electrode is drawn down from the upper part of the atrium (HRA) to the lower part (LRA).

the catheter tip has passed from the subclavian vein into the right atrium. If the catheter is kept full of bicarbonate solution, the position in the atrium and the passage through the ventricle can all be followed with reasonable confidence by observing the I.C.E.C.G. (Figs. 3.12 to 3.15).

A further useful application of this technique is in the analysis of difficult arrhythimas. The simultaneous recording of the atrial I.C.E.C.G. and the standard lead II greatly assists in the clarification of these abnormal rhythms by displaying the atrial E.C.G. in an unequivocal form.

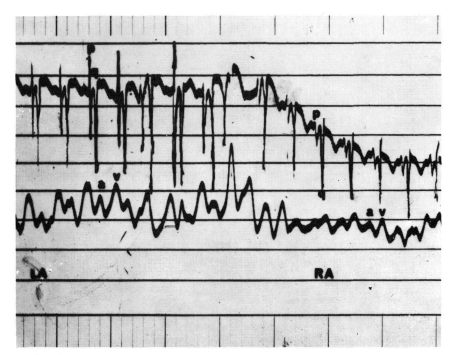

FIG. 3.13 Intracardiac electrocardiogram showing a withdrawal from left to right atrium through a foramen ovale. Note the abrupt change in the voltage and form of the P wave. Lower tracing shows pressure recorded from the catheter.

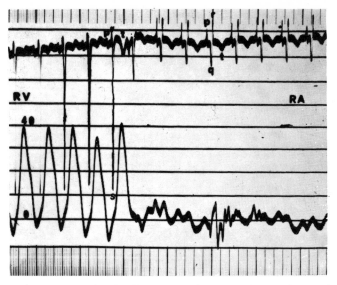

FIG. 3.14 Intracardiac electrocardiogram showing the change as the catheter is drawn back from the right ventricle to atrium. Note the great increase in P wave voltage and fall of S wave in atrium. Pressure trace below.

Bundle of HIS electrocardiogram

The recording of the intracardiac electrocardiogram from a series of electrodes placed along a cardiac catheter permits the study of the spread of depolarization through the endocardium. By suitable placing of the catheter across the tricuspid valve area it is possible to measure the components of atrio-ventricular conduction. The technique is yielding valuable information on the normal and disordered physiology. As yet it has only a limited application in the management of individual patients and remains essentially a research technique.

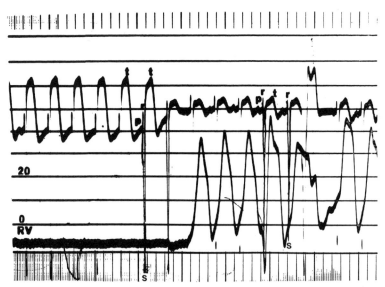

FIG. 3.15 Effect of disimpaction of catheter tip from ventricular wall on intracardiac electrocardiogram. The pressure tracing made with an end-hole catheter shows a sub-zero pressure while the catheter tip is obstructed by the ventricular wall. In this position the platinum ring electrode is applied to the muscle directly and shows a typical endocardial contact electrocardiogram with gross S–T elevation and a deep S wave. When drawn back the pressure change shows the moment of disimpaction of the tip of the catheter. The electrocardiogram changes to one typical of the cavity of the right ventricle with a small P wave, deep S wave, and no S–T elevation. Two complexes have been fully inked in, but most do not show the S wave well as the movement of the recording light beam was too fast to darken the recording paper.

References

Oxygen Analysis

BRINKMAN, R., COST, W. S., KOOPMAN, R. K. & ZIJLSTRA, W. G. (1949). Continuous observation on the percentage oxygen saturation of capillary blood in patients. *Archum. chir. neerl.* **1**, 184.

HOLLING, H. E., MACDONALD, L., O'HALLORAN, J. A. & VENNER, A. (1955). Reliability of spectrophotometric method of measuring blood oxygen. *J. appl. Physiol.* **8**, 249.

ROUGHTON, F. J. W. & SCHOLANDER, P. F. (1943). Microgasometric estimation of blood gases. *J. biol. Chem.* **148**, 541.

VEREL, D., SAYNOR, R. & KESTEVEN, A. B. (1960). A spectrophotometric method of estimating blood oxygen using the UNICAM SP 600. *J. clin. Path.* **13**, 361.

Dye Curves

NICHOLSON, J. W., III, BURCHELL, H. B. & WOOD, E. H. (1951). A method for the continuous recording of Evans blue dye curves in arterial blood and its application to the diagnosis of cardiovascular abnormalities. *J. Lab. clin. Med.* **38**, 588.

Symposium on Dye Dilution Curves (1962). *Circulation Res.* **10**, 377.

Other Tracer Techniques

ALAZRAKI, N. P., ASHBURN, W. L., HAGANA & FRIEDMAN, W. F. (1972). Detection of left-to-right cardiac shunts with the scintillation camera pulmonary dilution curves. *J. Nuclear Med.* **13**, 142.

CLARK, L. C., Jr. & BARGERON, L. M. (1959). Shunt detection with the hydrogen electrode. *Surgery,* **46**, 173.

ENNIS, J. T., WALSH, M. J. & MAHON, J. M. (1975). Value of infarct-specific isotope (^{99m}Tc-labelled stannous pyrophosphate) in myocardial scanning. *Br. Med. J.* **ii**, 517.

FLAHERTY, J. T., CANENT, R. V., BOINEAU, J. P., ANDERSON, P. A. W., LEVIN, A. R. & SPACH, M. S. (1967). Use of externally recorded radiosotope dillution curves for quantitation of left to right shunts. *Am. J. Cardiol.* **20**, 341.

LEVY, A. M., MONROE, R., HUGENPOLY, P. G. & NADAS, A. S. (1967). Clinical use of ascorbic acid as an indicator of right to left shunts with a note on other applications. *Br. Heart J.* **29**, 32.

NIXON, P. F. G., HAY, G. A., HEPBURN, F., SNOW, H. M. & ADDYMAN, R. (1963). Amphoretic technique for recording ascorbate dilution curves and blood flow pulses. *Br. Heart J.* **25**, 173.

SANDERS, R. L. & MORROW, A. G. (1959). Identification and quantitation of left to right shunts with Krypton 85. *Am. J. Med.* **26**, 508.

WEBER, P. M., REMEDIOS, L. V. DOS & JASKO, I. A. (1972). Quantitative radioisotopic angiocardiography. *J. Nuclear Med.* **13**, 815.

Intracardiac Electrocardiography

STENTIFORD, N. H. (1968). Increasing the safety of ventricular angiocardiography. *Clin. Radiol.* **19**, 192.

WATSON, H. (1962). Intracardiac electrocardiography in the investigation of congenital heart disease in infancy and the neonatal period. *Br. Heart J.* **24**, 144.

Intracardiac Phonocardiography

BEUREN, A. J. & APITZ, J. (1963). Intracardiac phonocardiography of the left heart by transseptal left heart puncture. *Am. Heart J.* **66**, 597.

JOLY, F., VOLTY, J. & CARLOTTÉ, J. (1966). Les bruits diastoliques auriculoventriculaires captés par le micromanomètre dans les insuffisances valvulaires pures du coeur gauche. 2e partie, insuffisance mitrale. *Archs. Mal. Coeur,* **59**, 1.

LUISADA, A. A., LIU, C. K., SZATOWSKI, J. & SLODKI, S. J. (1963). Intracardiac phonocardiography in 172 cases studied by left or right heart catheterization or both. *Acta cardiol.* **18**, 533.

PY, J. & BARDET, A. (1966). Phonocardiographie du rétrécissement mitrale. *Archs. Mal. Coeur,* **59**, 917.

SOULIÉ, P., BAQULARD, P., BOUCHARD, F., CORNU, C., LAURENS, P. & WOLFF, F. (1961). La cathétérisme du coeur au micromanomètre. Le son intracardiaque. *Archs. Mal. Coeur,* **54**, Suppl. 1.

TOURRAINE, A., DEYREUX, M., TARTULIER, M. & BLUM, J. (1964). Détection des petites communications interventriculaires par phonocardiographie endocavitaire. *Archs. Mal. Coeur,* **57**, 919.

4. Calculated Data

Surgical experience in treating patients suffering from heart lesions soon revealed a close relationship between surgical success and the state of the lungs. Patients with evidence of pulmonary artery hypertension fared badly compared with those with more normal lungs, whether the lesion was rheumatic damage to valves, or a congenital defect. The haemodynamic data obtained from cardiac catheterization (pressure and oxygen saturation measurements) offered a means of calculating the state of affairs in the pulmonary and systemic systems. The grave hazards of cardiac surgery, particularly in its early stages, lead to widespread use of these calculations in the selection of cases suitable for operation. The great importance of establishing the new techniques of open heart surgery as acceptably safe has perhaps led to an overemphasis of the value of these calculations as criteria.

Increasing experience of open heart techniques has shown the importance of a pre-operative assessment of left ventricular function, especially in patients with coronary artery disease. The particular hazard in operating on a patient with impaired left ventricular function is that at the end of the by-pass period the heart will be unable to sustain a sufficient systemic blood pressure. While measures such as balloon counterpaulsation allow temporary assistance to an inadequate left ventricle, ultimate surgical success and the quality of the result depend upon the capacity of the left ventricle to sustain an adequate output at rest and on exercise.

In this chapter the data and calculations derived from them are described. An attempt to assess their value and limitations is made later (Chapter 18).

Cardiac output and vascular resistance

The calculation of cardiac output, systemic and pulmonary vascular resistances requires the following data:

1. The oxygen uptake.
2. The pulmonary and systemic mean arterial pressures.
3. The oxygen saturations of mixed venous and arterial bloods, the pulmonary venous and pulmonary arterial saturations.

The measurement of (2) and (3) has been discussed.

Oxygen consumption

Oxygen consumption is usually measured by a spirometer, incorporating a carbon dioxide absorber. In another method, which is less convenient, the air expired over a measured interval is collected, the oxygen content estimated and the volume measured by a volume meter. In either case the following data are needed:

(a) Volume of oxygen consumed per minute.

(b) Temperature of gas measured (i.e. temperature of either the spirometer bell or of the gas passing through the volume meter).

(c) Barometric reading.

(d) Height and weight of subject if comparison by du Bois formula for surface area is intended.

The oxygen consumption per minute as measured is corrected to standard temperature and pressure (S.T.P. $0°C$, 760 mmHg + saturated water vapour pressure) by multiplying by the appropriate correction factor, obtained from Table A (p. 39).

Example:

Measured oxygen uptake 230 m/min
Barometric pressure 754·2 mmHg
Gas temperature 23°C
Correction factor from Table A, 0·89
∴ Oxygen consumption at S.T.P. $= 230 \times 0·89$
$= 204.$

Note that the temperature may range from about 17°C to as high as 27°C in temperate climates. This represents a variation of 10/273 or 4 per cent. The barometer may range from about 740 to 780 mmHg, about ± 3 per cent of the normal 760. Neglecting this correction in respect of either temperature or barometric pressure may bring an error of up to 3 per cent into this calculation.

Cardiac output

Cardiac output is measured either directly by the Fick method from catheter data, or by the injection of dyes or other tracers into the circulation. The Fick method is described first.

Fick method

The Fick method of calculating cardiac output is the most convincingly simple in the principle upon which it depends. The rate at which the oxygen is being consumed is divided by the quantity of oxygen removed from the blood by the body. The result must be the quantity of blood in which the oxygen was contained. Stated as an equation:

Cardiac output

$$= \frac{\text{Oxygen consumption}}{\text{Arterial-venous oxygen difference}}.$$

The measurement of oxygen consumption has been described above. The arterio-venous oxygen difference (A.-V.o_2 diff.) is obtained by estimating the O_2 content of blood samples from the systemic and pulmonary arteries and subtracting.

Example:

Oxygen uptake 160 ml/min

Systemic arterial O_2 content 211 ml oxygen/litre

Pulmonary arterial O_2 content 178 ml oxygen/litre

∴A.-V. oxygen difference 33 ml oxygen/litre

∴Cardiac output $= 160/33 = 4.85$ litres/min.

It will be noted that in the preceding calculation the O_2 *content* of blood is needed. When the percentage saturation is determined by haemoreflection or absorptiometry, the oxygen content of blood is easily calculated if the haemoglobin content of the samples is known. The calculation is based on the capacity of haemoglobin to combine with oxygen: 1 g of haemoglobin when fully saturated combines with 1.34 ml of oxygen.

Example:

Calculations of oxygen content from percentage saturation

Saturation: 73 per cent

Haemoglobin: 14.3 g per 100 ml

Oxygen content of sample

$$= \frac{73 \times 14.3 \times 10 \times 1.34}{100}\text{ml/litre}$$

$$= 140 \text{ ml oxygen per litre of blood.}$$

It should be noted that this calculation neglects the small quantity (about 1 per cent) of O_2 in physical solution in blood. Where a large number of samples are taken from the same patient, it is usual to measure the haemoglobin on only one and assume that no major difference between samples exists.

Cardiac output by dye dilution

A typical dye curve is shown in Figure 4.1. The initial deflection represents the change in the colour of the plasma, due to the first passage of the dye through the cuvette, and its area is a measure of the quantity of dye to pass the measuring point. Recirculation of dye prevents the return of the curve to the base line, but when the curve is replotted on semilogarithmic paper (Fig. 4.2) the initial rise and fall in concentration becomes linear, thus providing a precise measure of the transit time (T seconds) by extrapolation. In the time T seconds the blood passing the recording point is all labelled, for the first time, with the injected dye, although the concentration of the dye is varying continuously. The principle of the method is to determine the volume which this dye would label if it were uniformly mixed. Experimental work on models has

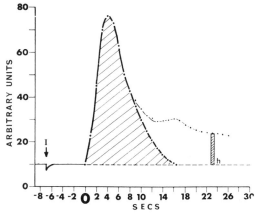

FIG. 4.1 A typical dye dilution curve. The indicator was injected at the time I, a downward deflection of the base line being produced by the event marker. At the time 0 the dye appears at the cuvette and describes the curve shown initially as a heavy interrupted line until the point on the downward curve is reached where the lighter line shows the curve recorded by the cuvette—this divergence indicates recirculation. The predicted area for the first circulation of dye is obtained from a second graph made by plotting the curve on semi-logarithmic paper (Fig. 4.2). Here the fall to base line is linear since the change in concentration is expotential. At h a sample is taken to measure the plasma concentration of dye (see text). In modern instruments the calculation of the area representing the volume of blood labelled on the first circuit (shown hatched) is done electronically.

shown that, if sufficiently frequent samples are taken from such a system, the mean concentration of dye in these samples is the same as that obtained by pooling the whole volume and mixing it up until the dye is evenly distributed.

The mass of dye injected (M mg) produces an average concentration in its first circulation of c mg per litre. The average height of the dye curve is a sample of this labelled volume. This volume is M/c litres. This passes the measuring point in T seconds. In one minute, a volume of $60/T \times M/c$ litres would pass the recording point. It is assumed that the sample curve recorded is a representative one, and that the calculation is therefore a measure of the cardiac output in litres per minute. When a continuous arterial sampling method is used the value of c may be estimated quantitatively by adding dilutions of dye to whole blood and passing them through the arterial cuvette. The patient's blood drawn off before the dye injection may be used for this, and many variables are thus standardized.

Some find the ear cuvette is a more convenient method of measurement. The ear should be rubbed with a vasodilator cream, the cuvette applied and allowed to stabilize with extraneous light excluded. After recording the dye curve, the quantity of c is most easily determined by

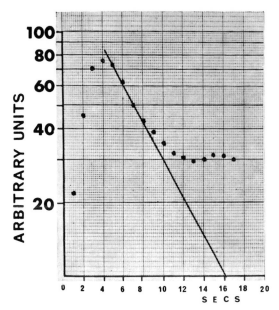

FIG. 4.2   The dye dilution curve shown in Fig. 4.1 plotted on semilogarithmic paper. The straight line is the line best fitting the initial fall from maximal concentration and the curve enclosing the hatched area on Fig. 4.1 is drawn by plotting the points on this line on the linear paper of Fig. 4.1. Note that time 0 is common to both graphs as the intersection with the base on this graph is the transit time used in calculating output. Although the whole curve has been plotted for this illustration, this is not necessary. Only the first four or five points after the peak concentration on Fig. 4.1 are needed to establish the necessary line.

taking a blood sample after the curve has stabilized. The height of the curve above the base line at this sample point is noted. The plasma concentration of the dye in the sample is measured, either after suitable extraction or prolonged centrifuging at high speeds.*

From this measurement, it is possible to deduce that h, the height of the curve when stable, is equivalent to a *plasma* concentration of x mg per litre. If the mean height of the dye curve is H, then the mean concentration of the dye in the labelled sample in its first transit under the recorder (c in the previous section) is Hx/h per litre. The equation for plasma flow is thus:

$$\frac{60}{T} \times \frac{Mh}{Hx} \text{ litres per minute.}$$

*Most dye samples can be measured accurately in whole plasma if the sample is first centrifuged at 3000 r.p.m. for 30 minutes, and the supernatant fluid then centrifuged for a further 30 minutes at 45° and 9000 to 13,000 r.p.m. The intermediate layer should be used, as this high speed spins sediment down and fat up. It is important to treat the blank similarly, and make up a standard, using dye diluted in the blank, by a micro technique. The Agla syringe is suitable for such microdilution.

This is readily converted into whole blood output by use of the haematocrit (it is assumed that there is no significant difference between arterial, venous and capillary haematocrits). If the packed cell volume is measured accurately, the equation becomes:

$$\text{C.O.} = \frac{60}{T} \times \frac{Mh}{Hx} \times \frac{100}{100 - \text{P.C.V.}} \text{ litres per minute.}$$

Comparison of direct arterial sampling techniques with those relying on ear oximetry show a reasonable agreement to within ±10 per cent for estimation of cardiac output.

Precision of measurement and attention to detail are essential in this technique. The apparatus used must be electrically stable, and its response linear. To give accurate, consistent results, the method should be in regular use. Occasionally performed output determinations are likely to be unreliable. The need for care is evident when a typical calculation is examined:

$$\text{C.O.} = \frac{60}{15} \times \frac{100 \times 2}{8 \times 40} \times \frac{100}{100 - 45}$$
$$= 4 \cdot 5 \text{ litres per minute.}$$

Here the transit time was 15 seconds. Conversion to 1 minute, multiplies any errors by four. An error of 0·1 seconds in calculating the transit time is therefore an error of 0·1/15 × 4, which equals 2·7 per cent. Similarly, a 1 mm error in the haematocrit is equivalent here to 1/45 × 4 or 9 per cent. In general, all measurements should be made by the most accurate method available. The average height of the curve (H) is most precisely measured, either by the average of repeated linear measurements or by cutting the curve carefully out and weighing the paper on a micro balance. Planimetry, while superficially attractive, is difficult, as the areas measured are usually too small for precise estimation by this technique. Haematocrit should be measured in duplicate by the method of Chaplin and Mollison (1952).

Computer estimation of cardiac output can be made by suitable apparatus. The output from the photocell is fed into an analyser which computes the area of the curve from the form of the curve. The instrument will provide an immediate estimate of output providing the curve height does not exceed the capacity of the computer. The curve should be recorded simultaneously on another instrument so that the computer estimate can be checked by direct measurement.

Thermodilution may also be used to measure output. The principle is similar to that of dye dilution. A measured quantity of normal saline at a known temperature is injected into the circulation and the temperature change is measured by a sensitive thermocouple. The change recorded is proportional to the volume of cold saline injected and the volume to which it has been added.

In a typical instrument a thermocouple is located on the end of a catheter in the main pulmonary artery or the outflow tract of the right ventricle. Saline is injected proximal to this in the inflow tract of the right ventricle or the right atrium. A curve similar to a dye dilution curve is recorded. The technique assumes that there is no significant warming of the saline in its passage down the catheter. Computer estimation is again available but as the output of a thermocouple is not linear the electronics have to be able to correct for this.

Calculation of intracardiac shunts

The calculation of intracardiac shunts is in principle a simple extension of the measurement of cardiac output by the Fick method. The blood flowing through the pulmonary or systemic circuit is calculated by an equation similar to that used for cardiac output, the samples being taken from the arteries and veins of the system examined. In the systemic system, the oxygen removed from the blood by the metabolism of the body is the numerator of the equation, while in the lung, the oxygen added to the blood by the lungs is used. In both cases this quantity is the oxygen consumption in ml per min.

Example:

Oxygen consumption 160 ml/min (same as oxygen uptake)

P.V. sample (assumed) 98 per cent saturated

P.A. sample (measured) 76 per cent saturated

Haemoglobin 12·8 g/100 ml (measured on a random sample).

1g. Haemoglobin combines with 1·34 ml. oxygen

The blood flow through the lung is calculated from the equation:

Pulmonary blood flow (litres/min)

$$= \frac{\text{Oxygen uptake (ml/min)}}{\text{P.V.}_{O_2} \text{ content}-\text{P.A.}_{O_2} \text{ content (ml/litre)}}$$

In many cases the pulmonary vein blood cannot be sampled. A saturation of 98 per cent is usually assumed and the O_2 content calculated from the haemoglobin of a venous blood sample. In practice, if the blood oxygen of the samples has been measured as saturation, the equation can be simplified so:

Pulmonary blood flow =

$$\frac{O_2 \text{ uptake}}{\text{(P.V.—P.A.) per cent saturation} \times 1\cdot34 \times \text{Hb. g./litre}}$$

Substituting the data in the example, we have:

Pulmonary blood flow (B.F.)

$$= \frac{160}{(98-76)/100 \times 1\cdot34 \times 12\cdot8 \times 10}$$

$$= \frac{160}{0\cdot22 \times 1\cdot34 \times 128}$$

$$= 4\cdot2 \text{ litres/min}$$

The systemic blood flow is calculated from the equation:

Systemic B.F.

$$= \frac{O_2 \text{ consumption}}{\text{A.-V. oxygen content}}$$

This may be simplified to:

Systemic B.F.

$$= \frac{O_2 \text{ consumption}}{\text{A.-V. per cent saturation} \times 1\cdot34 \times 10 \times \text{Hb. g. per cent}}$$

In practice, the main difficulty is deciding on a figure for the venous saturation, particularly when there is a left to right shunt (L–R) at atrial level. Suppose the samples obtained are:

Superior vena cava	64 per cent
High right atrium	68 per cent
Middle right atrium	78 per cent
Low right atrium	62 per cent
High inferior vena cava	68 per cent
Low inferior vena cava	68 per cent

This indicates a L–R shunt at atrial level. The low saturation (62 per cent) at the bottom of the atrium presumably indicates that the catheter lay in the stream of desaturated blood coming from the coronary sinus. In this case the mixed venous saturation is about 66 per cent, but no certain estimate of the level can be made, and the possible errors introduced by an error of even 2 per cent in this determination are discussed elsewhere (p. 154).

In the case considered we have:

Oxygen uptake 160 ml/min

Arterial sample 96 per cent saturated

Venous saturation 66 per cent

Haemoglobin 12·8 g/100 ml

$$\text{Systemic blood flow} = \frac{160}{(96-66) \text{ per cent} \times 12\cdot8 \times 10 \times 1\cdot34}$$

$$= \frac{160}{0\cdot30 \times 13\cdot4 \times 12\cdot8}$$

$$= 3\cdot11 \text{ litres/min.}$$

The ratio of pulmonary blood flow to systemic blood flow is therefore:

$$\frac{4\cdot2}{3\cdot11} = 1\cdot35:1$$

The inaccuracies of these calculations are so great that the figures in litres per min mean very little (p. 155). A simple calculation of shunt, while still inaccurate, is easily made from the blood saturations alone as the following calculations demonstrate:

Shunt

$$= \frac{\text{Pulmonary B.F.}}{\text{Systemic B.F.}}$$

$$= \frac{O_2 \text{ uptake}}{\text{(P.V.—P.A.)}_{O_2} \text{ content}} \quad \frac{\text{A.-V.}_{O_2} \text{ content}}{O_2 \text{ consumption}}$$

$$= \frac{\text{A.-V.}_{O_2} \text{ content}}{\text{(P.V.}-\text{P.A.)}_{O_2} \text{ content}}$$

$$= \frac{\text{A.-V.} \% \text{ saturation} \times 13 \cdot 4 \times \text{Hb}}{(\text{P.V.} - \text{P.A.}) \% \text{ saturation} \times 13 \cdot 4 \times \text{Hb}}$$

$$= \frac{\text{A.-V.}}{\text{P.V.} - \text{P.A.}} \% \text{ saturations}$$

Using these figures the shunt can be quickly calculated. For example, taking the figures already used in the preceding examples, we have

Arterial saturation	96 per cent
Venous saturation	66 per cent
Pulmonary venous saturation	98 per cent
Pulmonary arterial saturation	76 per cent

$\dfrac{\text{Pulmonary}}{\text{Systemic}}$ shunt

$$= \frac{\text{A.-V.}}{\text{P.V.} - \text{P.A.}} \text{ per cent saturation}$$

$$= \frac{96 - 66}{98 - 76}$$

$$= \frac{30}{22}$$

$$= 1 \cdot 4 : 1.$$

Methods for calculating shunts based on dye curves have been suggested, but are not in general use.

Vascular resistance

The arterial pressure in any system is mainly a product of the volume of blood passing through the blood vessels of the system and the resistance of the vessels to this flow. This resistance is primarily due to the tone of the arterioles or their number, i.e. high arterial pressure may result either from arteriolar vasoconstriction or from reduction in the size of the vascular bed as in pulmonary embolism. Other factors such as blood viscosity play a minor part. The vascular resistance is calculated from the formula

$$\text{Resistance} = \frac{\text{Mean arterial pressure}}{\text{Mean flow}}$$

In this formula the mean arterial pressure is the driving force, and the mean flow is either the cardiac output if there is no shunt, or the flow through the lung or systemic system as determined in the previous section. If the pressures and flow are expressed in conventional units (mmHg and litres/min) the quotient is in arbitrary units. These are usually converted to absolute units by multiplying by 80: thus

(total) Resistance

$$= \frac{\text{Mean pressure (mmHg)}}{\text{Flow litres/min}} \times 80 \text{ dyne sec cm}^5$$

A calculation of arteriolar resistance is made by subtracting the mean venous pressure from the mean arterial pressure:

Arteriolar resistance

$$= \frac{(\text{Mean arterial} - \text{mean venous}) \text{ pressure mm. Hg.}}{\text{Flow litres/min.}}$$
$$\times 80 \text{ dyne sec. cm}^5.$$

Normal values have been established by Barratt-Boyes and Wood (1958).

Total system resistance $= 1130 \pm 178$ dyne sec cm^5.
Total pulmonary resistance $= 205 \pm 51$ dyne sec cm^5.
Pulmonary arteriolar resistance $= 67 \pm 23$ dyne sec cm^5.

Assessment of left ventricular function

Methods of measuring cardiac output have been in use for over half a century and their intrinsic accuracy is well established. Further, the concept of output and vascular resistance is a simple one, representing the end product of cardiovascular function. In contrast, the function of the left ventricle is determined by many independent factors whose interaction is complex and may be difficult to assess. Similar clinical pictures of *left ventricular failure* may result from such different causes as *aortic stenosis* where the prime difficulty is the pressure needed to distend the thickened ventricle in diastole; *aortic incompetence* where a main factor may be the transmission of aortic diastolic pressure through the ventricle to the atrium; *failure of the ventricular wall to contract* adequately as a result of dyskinesis from nutritional failure or scarring in coronary artery disease, or diversion of its stroke volume into an aneurysm; *inadequate contraction* in thinning due to disease; or simply *inadequate nutrition* in an unconnected disease such as anaemia. The symptoms may even occur in conditions such as *mitral stenosis* where the ventricle is normal. Any assessment, therefore, may have to take into account a number of factors such as the state of the myocardium, the valves and coronary arteries before the significance of any observations on the ventricle can be appreciated.

Measurements reflecting function

Several methods for the assessment of left ventricular function are currently being explored. The ideal technique would provide by non-invasive methods a sufficiently reliable guide to the state of the left ventricle for a firm opinion as to the safety of surgery. Other desirable qualities are measurement in absolute units, ease of repetition so that progress can be measured, and simplicity of technique so that observations made in one diagnostic unit are readily acceptable in another in the same way that measurements of intra-cardiac pressure are so accepted. It is with these considerations in mind that the methods described should be criticized.

Non-invasive methods

SYSTOLIC TIME INTERVALS (S.T.I.)

The measurement of S.T.I. is the oldest and one of the simplest methods for the assessment of left ventricular

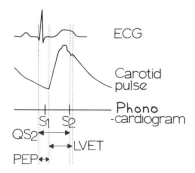

FIG. 4.3 Relations between the electrocardiogram, carotid pulse trace and phonocardiogram used in the calculation of systolic time intervals.

function. The technique, which has been continuously developed for over a century, utilizes a recording of the peripheral arterial pulse wave to infer the behaviour of the left ventricle. Reliable measurements may be made by simultaneously recording the electrocardiogram, the carotid pulse wave, and the aortic phonocardiogram at high speed. Weissler and Garrard (1971) provide an interesting historical review and clear description of the method. The cardiac cycle as recorded by this technique is divided by three events: The Q wave of the electrocardiogram which is taken to signal the onset of 'electromechanical systole', the onset of the rise in pressure in the arterial tracing indicating the beginning of the ejection phase, and the dicrotic notch (incisura) which terminates it (Fig. 4.3). The delay in the appearance of the arterial trace due to the time taken for it to reach the recording point on the carotid or subclavian artery is corrected by a simple technique described below. The point at which the pulse trace begins to rise may be more precisely defined by projecting the trace before and after its onset by straight lines as suggested by De Werf et al., 1975 (Fig. 4.4).

The cardiac systolic phase is in this way defined as electromechanical systole $(Q.S._2)$ which is subdivided into the pre-ejection phase (P.E.P.) and left ventricular ejection time (L.V.E.T.). $Q.S._2$ is derived from the phonocardiographic and electrocardiographic records, and P.E.P. calculated by subtracting the L.V.E.T. measured from the pulse trace thus correcting for the pulse delay. P.E.P. is thus a qualitative estimate of the isometric phase of left ventricular contraction while L.V.E.T. corresponds to the isotonic phase. In general, left ventricular failure is accompanied by a relative lengthening of the P.E.P.

A refinement of the method is to use the echocardiogram to record the valve movement instead of the phonocardiogram. The comparison of the parameters derived by this method with those obtained by phonocardiography showed a high correlation of $r > 0.97$, con-

C

firming the value of the simpler technique (Stephandouros and Witham, 1975). In addition, echocardiography does permit S.T.I. of the right ventricle (Hirschfeld et al., 1975).

The main disadvantage of this technique is the need to correct for the heart rate since the proportion of P.E.P. to L.V.E.T. varies with rate in normal hearts. Formulae for achieving this are given by Weissler and Garrard. De Werf et al., (1975) in a comparison of this indirect measurement of left ventricular function with direct measurements made with catheter-tip micromanometers discuss the limitations of the method. They found that despite close linear correlations between internally and externally measured S.T.I., there were significant differences dependent on heart rate. They also noted differences in the transmission times for upstroke and incisura of the pulse trace to that of the phonocardiogram, for example at a mean heart rate of 76, the transmission time of the upstroke exceeded that of the incisura by 6 msec. At 110 beats per minute the times were equal.

Wanderman et al. (1976) found in mitral valve incompetence, P.E.P. prolonged and L.V.E.T. shortened, presumably due to the leak prolonging the time needed to reach opening pressure and reducing the volume to be ejected.

ECHOCARDIOGRAPHY

Echocardiographic techniques are described in Chapter 5. The technique has been rapidly developed recently, and with the latest instruments a three dimensional picture of the cardiac valves and heart chambers can be built up from the records obtained. Measurements of systolic and diastolic size of the ventricle, the thickness of the ventricular muscle and valve cusps, and the rate at which the ventricular walls move can all be made. The measurements are obtained in absolute terms (cms) and the data satisfies the criteria defined earlier (p. 32). The main limitation of the technique is the difficulty in obtaining results in patients in whom lung disease such as emphysema interposes lung tissue between the surface of the chest and the heart since echoes are not satisfactorily recorded through lung tissue. The technique gives reliable results and is likely to become generally accepted as the most useful of the non-invasive techniques for assessing left ventricular function.

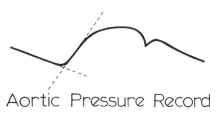

Aortic Pressure Record

FIG. 4.4 Extrapolation to identify the onset of the systolic rise in pressure as a point.

Invasive methods

All invasive methods depend upon information obtained by cardiac catheterization, and may be divided into those in which the primary data is *measurement of pressure* and those in which the data is primarily *angiographic*. In both, the objective, as in the non-invasive methods is to assess left ventricular function, and the interpretation of the data has to be considered in the context of the anatomical lesions which may be present.

Methods based on pressure measurement

VENTRICULAR DIASTOLIC PRESSURE

The ventricular diastolic pressure is the simplest measurement which may provide an index of left ventricular function. It is the filling pressure of the ventricle and is normally just below zero immediately after the opening of the mitral valve, rising as the ventricle fills to about 7 mmHg after atrial systole. The pressure at the end of diastole (end-diastolic pressure or E.D.P.) immediately after the atrial impulse is generally taken as the most significant point (Ross and Braunwald, 1961).

The interpretation of the value of the E.D.P. depends upon the nature of the disease affecting the heart. In cases in which the mitral and tricuspid valves are normal, the E.D.P. is a fair indicator of the degree of ventricular failure and so of the state of the ventricular muscle. In such cases the E.D.P. is consistent with the symptoms (chiefly dyspnoea) and the decision on whether surgical treatment is possible depends upon the diagnosis established by investigation. The problem in treatable cases is to balance the risk of surgery against the improvement in myocardial function which may result from operation, be it, for example, excision of a myocardial aneurysm or relief of an obstruction to a major coronary artery.

When valve lesions are present the findings must be related to these and to the state of the myocardium, thus, in mitral incompetence the E.D.P. is partly the result of the increased stroke volume and partly due to any myocardial disease such as infarction or rheumatism. A particularly dramatic situation may arise in acute destruction of the aortic valve by endocarditis. Here aortic reflux may be so gross as to cause the E.D.P. to equal aortic diastolic pressure. Premature closure of the mitral valve occurs and acute pulmonary oedema is an indication for emergency surgery to replace the aortic valve (Fig. 2.20). In favourable cases the results are good since the ventricular myocardium is normal—the E.D.P. being wholly a consequence of the torrential aortic regurgitation.

V-MAX

As the measurement of V-max has been advanced as a useful parameter for the assessment of left ventricular function, a description of the principle involved and assessment of its usefulness is desirable. The concept is a somewhat complex one—perhaps best approached historically.

In a series of elegant experiments Hill (1939) demonstrated that in striated voluntary muscle the work done in contracting against varying loads could be measured by a thermopile, the mechanical work done and the heat evolved being related. Heat was evolved in isometric and in isotonic contraction. Voluntary muscle has the property of allowing passive extension without increasing its tension, so any series of observations could begin at zero tension or 'pre-load'. The velocity with which contraction occurred varied with the load, being greatest at zero load and falling along a hyperbolic curve to a minimum velocity at the maximum load of which the muscle was capable. This curve of force against velocity is termed a force–velocity curve, the velocity of contraction being highest at $F = O$ and termed V-max (Fig. 4.5).

Hill constructed a theoretical model to illustrate the properties of the muscle in the preparation. This consisted of a contractile element (C.E.) in series with an elastic element (S.E.). This concept provided a simple image to take account of the curious properties of voluntary muscle—its extensibility without change in tension and its capacity to increase its tension without change in length. The primary contractility without load, V-max, appeared a useful parameter for determining the state of the contractile elements of muscle fibre and so for estimating its normality.

Abbott and Mommaerts (1959) and Sonnenblick (1962) investigated the properties of myocardial papillary muscle in an attempt to derive figures for V-max for cardiac muscle. They found that cardiac muscle differs fundamentally from skeletal muscle in that myocardial strips exhibit an intrinsic tone proportional to the degree to which they are passively stretched. It is therefore impossible to begin a series of measurements at V-max because the point of no tension is not attainable. V-max, however, can be estimated as a (theoretical) point

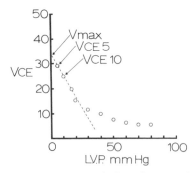

FIG. 4.5 Telation between velocity of contraction of the myocardial contractile elements (V_{CE}) and rise in left ventricular pressure from which V-max, V_{CE5} and V_{CE10} are derived.

of maximal velocity for the contractile elements of the muscle (V_{ce}-max) by making a series of measurements with different loads and projecting back along the hyperbolic curve obtained to the zero load point. Sonnenblick (1962) showed that a family of curves obtained by using different initial lengths all projected back to the same point, thus demonstrating the validity of the concept. Hill's simple model is clearly inadequate to explain the phenomena observed. The difficulties of this work and the problems of constructing models to illustrate it are discussed by Pollack (1970) and by Parmley et al. (1972).

The difficulties in extending the concept of V-max to the intact human heart are evident. In addition to the intrinsic difference in the matter of tone between skeletal and cardiac muscle, the heart does not contract like an experimental preparation responding to an electrical stimulus: the isovolumic contraction of the ventricle is a progressive event more akin to gastric peristalsis than to the global contraction of the urinary bladder (Spiller et al., 1975). Further, the muscle of the ventricular wall is a complex basket-like weave of interlacing fibres running in many directions. However, during the isometric phase of ventricular contraction it is reasonable to regard the rate of pressure change and the pressure developed within the ventricle as equivalent respectively to the rate of shortening of the contractile elements (S.E.) and the muscle force of the papillary muscle preparation. (The term 'isometric' is, of course, strictly applicable to the muscle strip experimental preparation. In the heart, the pre-ejection phase of ventricular systole is accompanied by a complex combination of movements and the hybrid word 'isovolumic' has been coined to describe it.)

In the intact human heart, an estimate of V-max is based upon measurements of the ventricular *pressure change* during the isovolumic phase of contraction and simultaneous measurements of the *rate of pressure change* (dp/dt) derived electronically from the ventricular pressure record. A variety of calculations has been proposed making use of these measurements, but in all of them the force-velocity curve (Fig. 4.5) is the underlying concept with ventricular pressure representing force and dp/dt the velocity of contraction of the contractile elements (C.E.).

To estimate V-max the left ventricular pressure is recorded by an intracavity transducer at high speed (200 cm/s) with simultaneous recording of dp/dt. V_{ce} is derived from the data by means of the formula.

$$V_{ce} = \frac{dp/dt}{32\,P}$$

The constant, 32, is the series elastic constant for myocardium determined by Parmley et al. (1968). V_{ce} is determined for a series of points on the isovolumic phase of the pressure rise and plotted against the cor-

responding intraventricular pressure on linear graph paper. The curve, which because of the tone of cardiac muscle cannot start at $P = 0$, is extrapolated back to P_0 to determine V-max. Any extrapolation of a curve is, of course, subject to error and some authors have preferred to take a point on the V_{ce}-pressure curve such as V_{ce} at 5 mm or at 10 mmHg pressure as less liable to error for purposes of comparison (Parmley et al., 1974; Kreulen et al., 1975).

Other parameters which have been used and which are based on the same concept are: V_{ce} at peak stress, in contrast to V-max which is V_{ce} at zero stress; peak V_{ce}; peak circumferential fibre velocity; and maximum dp/dt, (Gault et al., 1968; Falsetti et al., 1970 & 1971).

V-max is the most selective gauge of the state of cardiac muscle, providing an index of the contractile elements of the muscle fibre. Perhaps because of its selectivity it has not proved in practice to be superior to the cruder measurements of function. (It should be noted that Pollack (1970) has thrown doubt on the specificity of V-max as a measure of C.E.) In general, the left ventricular E.D.P. emerges from a series of studies as the simplest and more useful index of the performance of the left ventricle (Hugenholtz et al., 1970; Levine et al., 1970; Mason et al., 1971; Falsetti et al., 1971; Graham et al., 1971; Graber et al., 1972; Krayenbuel et al., 1973; Parmley et al., 1974; Peterson et al., 1974). In a comparison of several factors used to estimate left ventricular function (Kreulen et al., 1975) compared L.V.E.D.P., ejection fraction, left ventricular contraction patterns and V-max. They concluded that each of these could give an index of dysfunction in particular circumstances but that on the whole V-max was the least sensitive index.

PEAK VENTRICULAR DP/DT

The measurement of ventricular dp/dt has been mentioned in the section describing V-max. Ventricular pressure change is measured by a catheter-tip manometer and a differentiating electronic circuit derives the rate of change in pressure (Fig. 2.21). The maximum rate of change achieved might reasonably be expected to give a useful index of the state of ventricular muscle. The measurements are easily made, and the results are obtained in absolute units—mmHg/sec, and have been shown convincingly to be related to the contractile state of the ventricles. Thus, the administration of muscle stimulants increases the maximal dp/dt while depressant drugs or hypoxia depress it.

Observations on normal hearts, however, show that maximal dp/dt is affected by many factors. The maximal rate of ventricular contraction usually occurs immediately before the opening of the ventricular exit valve—aortic or pulmonary. The opening time is therefore related to the *aortic and diastolic pressure* (when ventricular and aortic pressures equalize). A rise in the end diastolic aortic pressure delays the opening of the valve. This is associated with a rise in the maximal dp/dt.

Similarly, a rise in the *ventricular filling pressure* increases maximal dp/dt. A rise in the ventricular end-diastolic pressure such as that caused by exercise or leg raising in the recumbent normal subject will cause increased ventricular filling and a rise in the maximal dp/dt.

Sustained arterial hypertension has also been shown to increase maximal dp/dt (Wallace *et al.*, 1963). The mechanism here appears to be neurogenic.

Finally, maximal dp/dt is affected by *heart rate,* increasing with tachycardia and falling with bradycardia.

The problems set by this dependence of dp/dt upon the conditions of ventricular work are discussed in detail by Mason *et al.* (1969). A number of possible ways of producing a derivative of dp/dt which would have an absolute value as a basis for comparison with a normal have been suggested. These include the time from initial contraction to peak dp/dt; peak dp/dt as a function of a variety of ventricular-pressure fractions including end-diastolic pressure and peak dp/dt related to ventricular end-diastolic volume. None has emerged convincingly as a generally accepted basis for comparing cases. The measurement is accepted as a valid index of contractility but is mainly of use in acute observations.

Methods based on cardioangiography

Of all the invasive methods of assessing left ventricular function the evidence from the angiocardiogram is perhaps the most convincing. The pattern of contraction is observed on cine film during a slow injection of contrast medium (15 ml/s), the electrocardiogram being monitored to confirm the absence of extrasystoles. Much early work on the contraction pattern of the ventricle was done using biplane cine angiography (Dodge *et al.*, 1960; Brun *et al.*, 1966; Kennedy *et al.*, 1966). The normal end-diastolic volume of the left ventricle was found to correlate poorly with age, sex, body-area or weight. The method using biplane film is time consuming and exposes the patient to unnecessary radiation since single plane filming provides a sufficiently accurate measurement (Sandler and Dodge, 1968).

The right anterior oblique (R.A.O.) projection centred over the ventricle is now usually employed as this displays the ventricle best. With a little experience the performance can be assessed by eye—the rapid contraction to a small end-systolic volume of a normally contracting ventricle contrasting with a poor emptying and inadequate contraction in severe disease. Multiple projections may be needed to display, adequately, areas of akinesia, paradoxical movement or aneurysm formation.

A number of methods of quantitating the contraction of the ventricle have been suggested. All provide a measurement of end-systolic size and a ratio of end-diastolic to end-systolic size. Most, directly or indirectly, provide an index of the area visualized on the cine film and so of volume, the left ventricle being approximately an ellipsoid, circular in sections in the plane at right angles to the axis between the apex and aortic valve. The measurements thus provide figures which are meaningful—corresponding to stroke volume (the difference between end-diastolic and end-systolic area) and to muscle efficiency (end-systolic volume). The analogy with Starling's law is evident.

The inverse square law, of course, applies to the conditions in which the angiocardiography is performed. The X-ray beam may be considered as having a point source and the true size of the ventricle is exaggerated by the beam. The true end-systolic area can only be computed if the relative positions of the origin, the ventricle and the image are known.

Determining this accurately is difficult. However, these conditions do not apply to the ratio of the end-systolic to end-diastolic volumes since the correction for the inverse square law applies equally to both measurements and does not affect the ratio. In practice, therefore, the *ejection fraction* as this ratio is called, is usually the only parameter calculated.

Determination of the ejection fraction may be made either by calculating the *area* of the cavity of the left ventricle in systole and diastole or by *measurement of selected axes.*

The area is most easily measured by an electronic planimeter. This expensive apparatus consists of a television monitor on which the cine angiogram is displayed. The maximal and minimal ventricular sizes are selected and the ventricle outlined with an electronic pencil at these points. The apparatus computes the areas and the ratio between them.

A more laborious but vastly less expensive technique is to determine the areas with a mechanical planimeter.

The method using *axes* is simpler, providing a linear measurement proportional to the area. The long axis of the ventricular cavity is measured in systole and in diastole and to this is added either the single maximal transverse axis at right angles to the long axis or two axes are taken at one-third of the long axis from either end.

AORTIC BLOOD VELOCITY

The velocity with which blood passes up the aorta is a result of several factors. When the anatomy is normal, these are primarily the ejection of blood by the ventricle, the diameter of the aorta and the degree of elastic recoil. The ventricular ejection is dependent on pressure gradients, heart rate and venous return. Measurement of flow rates is further complicated by the recoil which follows closure of the aortic valves, when the direction of flow may be briefly reversed, and by the observation that the rate of flow is not uniform over the cross-section of the aorta, being less close to the walls (Schultz, 1972). The value of the observation is greatly complicated in the presence of valve lesions, stenosis of the aortic valve leading the slowing of flow with abnormal turbulence, aortic incompetence distorting the normal effects due to valve closure, and mitral-valve stenosis reducing the cardiac output without having any direct effect upon left ventricular function. Measurements of aortic blood velocity, therefore, may be expected to have a limited usefulness in gauging the function of the left ventricle.

Aortic blood velocity can be measured by electromagnetic flow meter, Doppler ultrasound, or by differential-pressure measurement. The last makes use of a double lumen catheter with two outlets 5 cm apart. Flow velocity is computed electronically from the recordings of pressure (Barnett *et al.,* 1961; Porje and Rudewald, 1961). A critical discussion of the value of these techniques will be found in *Cardiovascular Fluid Dynamics* (1972). A useful discussion of the value of aortic blood velocity and other measurements in the assessment of left ventricular function will be found in the paper by Kolettis *et al.* (1976).

Combinations of invasive and non-invasive techniques

Several of the techniques described above have been used in combination to define aspects of left ventricular function. Agress and Wegner (1968) have suggested a technique for predicting stroke volume from the ratio of the isovolumic contraction time to the ejection time. The I.C.T. was derived from the electrocardiogram and aortic-pressure trace, the E.T. from the aortic trace. Hermann *et al.* (1969) have assessed myocardial contractility as a ratio of maximal ventricular dp/dt to integrated isovolumic stress, a parameter calculated from the integrated pressure change during the isovolumic phase of contraction, and the ventricular dimensions determined angiographically. Falsetti *et al.* (1970) have made somewhat similar calculations more simple by using a transverse diameter of the ventricle determined angiocardiographically. Gibson and Brown (1976) have used echocardiography, pressure measurement and angiocardiography to demonstrate the use of simultaneous echocardiography, with pressure measurement to assess left ventricular function. From the data, pressure-dimension loops may be derived to provide a graphic display of the quality of left ventricular function.

Whatever method is employed, the result is a useful measure of left ventricular function, a high ejection fraction being associated with good function and a low ejection fraction with poor function (Dodge and Baxley, 1969). The angiocardiogram does not cause any significant disturbance of ventricular contraction (Carleton, 1971; Hammermeister and Warbrasse, 1973).

The evaluation of left ventricular function is important for any pre-operative or post-operative assessment. The review presented here is brief and could be greatly extended. A useful review of the difficulties in this field is provided by Sandler and Alderman (1974). The work of Kreulen *et al.* (1975) compares a number of techniques. Studies comparing echocardiography with other methods of assessing left ventricular function will be found in the work of Ludbrook *et al.* (1973) and of Stack *et al.* (1976). Other useful papers are those of Naqvi *et al.* (1976), Rackley (1976) and of Noble (1972). Eddleman *et al.* (1977) found S.T.I. measurements correlated poorly with angiographic determination of L.V. Ejection fractions. Recent developments in the construction of echocardiographic apparatus are likely to provide a reliable noninvasive technique for accurate measurement of ejection fractions.

References

ABBOTT, B. C. & MOMMAERTS, W. F. H. M. (1959). Study of inotropic mechanisms in the papillary muscle preparation. *J. Gen. Physiol.* **42**, 553.

AGRESS, C. M. & WEGNER, S. (1968). Determination of stroke volume from left ventricular isovolumetric contraction and ejection times. *Jap. Heart J.* **9**, 339.

BARNETT, G. O., GREENFIELD, J. C. & FOX, S. M. (1961). The technique of estimating the instantaneous aortic blood velocity in man from the pressure gradient. *Am. Heart J.* **62**, 359.

BARRATT-BOYES, B. G. & WOOD, E. H. (1958). Cardiac output and related measurements in healthy subjects. *J. Lab. Clin. Med.* **51**, 72.

CHAPLIN, J. G. & MOLLINSON, P. L. (1952). Correction for plasma trapped in the red cell column of the haematocrit. *Blood* **7**, 1227.

DE WERF, F. V., PIESSENS, J., KESTELOOT, H. & DE GEEST, H. (1975). A direct comparison between internally and externally measured left ventricular systolic time intervals. *Acta Cardiologica* **30**, 171.

DODGE, H. T. & BAXLEY, W. A. (1969). Left ventricular volume and mass and their significance in disease. *Am. J. Cardiol.* **23**, 528.

DODGE, H. T., SADLER, H. H., BALLEW, D. M. & LORD, J. D. (1960). The use of biplane angiocardiography for the measurement of the left ventricle in man. *Am. Heart J.* **60**, 762.

EDDLEMAN, E. E., JR., SWATZELL, R. H., JR., BANCROFT, W. H., JR., BALDONE, J. C., JR. & TUCKER, M. S. (1977). The use of systolic time intervals in predicting left ventricular ejection fraction in ischaemic heart disease. *Am. Heart J.* **93**, 450.

FALSETTI, H. L., MATES, R. E., GRANT, C., GREENE, D. G. & BUNNELL, I. L. (1970). Left ventricular wall stress calculated from one-plane cineangiography. *Circ. Res.* **26**, 71.

FALSETTI, H. L., MATES, R. E., GREEN, D. G. & BUNNELL, I. L. (1971). V-max as an index of contractile state in man. *Circulation* **43**, 467.

GAULT, J. H., ROSS, J. J. & BRAUNWALD, E. (1968). Contractile state of the left ventricle in man. Instantaneous tension–velocity–length relations in patients with and without disease of the left ventricular myocardium. *Circ. Res.* **22**, 451.

GIBSON, D. G. & BROWN, D. J. (1976). Assessment of left

ventricular systolic function from simultaneous echocardiographic and pressure measurements. *Br. Heart J.* **38**, 8.

GORLIN, R. & GORLIN, S. G. (1951). Hydraulic formula for calculation of area of stenotic mitral valve, other cardiac valves and central circulatory shunts. *Am. Heart J.* **41**, 1.

GRABER, J. D., CONTI, C. R., LAPPE, D. L. & ROSS, J. R. (1972). Effect of pacing, induced tachycardia and myocardial ischaemia on ventricular pressure-velocity relationships in man. *Circulation* **46**, 74.

GRAHAM, T. P., JARMAKANI, J. M., CANENT, R. V. & ANDERSON, P. A. W. (1971). Evaluation of left ventricular contractile state in childhood. *Circulation* **44**, 1043.

HAMMERMEISTER, K. E. & WARBASSE, J. R. (1973). Immediate haemodynamic effects of cardiac angiography in man. *Am. J. Cardiol.* **31**, 307.

HERMANN, H. J., SINGH, R. & DAMMANN, J. F. (1969). Evaluation of myocardial contractility in man. *Am. Heart J.* **77**, 755.

HILL, A. V. (1939). Heat of shortening and dynamic constants of muscle. *Proc. Roy. Soc.(B)* **126**, 136.

HIRSCHFELD, S., MEYER, R., SCHWARTZ, D. C., KORFHAGEN, J. & KAPLAN, S. (1975). Measurement of right and left ventricular systolic time intervals by echocardiography. *Circulation* **51**, 304.

HUGENHOLT, R. G., ELLISON, R. C., URSCHEL, C. W., MIRSKY, I. & SONNENBLICK, E. H. (1970). Myocardial force-velocity relationships in clinical heart disease. *Circulation* **41**, 191.

KENNEDY, J. W., BAXLEY, W. A., FIGLEY, M. M., DODGE, H. T. & BLACKMAN, J. R. (1966). Quantitative angiocardiography. 1. The normal left ventricle in man. *Circulation* **34**, 272.

KOLETTIS, M., JENKINS, B. S. & WEBB-PEPLOE, M. M. (1976). Assessment of left ventricular function by indices derived from aortic flow velocity. *Br. Heart J.* **38**, 18.

KREULEN, T. H., BOVE, A. A., McDONOUGH, M. T., SANDS, M. J. & SPANN, J. F. (1975). The evaluation of left ventricular function in man. A comparison of methods. *Circulation* **51**, 677.

LEVINE, H. J., McINTYRE, K. M., LIPANA, J. G. & BING, O. H. L. (1970). Force-velocity relations in failing and non-failing hearts of subjects with aortic stenosis. *Am. J. Med. Sci.* **259**, 79.

LUDBROOK, P., KARLINER, J. S., PETERSON, K., LEOPOLD, G. & O'ROUKE, R. A. (1973). Comparison of ultrasound and cineangiographic measurements of left ventricular performance in patients with and without wall motion abnormalities. *Br. Heart J.* **35**, 1026.

MASON, D. T., SPANN, J. F., ZEUS, R. & AMSTERDAM, E. A. (1971). Comparison of the contractile state in the normal, hypertrophied and failing heart in man. *Cardiac Hypertrophy* ed. Albert, N. Acad. Press, N.Y.

NAQVI, S. Z., CHISHOLM, A. W., STANDEN, I. R. & SHANE, S. I. (1976). Relative insensitivity of isovolumic phase indices in the assessment of left ventricular function. *Amer. Heart J.* **91**, 577.

NICHOLSON, J. W. & WOOD, E. H. (1951). Estimation of cardiac output and Evans blue space, using an oximeter. *J. Lab. clin. Med.* **38**, 588.

NOBLE, M. I. M. (1972). Problems concerning the applications of mechanics to the determination of contractile state in man. *Circulation,* **45**, 252.

PARMLEY, W. W., CHUCK, L. & SONNENBLICK, E. H. (1972). Relation of V-max to different models of cardiac muscle. *Circ. Res.* **30**, 34.

PARMLEY, W. W., SPANN, J. F., TAYLOR, R. R. & SONNENBLICK, E. H. (1968). The series elasticity of cardiac muscle in hyperthyroidism, ventricular hypertrophy and heart failure. *Proc. Soc. Exp. Biol. Med.* **127**, 606.

PARMLEY, W. W., TOMODA, H., FORRESTER, J. S. & SWAN, H. J. C. (1974). Dissociation of pump performance and contractility in patients with acute myocardial infarction. *Clin. Res.* **22**, 111.

PETERSON, K. C., SLKOVEN, D., LUDBROOK, P., UTHER, J. B. & ROSS, J. R. (1974). Comparison of isovolumic and ejection phase indices of myocardial performance in man. *Circulation* **49**, 1088.

POLLACK, G. H. (1970). Maximum velocity as an index of contractility in cardiac muscle. *Circ. Res.* **26**, 111.

PORGÉ, I. G. & RUDEWALD, B. (1961). Haemodynamic studies with differential pressure technique. *Acta physiol. scand.* **51**, 116.

RACKLEY, C. E. (1976). Quantitative evaluation of left ventricular function by radiological techniques. *Circulation* **54**, 802.

SANDLER, H. & ALDERMAN, E. (1974). Determination of left ventricular size and shape. *Circ. Res.* **34**, 1.

SANDLER, H. H. & DODGE, H. T. (1968). The use of single plane angiocardiograms for the calculation of left ventricular volume in man. *Am. Heart J.* **75**, 325.

SCHULTZ, D. L. (1972). *Cardiovascular Fluid Dynamics*, Acad. Press, Ch. 9.

SIMON, H., KRAYENBUEHL, H. P., RUTISHAUSER, W. & PRETTER, B. O. (1970). The contractile state of the hypertrophied left ventricular myocardium in aortic stenosis. *Am. Heart J.* **79**, 587.

SONNENBLICK, E. H. (1962). Force-velocity relations in the mamalian heart muscle. *Am. J. Physiol.* **202**, 931.

SPILLER, F., KREUZER, H. & MORITZ-RAHN, G. (1975). Geometrische Änderungen des linken Ventrikels während der isovolumetrischen Kontraktion bei Gesunden und Koronarkranken. *Zeitschrift für Kardiologie* **64**, 1004.

STACK, R. S., LEE, C. C., REDDY, B. P., TAYLOR, M. L. & WEISSLER, A. M. (1976). Left ventricular performance in coronary artery disease evaluated with systolic time intervals and echo-cardiography. *Amer. J. Cardiol.* **37**, 331.

STEPHANDOUROS, M. A. & WITHAM, A. C. (1975). Systolic time intervals by echocardiography. *Circulation* **51**, 114.

Symposium on Dye Dilution Curves (1962). *Circ. Res.* **10**, 377. See also the references to Chapter 17.

WANDERMAN, K. L., GOLDBERG, M. J., STACK, R. S. & WEISSLER, A. M. (1976). Left ventricular performance assessed by S.T.I. and echocardiography. *Am. J. Cardiol.* **38**, 831.

WEISSLER, A. M. & GARRARD, C. L., Jr. (1971). Systolic time intervals in cardiac disease. I & II. *Modern Concepts of Cardiovascular Disease* **40**, 1–8.

Table A reducing to 0°C and 760 mmHg 1 litre of air from 10° to 25°C and 740 to 760 mmHg, saturated with water vapour.
(From Meakins, J. C. and Davies, H. Whitridge (1926). Respiratory Function in disease, Edinburgh: Oliver and Boyd.)

BAROMETER

Temperature	29·13 740	29·17 741	29·21 742	29·25 743	29·29 744	29·33 745	29·37 746	29·41 747	29·45 748	29·49 749	29·53 750	29·57 751	29·60 752	29·64 753	29·68 754	29·72 755	29·76 756	29·80 757	29·84 758	29·88 759	29·92 760
10	927·7	928·9	930·2	931·4	932·6	933·9	935·1	936·4	937·6	938·9	940·4	941·6	942·9	944·2	945·4	946·6	947·9	949·2	950·5	951·8	953·0
11	923·6	924·8	926·1	927·3	928·5	929·8	931·0	932·3	933·5	934·8	936·3	937·5	938·8	940·1	941·3	942·5	943·8	945·1	946·4	947·7	948·9
12	919·5	920·5	921·8	923·0	924·2	925·5	926·7	928·0	929·3	930·5	931·8	933·1	934·3	935·6	936·8	938·0	939·4	940·7	942·0	943·3	944·4
13	915·4	916·7	918·0	919·2	920·4	921·7	922·9	924·2	925·4	926·7	928·0	929·2	930·4	931·7	932·9	934·1	935·3	936·8	938·1	939·4	940·5
14	911·3	912·6	913·9	915·1	916·3	917·6	918·8	920·1	921·3	922·6	923·8	925·0	926·2	927·6	928·8	930·0	931·3	932·6	933·9	935·2	936·2
15	907·1	908·4	909·7	910·9	912·1	913·4	914·6	915·9	917·1	918·4	919·6	920·8	922·0	923·3	924·5	925·7	927·1	928·4	929·7	931·0	932·0
16	902·9	904·2	905·5	906·7	907·9	909·2	910·4	911·7	912·9	914·2	915·4	916·6	917·8	919·1	920·3	921·5	922·8	924·1	925·4	926·7	927·8
17	898·7	900·0	901·3	902·5	903·7	905·0	906·2	907·5	908·7	910·0	911·1	912·3	913·5	914·8	916·0	917·2	918·5	919·8	921·1	922·4	923·5
18	894·5	895·8	897·1	898·3	899·5	900·8	902·0	903·3	904·5	905·8	906·8	908·0	909·2	910·5	911·8	913·0	914·2	915·5	916·8	918·1	919·2
19	890·2	891·5	892·7	893·9	895·1	896·4	897·6	898·9	900·1	901·2	902·5	903·7	904·9	906·2	907·4	908·6	909·9	911·2	912·5	913·8	914·8
20	885·9	887·2	888·4	889·6	890·8	892·1	893·3	894·6	895·8	897·1	898·1	899·3	900·5	901·7	902·9	904·1	905·3	906·5	907·7	908·9	910·4
21	881·8	883·0	884·3	885·5	886·7	888·6	889·2	890·5	891·7	893·0	894·0	895·2	896·4	897·7	898·9	900·1	901·3	902·6	903·9	905·2	906·2
22	877·1	878·3	879·5	880·7	881·9	883·2	884·4	885·7	886·9	888·2	889·0	890·2	891·4	892·9	894·1	895·3	896·6	897·9	899·2	900·5	901·4
23	872·6	873·8	875·0	876·2	877·4	878·7	879·9	881·2	882·4	883·7	884·7	885·9	887·1	888·4	889·5	890·8	892·0	893·3	894·6	895·9	896·9
24	868·1	869·3	870·6	871·8	873·0	874·3	875·5	876·8	878·0	879·3	880·1	881·3	882·5	883·8	885·0	886·2	887·5	888·8	890·1	891·4	892·3
25	863·5	864·7	865·9	867·1	868·3	869·6	870·8	872·1	873·3	874·5	875·7	876·9	878·1	879·3	880·5	881·7	882·9	884·2	885·5	886·8	887·9

BAROMETER

Temperature	29·96 761	30·00 762	30·04 763	30·08 764	30·12 765	30·16 766	30·20 767	30·24 768	30·28 769	30·31 770	30·35 771	30·39 772	30·43 773	30·47 774	30·51 775	30·55 776	30·59 777	30·63 778	30·67 779	30·71 780
10	954·3	955·6	956·8	958·0	959·3	960·6	961·8	963·1	964·4	965·7	967·0	968·3	969·6	970·8	972·1	973·3	974·6	975·9	977·1	978·4
11	950·2	951·5	952·7	953·9	955·2	956·5	957·7	959·0	960·3	961·6	962·8	964·1	965·4	966·6	967·9	969·1	970·4	971·7	972·9	974·2
12	945·7	947·0	948·2	949·4	950·7	951·9	953·1	954·4	955·7	957·0	958·2	959·5	960·8	962·0	963·3	964·5	965·8	967·1	968·3	969·6
13	941·8	943·1	944·3	945·5	946·6	948·1	949·3	950·6	951·9	953·1	954·3	955·6	956·9	958·1	959·4	960·6	961·9	963·2	964·4	965·7
14	937·6	938·9	940·1	941·3	942·6	943·8	945·0	946·3	947·6	948·8	950·1	951·3	952·6	953·8	955·1	956·3	957·5	958·8	960·0	961·3
15	933·3	934·6	935·8	937·0	938·2	939·5	940·7	942·0	943·2	944·4	945·8	947·0	948·3	949·6	950·8	952·0	953·2	954·5	955·7	957·0
16	929·1	930·4	931·6	932·8	934·0	935·2	936·4	937·7	938·9	940·1	941·4	942·6	943·9	945·2	946·4	947·6	948·8	950·1	951·3	952·6
17	924·7	926·0	927·2	928·5	929·7	930·9	932·1	933·4	934·6	935·8	937·1	938·3	939·6	940·9	942·1	943·3	944·5	945·8	947·0	948·3
18	920·4	921·7	922·9	924·2	925·4	926·6	927·8	929·1	930·3	931·5	932·7	933·9	935·2	936·5	937·7	938·9	940·1	941·4	942·6	943·9
19	916·0	917·2	918·4	919·7	920·9	922·2	923·4	924·7	925·9	927·1	928·3	929·5	930·8	932·0	933·2	934·4	935·6	936·9	938·1	939·4
20	911·6	912·8	914·0	915·2	916·5	917·7	918·9	920·2	921·4	922·6	923·8	925·0	926·3	927·5	928·8	930·0	931·2	932·5	933·7	935·0
21	907·4	908·6	909·8	911·1	912·3	913·5	914·7	916·0	917·2	918·4	919·6	920·8	922·1	923·3	924·5	925·7	926·9	928·2	929·4	930·7
22	902·6	903·8	905·9	906·3	907·5	908·7	909·9	911·2	912·4	913·6	914·8	916·0	917·2	918·4	919·7	920·9	922·1	923·4	924·6	926·0
23	898·0	899·2	900·4	901·7	902·9	904·1	905·3	906·6	907·8	909·0	910·2	911·4	912·6	913·8	915·1	916·3	917·5	918·8	920·0	921·3
24	893·4	894·6	895·8	897·1	898·3	899·5	900·7	902·0	903·2	904·4	905·6	906·8	908·0	909·2	910·4	911·6	912·8	914·0	915·2	916·5
25	888·9	890·1	891·3	892·6	893·8	895·0	896·2	897·4	898·6	899·8	900·9	902·1	903·3	904·5	905·7	906·9	908·1	909·3	910·5	911·7

5. Echocardiography

Cardiac ultrasound or echocardiography has gained wide acceptance as a diagnostic technique since its introduction to this field by Edler and Hertz in 1954. The technique has the obvious advantage in being non-invasive. The examination can be rapidly performed, does not require the patient's admission to hospital and can be repeated without any known hazard to the patient.

Echocardiography is a developing technique and rapid advances are being made both in the instrumentation and in the range of its application to cardiology. While echocardiography remains complementary to other diagnostic methods used in investigation of the cardiovascular system, the information obtained is increasingly demanded in the pre-operative assessment of congenital and acquired heart disease.

Understanding a few basic principles is necessary to appreciate the capabilities and the limitations of echocardiography. The term 'ultrasound,' by definition, refers to frequencies of sound higher than the audible range i.e. over 20,000 cycles per second. In practice, a range of $1-5 \times 10^6$ cycles per second (1–5 megaHz) is used in echocardiography. The ultrasound is produced by applying an alternating current to a piezoelectric crystal which expands and contracts with the changing polarity. This change of shape produces sound waves. Conversely, the same crystal when struck by a sound wave produces an electrical impulse. The same crystal, thus, acts as both the transmitter and the receiver of ultrasound. In clinical use, the ultrasound is transmitted for one microsecond and this short pulse is repeated 1,000 times every second. The crystal therefore transmits the ultrasound for one-thousandth of a second every second, and acts as a receiver for 99·9 per cent of the time.

When a beam of ultrasound strikes a tissue interface, some of it is reflected, some absorbed and some is transmitted. It is important to remember that air is a poor transmitter of ultrasound and therefore a contact medium such as a water-soluble jelly is necessary to exclude air between the transducer and the patient's skin. The time between the initial pulse and a returning echo from a reflecting surface is a function of the depth of that surface. The echo is represented on the face of a cathode ray oscilloscope as a peak whose amplitude is proportional to the intensity of the returning echo. This amplitude-modulated representation is called the A-mode or A-scope display. The same information can also be represented as a series of dots where the brightness of the dot corresponds to the intensity of the echo. This brightness-modulated display is called the B-mode. The B-mode display can be swept across the face of the oscilloscope on a time-base to provide a time-motion display or the M-mode, which is the method used in cardiac examinations.

The information on the face of the oscilloscope can be recorded on a Polaroid film or a strip-chart recorder. Recording on the Polaroid film has obvious limitations as the record covers only a few heart beats (Fig. 5.1). Spatial relationships of different structures and continuous records from one area of interest to another can be obtained only by using a continuous recording method such as a strip-chart recorder. A strip-chart recorder, therefore, is considered an essential part of the equipment to obtain maximum information from every examination (Fig. 5.2). The electrocardiogram is simultaneously recorded with all cardiac ultrasound examinations.

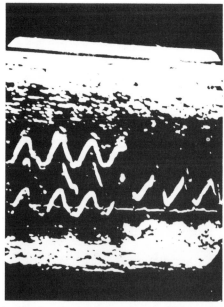

FIG. 5.1 A polaroid print of a continuous scan from the aortic to the mitral area showing limitations of this mode of recording.

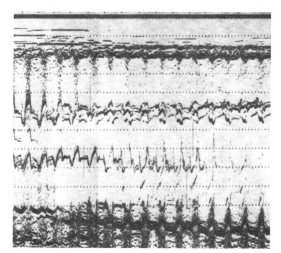

FIG. 5.2 A continuous scan similar to Fig. 5.1 recorded on a strip-chart recorder. The relationship of various structures is easily demonstrated. The quality of recording is also superior.

The examination is carried out with the patient in the supine position with the head of the bed raised about 30–40°. In some cases it is necessary to turn the patient partly on the left side to improve the quality of the trace. Occasionally, it may also be necessary to ask the patient to hold his breath in expiration during the recording. In spite of these precautions, echographic examination may be very difficult or impossible in some instances. For example, in obese patients there is attenuation of the beam by the thick chest wall and this can result in failure to obtain a diagnostic examination. Also, any air between the transducer and the heart will reduce the quality of the examination. Thus, in emphysematous patients any lung tissue interposed between the transducer and the heart can make the examination virtually impossible. In such patients, we have found a substernal approach with the transducer placed in the midline in the region of the xiphisternum, extremely useful. Chest deformities such as depressed sternum also cause difficulties due to displacement or rotation of the heart.

For a routine examination, the transducer is usually placed in the fourth left interspace close to the sternal edge. Sometimes it may be necessary to place the transducer in the fifth or in the third left interspace. In our department, a routine examination consists of many cardiac cycles to show the mitral, aortic and tricuspid valves. The anterior heart wall, the interventricular septum and the posterior left ventricular wall are also routinely demonstrated. The results are recorded on a strip-chart recorder using direct print paper. Using this technique, the ultrasonic beam can be angled from the base of the heart to the apex of the left ventricle, thus outlining the areas of interest (Fig. 5.3).

With the beam directed medially and superiorly, the anterior heart wall and the anterior ventricle, the root of the aorta, the aortic valve cusps and the cavity of the left atrium are demonstrated. Change of angulation slightly downwards and laterally (position 2) results in the beam passing through the right ventricle, the interventricular

ECHOCARDIOGRAPHIC EXAMINATION OF THE HEART

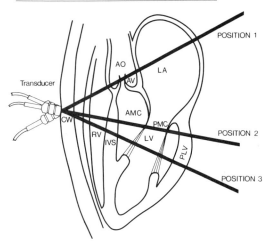

AV   AORTIC VALVE
PLV   POSTERIOR LEFT VENTRICULAR WALL
PMC   POSTERIOR MITRAL CUSP
AMC   ANTERIOR MITRAL CUSP
LV   LEFT VENTRICLE
LA   LEFT ATRIUM
AO   AORTA
IVS   INTER VENTRICULAR SEPTUM
RV   RIGHT VENTRICLE
CW   CHEST WALL   a

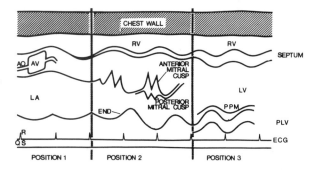

AO   AORTA   LV   LEFT VENTRICLE
AV   AORTIC VALVE   PLV   POSTERIOR LEFT VENTRICULAR WALL
END   ENDOCARDIUM   PPM   POSTERIOR PAPILLARY MUSCLE
LA   LEFT ATRIUM   RV   RIGHT VENTRICLE   b

FIG. 5.3 (a) Sagittal section of the heart showing the normal anatomical relationship of the cardiac chambers and the mitral and aortic valves. The ultrasonic beam is directed along positions 1, 2 and 3 to outline the areas of interest. (b) Diagrammatic representation of the trace which is obtained when the ultrasonic beam traverses the heart from position 1 to position 3. Note: The anterior aortic wall is continuous with the septum and the posterior aortic wall continues as the anterior mitral leaflet in position 2.

septum, and the anterior and posterior leaflets of the mitral valve and the posterior wall of the left ventricle. Angulation into the cavity of the left ventricle (position 3) shows the interventricular septum and the posterior left ventricular wall at the level of the posterior papillary muscle.

Identification of the different cardiac echoes is achieved by recognition of their relative positions, their characteristic motion pattern and by knowing the position of the transducer during recording.

Mitral valve

The mitral valve is the most important structure outlined in the ultrasound examination of the heart. Its recognition is important both in the assessment of mitral valve disease and as a landmark for obtaining recordings of other intracardiac structures.

The anterior leaflet of the mitral valve has the greatest amplitude of movement amongst the cardiac structures and usually lies at a depth of between 5 and 10 cm from the anterior chest wall. A normal anterior leaflet of the mitral valve shows a characteristic M-shaped trace and the posterior leaflet shows the mirror image or W-shaped trace (Fig. 5.4). The mitral valve opens rapidly at the beginning of diastole (upward deflection) to its fully open position. This is followed by a phase of rapid ventricular filling and equalisation of the atrial and ventricular pressures, resulting in partial closure of the mitral valve. The rate at which this initial posterior movement takes place is called the *diastolic closure rate* (D.C.R.) (Fig. 5.5). This is followed by re-opening of the mitral valve with the atrial systole. At the onset of ventricular systole, the mitral valve closes rapidly and completely (downward deflection). During systole, the anterior and posterior leaflets of the mitral valve stay together to form two parallel echoes which move anteriorly through a smooth gradient. This anterior movement during systole is due to the movement of the whole heart during this part of the cardiac cycle. Any opening movement of the anterior

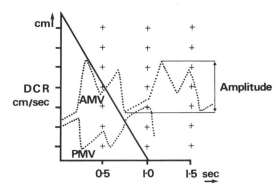

FIG. 5.5 The diastolic closure rate (D.C.R.) and the amplitude of movement of the anterior mitral valve (A.M.V.) are measured as shown here. P.M.V. denotes posterior mitral valve.

leaflet of the mitral (or tricuspid) valve is towards the transducer and is represented on the recording as an upwards deflection. Movement away from the transducer, downward deflection, denotes closure of the anterior leaflet of the mitral (or tricuspid) valve.

It is important to record the echoes from the anterior and posterior leaflets simultaneously in both normal and diseased mitral valves. When carrying out the examination of the mitral valve, it is important to vary the angulation of the beam in order to record the maximum amplitude and the maximum opening of the mitral valve. The normal amplitude of movement is between 2 and 3 cm, and the initial rate of opening should be greater than 300 mm/s. If the recording is obtained near the base of the mitral cusps the amplitude of movement will appear to be reduced. The diastolic closure rate may also be found to be reduced. A 'false' diagnosis of mitral stenosis will thus result (Fig. 5.6).

Mitral stenosis

In mitral stenosis, the leaflets are thickened and may show a diminished range of movement. The mitral valve orifice is reduced, the left atrial pressure remains high throughout diastole and the valve remains open throughout diastole (Fig. 5.7). The diastolic closure rate is reduced. This reduction in the *diastolic closure rate* is related to mitral stenosis but the severity of the stenosis cannot be reliably assessed (Nichol *et al.*, 1977). Table 5.1 shows the commonly accepted figures of D.C.R. for different degrees of stenosis.

Diminished D.C.R. is also seen with other causes of reduced ventricular filling and in poor left ventricular compliance. The diagnosis of mitral stenosis should not, therefore, be made without demonstrating movements of the posterior leaflet of the mitral valve.

The posterior leaflet of the mitral valve shows a W-shaped trace. Its amplitude is not as great as that of the anterior leaflet. In mitral stenosis this relationship is

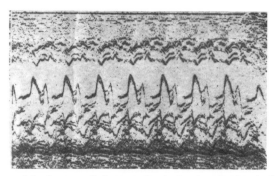

FIG. 5.4 A trace of the normal mitral valve showing both leaflets moving in the opposite direction in diastole and coming together in systole.

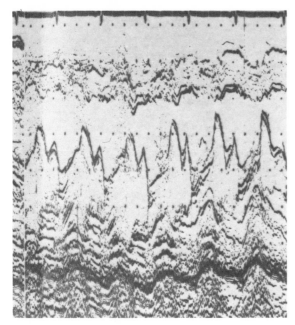

FIG. 5.6 Trace of a normal mitral valve. Examination near the base of the anterior mitral leaflet (left half of the trace) shows reduced amplitude of movement and may be mistaken for a stenosed valve. Normal movement of both leaflets is seen on the right.

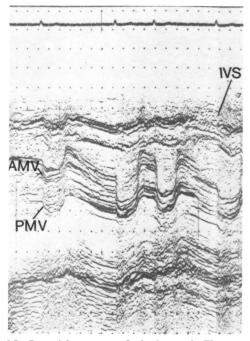

FIG. 5.7 Record from a case of mitral stenosis. The posterior leaflet moves in the same direction as the anterior leaflet in diastole. Multiple, thick, continuous echoes from both leaflets indicate calcification in the valve. A.M.V., anterior mitral valve; P.M.V., posterior mitral valve; I.V.S., interventricular septum.

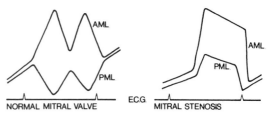

FIG. 5.8 Diagram showing the altered movement of the posterior mitral leaflet in the presence of mitral stenosis. A.M.L., anterior mitral leaflet; P.M.L., posterior mitral leaflet.

lost, and the posterior leaflet moves in the same direction as the anterior leaflet (Fig. 5.8). In diastole, therefore, the two leaflets of a stenosed mitral valve move in a parallel fashion. There is no clear explanation as to why the posterior leaflet should change its pattern of movement in mitral stenosis. It is possible that the fibrosed posterior leaflet does not move at all and the observed anterior movement is apparent rather than real; nevertheless, this observation is of great diagnostic significance in mitral stenosis. When the D.C.R. is diminished due to other causes such as pulmonary hypertension and poor left ventricular compliance, the posterior leaflet continues to move in a normal manner. The recording of a normal posterior leaflet in such cases will avoid 'false' diagnosis of mitral stenosis (Fig. 5.9). Occasionally, the posterior leaflet may continue to move normally with a stenosed mitral valve, but it will show fibrosis.

From the recording of the mitral valve, it is also possible to measure the mobility or *pliability of the anterior leaflet*. This is measured from the fully-closed position of the anterior leaflet to its fully open position (upward deflection). This is called the amplitude of movement of the mitral valve (Fig. 5.5). The *rate of opening* can also be measured from this upward deflection. The information about the amplitude of movement of the

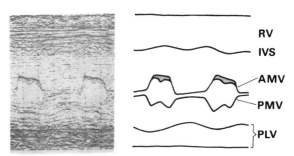

FIG. 5.9 Diminished diastolic closure rate in a case of severe pulmonary hypertension. The posterior mitral leaflet (P.M.V.) shows normal W-shaped trace, thus excluding mitral stenosis. R.V., right ventricle; I.V.S., interventricular septum; A.M.V., anterior mitral valve; P.M.V., posterior mitral valve; P.L.V., posterior left ventricular wall.

mitral valve is of some value in the surgical management of the stenosed mitral valve. A stenosed valve which shows a normal amplitude (over 2 cm) may be suitable for closed mitral valvotomy.

The echogram also provides useful information about the presence of *calcification* in the valve. In fact, the echogram detects calcification more reliably than fluoroscopic screening of the heart with an image intensifier. Calcification is recognized by the presence of multiple, thick echoes from the anterior leaflet which appear as parallel lines particularly in diastole. A *thickened fibrosed valve* also produces multiple echoes which are usually distinguishable from those of a calcified valve by a discontinuous and speckled appearance (Fig. 5.10). A further characteristic appearance is seen in cases with *vegetations* on the free margin of the anterior leaflet of the mitral valve which are evident mainly in the diastolic phase of the movement (Fig. 5.11).

Mitral incompetence

Whereas echography provides reliable evidence of mitral stenosis, it is less certain in the assessment of mitral incompetence. It used to be believed that the incompetent valve had an increased amplitude of movement and a more rapid D.C.R. compared to the normal. This is occasionally true but the changes are not specific and a

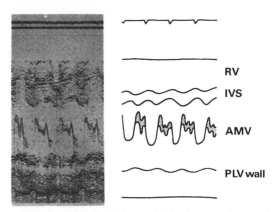

FIG. 5.11 Irregular, multiple, speckled echoes on the anterior mitral leaflet due to vegetations. Multiple echoes are also seen in the region of the posterior mitral leaflet. R.V., right ventricle; I.V.S., interventricular septum; A.M.V., anterior mitral leaflet; P.L.V., posterior left ventricular wall.

normal mitral valve can also exhibit the same signs. Increased D.C.R. is found in any type of high stroke volume, and thus may be observed in a number of conditions in which the rate of flow through the mitral valve is increased.

There are also other non-specific signs such as increased end-diastolic diameter of the left ventricle, and an enlarged left atrium which may suggest the diagnosis of mitral incompetence. Where there is clinical suspicion of mitral incompetence, these findings would help to confirm the diagnosis.

RHEUMATIC MITRAL INCOMPETENCE
This diagnosis can be made from the echogram by demonstration of certain features. The trace shows multiple thick echoes from the mitral valve leaflets, reflecting the fibrosis or calcification which may be present. Often the left ventricular cavity is large and the two leaflets of the valve are easy to outline. The amplitude of movement may be normal or often reduced.

PROLAPSE OF THE MITRAL VALVE
Mitral insufficiency associated with a prolapsed valve is clinically suspected when there is a late systolic murmur and a late systolic click. The echographic findings correlate well with these clinical observations. In systole, the two leaflets of a normal mitral valve stay together and are seen on the echogram as two parallel lines, which move anteriorly with a smooth gradient. In a prolapsed valve there is a sharp posterior movement of both leaflets, but the posterior leaflet may show greater displacement. These changes are seen in late systole (Fig. 5.12) and are specific to this condition. It is important to outline both leaflets of the mitral valve and not to confuse the movements of the posterior cusp with that of the posterior chordae. A continuous scan from the left

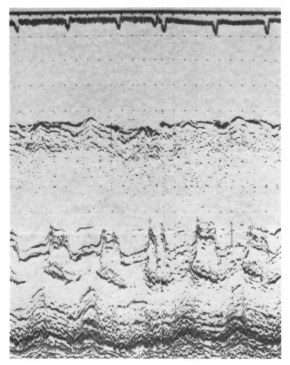

FIG. 5.10 Fibrosed mitral valve. The amplitude of movement is reduced and the trace from both leaflets gives a speckled appearance. No evidence of mitral stenosis.

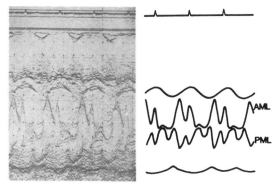

FIG. 5.12 Prolapse of the mitral valve. The two leaflets of the mitral valve come together at the onset of systole, but then show sharp posterior movement and separation. A.M.L., anterior mitral leaflet; P.M.L., posterior mitral leaflet.

ventricle to the left atrium is also necessary to demonstrate the bulging of the leaflets into the left atrium in systole.

RUPTURED CHORDAE

This condition can also be demonstrated on the echogram. Ruptured chordae of the anterior cusp show a characteristic pattern with a large amplitude of movement and coarse flutter of the anterior leaflet in diastole.

When the chordae of the posterior leaflet are ruptured, the leaflet separates from the anterior leaflet in early systole and also shows paradoxical (i.e. anterior) movement in early diastole.

Mitral-valve trace in other conditions

AORTIC INCOMPETENCE

The trace of the anterior leaflet of the mitral valve can show indirect evidence of this condition. The jet of blood which returns from the incompetent aortic valve into the left ventricle produces various changes in the mitral valve trace. The most common of these findings is the flutter of the anterior leaflet. This flutter is seen as fine oscillation of the leaflets in diastole. The flutter does not correlate with the presence of an Austin–Flint murmur nor does it correlate well with the degree of aortic regurgitation.

Another sign which may be present in cases of severe aortic regurgitation is premature closure of the mitral valve. The mitral valve opens normally in early diastole but closes rapidly and prematurely and remains closed for the remainder of the diastole.

HYPERTROPHIC OBSTRUCTIVE CARDIOMYOPATHY

This is discussed more fully later. The mitral valve trace shows a specific abnormality in cases of this cardiomyopathy. This is called systolic anterior movement and is recorded in mid-systole. The leaflets bulge upwards in

this part of the cardiac cycle. The anterior movement may be so marked that the leaflets come into contact with the septum. The changes correlate well with the narrowed outflow tract of the left ventricle. The leaflets return to the baseline before the normal opening of the valve in diastole. 'False' anterior systolic movement is seen if a recording is obtained near the base of the valve as the trace then reflects the movements of the mitral ring. This 'false' echo does not return to the baseline prior to the full opening of the valve.

Aortic valve

The aortic root and the aortic valve can be recorded by directing the beam of ultrasound towards the base of the heart (Fig. 5.3, position 1).

The aortic root shows up as two parallel echoes which move sharply anteriorly during systole and gradually move posteriorly during diastole. They are easy to recognize on the screen by their intensity or 'brightness' and their pattern of movement.

The cusps of the aortic valve are more difficult to record than the mitral valve cusps. Careful technique and patience, however, can result in obtaining these echoes in a very high percentage of cases.

Slender cusp echoes are seen within the parallel echoes of the aortic root. At the onset of systole, aortic cusps separate rapidly to lie against the wall of the aorta to form a box-like or diamond-shaped configuration. Rapid closure occurs at the end of systole and the cusps are seen as two thin lines which occupy a mid-aortic position (Fig. 5.13). The anterior-cusp echo arises from the right coronary cusp and the posterior-cusp echo from the non-coronary cusp.

The aortic root diameter in normal patients ranges between 19 and 25 mm. The aortic valve cusp separation is normally between 16 and 23 mm.

AORTIC STENOSIS

The diagnosis of aortic stenosis can be made with echography but the degree of accuracy does not approach that achieved in the assessment of mitral stenosis. This is

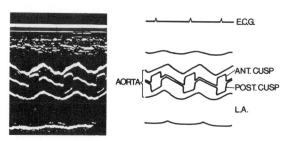

FIG. 5.13 Normal aortic valve. Anterior (right coronary) cusp and posterior (non-coronary) cusp are seen in systole and diastole. L.A., left atrium.

particularly true of congenital aortic stenosis as the leaflets are thin and their separation is within the normal range.

Two signs of aortic stenosis are recognized on echocardiographic recordings. Firstly, the presence of thick, multiple echoes of high intensity in diastole indicates fibrosis or calcification of the aortic valve. In the presence of heavy calcification these echoes may persist throughout the cardiac cycle and make the recording of cusp echoes very difficult or impossible (Fig. 5.14). The echogram is more sensitive at detecting aortic valve calcification then fluoroscopy.

The other sign which may be recorded from the stenosed aortic valve is reduced separation of the valve cusps. The cusps of the normal valve attain their maximum separation at the onset of the ventricular systole, and lie parallel to the walls of the aorta. In a stenosed valve, some separation of the valve cusps is seen in systole but their maximum excursion does not take them to the inner margins of the aortic walls. A valve-cusp separation of less than 16 mm is strongly suggestive of aortic stenosis.

Feigenbaum (1972) stated that if the echogram shows normal separation of the valve cusps, aortic stenosis is excluded. This is not our experience and other workers (Feizi et al., 1974) have also found that reduced cusp separation is not always seen in proven cases of aortic stenosis.

AORTIC REGURGITATION

The presence of aortic regurgitation may be suspected from the mitral valve trace as described previously.

The trace of the aortic root and the aortic valve may also be of some help in confirming this diagnosis. Dilatation of the aortic root (diameter greater than 25 mm) is sometimes seen when aortic incompetence is present.

Thickening of the cusps may also be recognized from

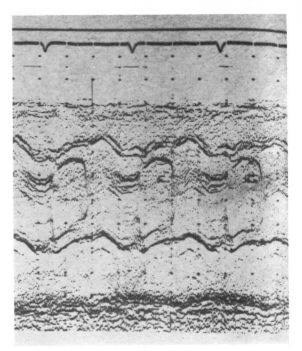

FIG. 5.15   Vegetations on the aortic valve cusps. Multiple linear echoes are seen in the anterior half of the aorta during diastole.

the trace. Sometimes, a *coarse flutter* of the cusps is seen during systole, but this sign is present with a number of other conditions such as hypertrophic obstructive cardiomyopathy and in normal echograms.

It has been stated (Feizi et al., 1974) that separation of the aortic valve cusps in diastole can be a pathognomonic sign of aortic regurgitation. We have not found this to be a useful sign.

BACTERIAL ENDOCARDITIS OF THE AORTIC VALVE

Echocardiography can provide useful information in the diagnosis of endocarditis involving the aortic valve.

Irregular thickening of the valve cusps may be seen in systole. Multiple linear echoes in diastole, especially with clinical observation of aortic regurgitation of recent onset, are highly suggestive of vegetations on the aortic valve (Fig. 5.15). Calcification of the aortic valve usually produces very dense echoes which persist throughout the cardiac cycle. Bulky valvular vegetations may appear as dense echoes which fill the aortic root in diastole (Wray, 1975).

Tricuspid valve

Echocardiography is useful in detection of disease involving the tricuspid valve. The valve lies more medially than the mitral valve and medial angulation of the transducer is therefore necessary. Turning of the patient to the

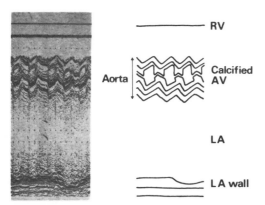

RV

Aorta
Calcified
AV

LA

L A wall

FIG. 5.14   Calcified stenosed aortic valve. The left atrium is enlarged due to mitral valve disease. R.V., right ventricle; A.V., aortic valve; L.A., left atrium.

left to bring the valve out laterally from behind the sternum is often advisable.

The trace of the tricuspid valve closely resembles that of the mitral valve. The anterior leaflet produces an M-shaped trace. The posterior leaflet is not often recorded but its trace also resembles that of the posterior cusp of the mitral valve (Fig. 5.16). The tricuspid valve lies much closer to the anterior chest wall than the mitral valve. Its average depth from the surface is 3–5 cm. The valve echo is easier to record when there is right ventricular volume overload. In such patients its trace can be easily mistaken for the mitral-valve trace. It is useful to remember, therefore, that the tricuspid valve lies much more anteriorly and no septal echo can be recorded in front of it. Stenosis and incompetence of the tricuspid valve produce echographic changes similar to those seen in a mitral trace with mitral valve disease.

Flutter of the tricuspid valve may be seen in pulmonary valve incompetence. Delayed and prolonged closure of the tricuspid valve is seen with raised end-diastolic pressure of the right ventricle.

In congenital heart disease, the trace of the tricuspid valve shows a characteristic abnormality in Ebstein's Anomaly. The valve shows increased amplitude of movement and delayed closure.

Pulmonary valve

The pulmonary valve is the most difficult valve in the heart from the echographic viewpoint. It lies relatively high in the chest with a possibility of some lung being interposed between the transducer and the valve. The examination is usually carried out with the transducer

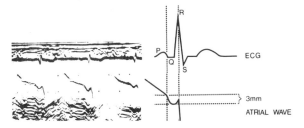

FIG. 5.17 Posterior leaflet of the normal pulmonary valve.

in the second left interspace, and the ultrasound beam is directed upwards and laterally towards the left shoulder. The anterior cusp of the pulmonary valve lies parallel to the beam of ultrasound and therefore its movements cannot be recorded. The posterior leaflet is easier to outline as its movements are perpendicular to the ultrasonic beam. But even here, the record is best seen in diastole. The valve is easier to record in children and young adults.

The pulmonary valve is a thin structure and responds to small gradients of pressure between the right ventricle and the pulmonary artery. In the closed position, during diastole, the valve lies nearly horizontally. There is slight posterior motion as the whole heart moves posteriorly during diastole. The important movement for echocardiographic diagnosis is abrupt posterior movement which takes place in late diastole prior to the onset of the ventricular systole. This is called the 'A' wave and coincides with the atrial systole or 'P' wave of the electrocardiogram. The 'A' wave is attributed to the movement of the pulmonary valve due to the small increase in right ventricular pressure which results from atrial systole. The 'A' wave varies with respiration, being at its deepest in inspiration. The valve returns to the neutral position before it opens fully at the onset of ventricular systole— the normal 'A' wave has an average depth of 3 mm (Fig. 5.17).

In pulmonary stenosis, the pulmonary artery pressure is low and remains so throughout the cardiac cycle. The atrial systole is, therefore, sufficient to produce doming of the pulmonary valve leaflets.

The pulmonary valve trace in pulmonary stenosis therefore shows a deep 'A' wave—usually deeper than 7 mm. Following the deep 'A' wave the leaflets fail to return to the neutral position. There is some evidence (Weyman et al., 1974) to show that the depth of the 'A' wave correlates well with the degree of stenosis. In pulmonary infundibular stenosis in addition to the 'A' wave there is also fine flutter of the valve leaflet.

Pulmonary hypertension also provides a detectable change on the trace of the pulmonary valve. The pulmonary artery pressure remains high in diastole and the atrial systole is insufficient to produce any movement of

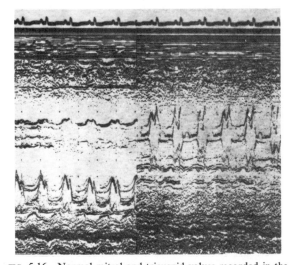

FIG. 5.16 Normal mitral and tricuspid valves recorded in the same patient. The pattern of movement of the anterior and posterior leaflets of both valves is similar. The tricuspid valve (on the right) is nearer the chest wall. The mitral valve has the interventricular septum in front of it.

the closed pulmonary valve. In pulmonary hypertension, the 'A' wave is absent and the valve remains in the horizontal position before it opens fully with the ventricular systole.

Examination of the interventricular septum

Demonstration of the septum should be included in every echographic examination of the heart. This gives useful information not only about the position, the thickness and movements of the septum itself, but also about the size and the function of the right and left ventricles.

The interventricular septum appears as a set of parallel lines on the echocardiogram. It usually behaves as a part of the left ventricle so that in systole it moves posteriorly to approach the anteriorly moving posterior left ventricular wall. In diastole, the two move away from each other as the ventricle relaxes. Proper setting of the ultrasound machine controls is essential to outline both sides of the septum. The depth-compensation setting should be set at its maximum and just to the left of the proximal margin of the septum. Very little near-gain should be used. If the near-gain is high, both the echo from the anterior right ventricular wall and the one from the right side of the septum are obliterated in a mass of continuous lines.

The normal septum is 9–10 mm thick. Its movement is not as great as that of the posterior wall of the left ventricle. Increased movement of the septum is usually seen in the volume overloads of the left and right ventricles. In left ventricular overload, as in mitral or aortic insufficiency, the septal movement is exaggerated but otherwise normal. On the other hand, with right-ventricular overload the exaggerated movement of the septum is reversed. Thus, the septum moves anteriorly in systole and posteriorly in diastole (Fig. 5.18). This abnormal movement of the septum is seen in atrial septal defect and tricuspid insufficiency.

The septal motion may be reduced following an antero-septal myocardial infarct. Reduced septal motion may also be recorded due to faulty technique. The two sides of the septum can be recorded from the region of the atrio-ventricular junction to the apex of the left ventricle. The septal movements near to the atrio-ventricular junction are reduced and may indeed be paradoxical. The septal thickness may also vary slightly. Septal thickness and movements should be assessed at, or just below, the tip of the mitral valve cusps. This is also the area in which the right and the left ventricular diameters are measured. Any comparison between the septal thickness and the posterior left ventricular wall is also made in this area.

The demonstration of the septum is extremely useful in the differential diagnosis of congenital heart disease. As the septum may be difficult to outline by any other method of investigation, time spent in showing the

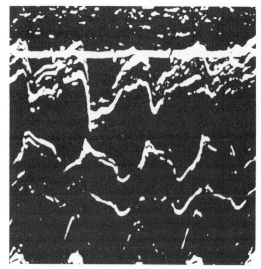

FIG. 5.18 Increased and paradoxical movement of the septum in a case of atrial septal defect. The septum moves anteriorly in systole.

position and the movement of the interventricular septum in infants and children can be highly rewarding.

Pericardial effusion

One of the earliest applications of ultrasound in clinical cardiology was in the detection of pericardial effusion (Feigenbaum, 1965). Early claims of its usefulness have been substantiated and echocardiography is now established as the investigation of choice in the diagnosis of pericardial effusion.

The technique depends on the fact that fluid is transonic and appears on the trace as an echo-free area. The normal pericardial space between the visceral and parietal layers of pericardium contains a small amount of fluid, but this is indistinguishable ultrasonically. In patients with pericardial effusion, as fluid accumulates between the two layers, an echo-free space can be demonstrated between the visceral and parietal pericardium (Fig. 5.19).

In the normal echogram, the anterior right ventricular wall is in close contact with the chest wall and there is no real separation between the echoes produced by the two structures. Similarly, the posterior left ventricular wall is formed by a group of echoes which represents from within outwards: the endocardium, the myocardium, the visceral pericardium (epicardium) and the parietal pericardium. The epicardial (visceral) echo moves normally with the myocardial echo. The pericardial echo is relatively less mobile.

Though the theory behind the detection of the pericardial fluid is simple and the examination is easy to perform, there are several pitfalls which lead to false-positive and false-negative diagnoses. First of all, it is

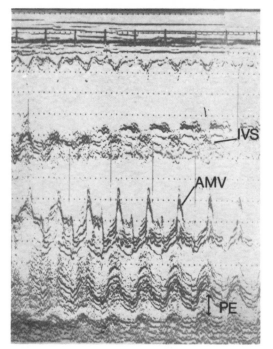

FIG. 5.19 A continuous scan from the base of the heart towards the apex of the left ventricle to demonstrate pericardial effusion. No fluid is present behind the left atrium (left of the trace). The amount of fluid increases gradually towards the apex of the left ventricle. No evidence of effusion anteriorly. I.V.S., interventricular septum; A.M.V., anterior mitral valve; P.E., pericardial effusion.

necessary to take care to outline and identify the cardiac structures, mentioned above i.e. right ventricular wall, posterior left ventricular endocardium, myocardium and the two layers of pericardium. It is also necessary to outline the interventricular septum and the mitral valve, as this ensures that the beam of ultrasound is not directed too medially. Undue medial angulation of the beam results in a false-positive diagnosis as the medial part of anterior right ventricular wall moves more vigorously and gives the impression of an echo-free space in the front.

The correct setting of the controls is essential to avoid errors in examination. High 'gain' can produce echoes within the fluid and therefore the separation between the two layers of the pericardium may be missed.

It is helpful to obtain a continuous scan from the base of the heart to the apex of the left ventricle in order to confirm the presence of pericardial effusion. When the beam is directed medially, there may be increased movement of the anterior right ventricular wall but at the same time the posterior wall is formed by the left atrium. No fluid can collect behind the central portion of the left atrium as the pericardium is reflected on to the pulmonary veins which enter the left atrium. As the beam is directed

downwards and laterally, the septum and the mitral valve echoes come into view. Any pericardial fluid will first be seen in this area as there will be some separation of the two layers of the pericardium. Further angulation of the transducer towards the apex of the left ventricle should result in increasing the separation between the pericardial echoes as fluid tends to collect in the dependent part round the left ventricular apex.

There has been some discussion in the literature as to whether the fluid is diagnosed more accurately by concentrating on the anterior heart wall or the posterior heart wall. There is little doubt that small amounts of pericardial fluid collect in the dependent parts i.e. posteriorly in the supine or semi-recumbent patient. The early diagnosis of effusion is therefore more likely by examining the posterior wall. As fluid increases it is easier to show it anteriorly. This leads to the question of whether it is possible to quantitate the amount of pericardial fluid using echocardiography.

A recent study (Horowitz et al., 1974) has attempted to evaluate the sensitivity of echocardiography in detecting and quantitating pericardial fluid. Patients undergoing cardiac surgery had echograms on the day prior to their operation. All fluid was aspirated and measured during the operation. It was found that when a persistent echo-free space is demonstrated between the two layers of the posterior pericardium, the lower limit of detectable fluid is 20 ml.

In patients with very large effusions, the whole heart may move excessively on the echogram trace. This is called the 'swinging' heart as the position of the heart in relation to the anterior chest wall varies from one cardiac cycle to another (Fig. 5.20).

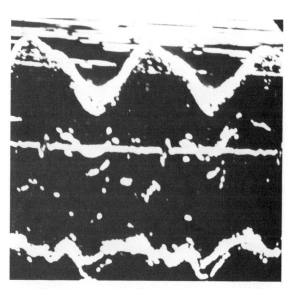

FIG. 5.20 Massive pericardial effusion with a 'swinging' heart. Fluid is seen both anteriorly and posteriorly.

Echographic examination is also useful in following the clinical course of patients with pericardial effusions. The efficacy of treatment, medical or surgical, can be assessed by comparing traces obtained at intervals.

The reliability and accuracy of echocardiography in detecting pericardial effusions is dependant on careful technique.

Hypertrophic obstructive cardiomyopathy

This condition is called idiopathic hypertrophic sub-aortic stenosis (I.H.S.S.) in the U.S.A. and muscular subaortic stenosis (M.S.S.) in Canada.

The disease spectrum is characterized by septal hyper-trophy and narrowing of the outflow tract of the left ventricle. Echocardiography has proven valuable in initial assessment of this group of diseases and also in the evaluation of medical and surgical treatment of this condition.

It was known from angiography studies (Simon *et al.*, 1967) that re-opening of the anterior mitral leaflet in mid-systole was an important component of the out-flow tract obstruction. Echocardiography confirmed this abnormal anterior systolic movement of the mitral valve. In systole, the two leaflets of the normal mitral valve appear as two parallel lines which show a gentle anterior gradient as the whole mitral annulus moves anteriorly. Abnormal systolic anterior motion (S.A.M.) is character-ized by a sharp movement of the anterior leaflet towards the septum in mid-systole, producing a hump on the trace (Fig. 5.21). When true systolic anterior motion is present, the leaflet returns to the normal position before full re-opening takes place at the beginning of diastole. 'False' systolic anterior motion can be produced by inadequate technique when the mitral valve is examined near its base. The leaflet does not return to the normal position in such traces (Fig. 5.22), and examination with angulation of the beam downwards usually shows a normally moving mitral valve.

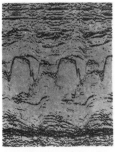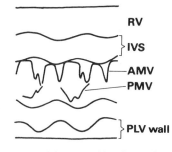

RV

IVS

AMV

PMV

PLV wall

FIG. 5.21 A trace from a case of hypertrophic obstructive cardiomyopathy. There is marked thickening of the septum, anterior systolic movement of the mitral valve, and reduced diastolic closure rate. R.V., right ventricle; I.V.S., inter-ventricular septum; A.M.V., anterior mitral valve; P.M.V., posterior mitral valve; P.L.V., posterior left ventricular wall.

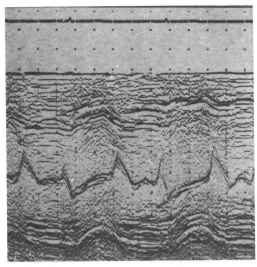

FIG. 5.22 'False' systolic anterior movement of the mitral valve. On the left of the trace, there is some upward bowing of the closed mitral valve in systole. On the right, the normal smooth gradient of the valve cusps is seen in systole.

S.A.M. used to be considered a pathognomonic sign of H.O.C.M. but it is now known to occur in other con-ditions. Nonetheless, its demonstration together with the other features, confirms the presence of left ventricular out-flow tract obstruction.

When the outflow tract of the left ventricle is markedly narrowed, the anterior leaflet of the mitral valve touches the septum in its fully open position and remains in contact with the septum for the greater part of the diastole. In some patients, these features are only seen after provocative tests such as sublingual administration of isoprenaline.

The echogram may also show a diminished D.C.R. of the anterior leaflet of the mitral valve due to poor left ventricular compliance. The posterior leaflet will show normal movement, thus excluding the possibility of mitral stenosis.

Hypertrophy of the septum is another feature of this condition which is demonstrable with echocardiography. Echocardiography has also played an important part in studies on families of the patients with asymmetric septal hypertrophy. These studies (Henry *et al.*, 1973) have con-cluded that the disease entity is transmitted as an auto-somal dominant trait and can exist in a pre-clinical form.

The interventricular septum is disproportionately thickened compared to the posterior left ventricular wall. The ratio of the thickness of the septum to that of the left ventricular wall (measured at the level of the posterior mitral leaflet) of greater than 1·5 is highly suggestive of hypertrophic obstructive cardiomyopathy. It is probably unwise to use this ratio as the sole criterion of disease in

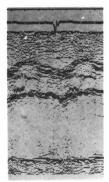

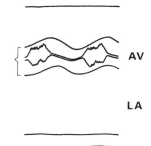

FIG. 5.23 Aortic valve trace in hypertrophic obstructive cardiomyopathy. There is flutter of the valve cusps and partial closure in mid-systole. A.V., aortic valve; L.A., left atrium.

the absence of clinical and electrocardiographic features.

The trace of the aortic valve may show two non-specific features of out-flow tract obstruction of the left ventricle. High frequency flutter (vibrations) of the aortic valve cusps is seen in systole. There may also be mid-systolic, premature closure of the aortic valve reflecting the reduced blood flow across the valve (Fig. 5.23).

Left ventricle

There is considerable interest and dispute about the use of ultrasound in the assessment of left ventricular function.

Examination of the left ventricle is carried out by directing the beam of ultrasound just below the tip of the anterior leaflet of the mitral valve (position 3). It is best to have some valve echoes in view so that the plane of measurement is sufficiently well-defined to be reproducible. In case of difficulty, turning the patient to the left or using a different interspace may improve the quality of the trace. For a valid and reproducible examination, the following criteria should be present on the trace: (1), both sides of the septum; (2), some echoes from the anterior and posterior leaflets of the mitral valve; (3), endocardial and pericardial echoes from the posterior left ventricular wall. It is probably wise to note the rib-interspace from which the recording has been obtained. Using this technique (Fig. 5.24) one should be able to record the end-diastolic diameters of the right and left ventricles—both measured at the peak of the Q.R.S. complex of the electrocardiogram. The end-systolic diameter is measured as the smallest diameter when the septum and posterior wall of the left ventricle approach each other. The septal thickness and the thickness of the posterior left ventricular wall are also measured.

The average amplitude of movement of the posterior wall of the left ventricle is 1 cm. Reduced movement (less than 5 mm) may indicate coronary artery disease,

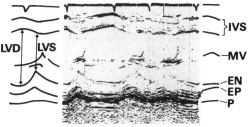

FIG. 5.24 Measurement of the internal dimensions of the left ventricle in systole and diastole. L.V.D., left ventricular end-diastolic diameter; L.V.S., left ventricular end-systolic diameter; I.V.S., interventricular septum; M.V., mitral valve; E.N., endocardium; E.P., epicardium (visceral pericardium); P., pericardium (parietal).

myocardial infarction, myopathy or cardiac failure. Excessive movement is usually seen with left ventricular volume overload and as a compensatory phenomenon when dyskinetic segments are present in other parts of the left ventricle. Paradoxical movement may be observed in the presence of a left ventricular aneurysm.

To obtain an overall view of the state of the left ventricle it is essential to carry out a continuous scan from the aortic root to the apex of the left ventricle. This is done by changing the direction of the ultrasound beam from position 1 to position 3 and beyond. Slow scanning speeds should be used on the strip-chart recorder. In a normal ventricle, the septum and the posterior wall show increased movement as the scan approaches the apex. There is also narrowing of the cavity of the ventricle as one would expect in a normal ventricle (Fig. 5.25). Continuous scans should be obtained from as many interspaces as possible to examine the whole of the left ventricle.

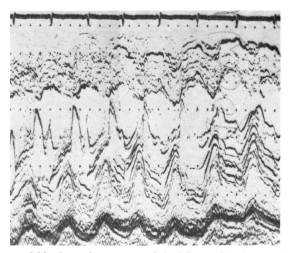

FIG. 5.25 A continuous scan of the left ventricle. Increased movements of the septum and the posterior wall are seen towards the apex (right of the trace). There is also tapering of the left ventricular cavity.

Assessment of left ventricular function

There is little doubt that with careful technique, accurate measurements of the end-systolic and end-diastolic dimensions of the left ventricle can be obtained on most patients. Several workers (Feigenbaum *et al.,* 1969; Popp and Harrison, 1970; Gibson, 1971) have calculated left ventricular volumes from the end-systolic and end-diastolic diameters. These derived volumes have been shown to have a good correlation with the results obtained from angiocardiographic measurements. Most formulae use a prolate ellipse as the model for calculating the volume of the left ventricle from echographic measurements. The long axis (L) of the ventricle is assumed to be twice the length of the short axis (D.).

Hence the formula $V = \frac{\pi}{6} LD^2$. But $L = 2D$.

$$\therefore \ V = \frac{\pi}{6} 2D \times D^2 = \frac{2\pi}{6} D^3 \simeq D^3$$

The volume is therefore proportional to the cube of the short axis, which is measured by echography. . In uniformly contracting ventricles, which are of normal shape, these assumptions are valid and the volume measurements are probably accurate. However, as the ventricle enlarges, its shape approaches that of a sphere and the conventional ellipse formula no longer applies. In addition, with segmental disease of the ventricle, as in coronary artery disease, the measurements taken in one area of the ventricle are not truly representative of the state of the whole ventricle. Linhart *et al.* (1975), have concluded that it is not possible to predict accurately, the end-diastolic and end-systolic volumes and, hence, the stroke volume. In spite of this, echocardiography has the merit of reproducing the same measurements in the same patient under varying conditions. It is, therefore, suitable for following the clinical course of any individual patient. Response to therapy, medical or surgical, can be assessed.

Echocardiography may also be useful in measuring the ejection fraction of the left ventricle. Linhart *et al.,* (1975) state that it is not necessary to measure volumes to derive ejection fraction as it can be measured in terms of the shortening of the minor axis.

Ludbrook *et al.* (1973), have shown that the mean velocity of circumferential fibre-shortening may be useful in assessing the ventricular performance in patients with coronary artery disease. Systolic time intervals can also be measured.

Feigenbaum (1975) has reviewed the rôle of echocardiography in the examination of the left ventricle.

Left atrium

Directing the beam of ultrasound along position 1 (Fig. 5.3) as in the examination of the aorta and the aortic valve, also results in demonstration of the left atrial cavity. The wall of the left atrium can be recognized by its pattern of movement. Thus, in systole, it moves posteriorly (away from the transducer), whereas, the left ventricular wall moves anteriorly. Also, the range of movement of the left atrial wall is much less than that of the left ventricular wall.

The left atrial cavity is measured between the posterior aortic wall and the posterior left atrial wall at the end of systole. Hirata *et al.* (1969), measured the left atrial size using this method and compared the results with the area of left atrium obtained from angiocardiograms. Extremely good correlation was shown.

The echographic dimensions of the normal left atrium vary from 2–4 cm. This range is rather wide and is obviously dependent on the overall heart size in any individual. The absolute dimension of the left atrium has not been found to be of value in excluding left atrial enlargement. In several patients with severe mitral valve disease, the left atrium has been found to be less than 4 cm in diameter. Brown *et al.* (1974), have therefore suggested that the left atrial diameter should be compared with the aortic root. The normal left atrial/aortic root ratio is less than 1·17. We have found this to be an extremely useful guide to assessing left atrial enlargement.

LEFT ATRIAL TUMOURS

Left atrial myxoma is the most common tumour arising from the heart. The tumour is often pedunculated and can prolapse into the left ventricular cavity during diastole. This obstruction of the mitral valve orifice can, therefore, produce clinical signs of mitral stenosis.

Echocardiography has proved extremely valuable in diagnosing these tumours. The trace of the mitral valve shows a characteristic abnormality. As the tumour prolapses into the left ventricle, the valve leaflets are held open throughout the diastole. The diastolic closure rate may, therefore, be diminished and may suggest the diagnosis of mitral stenosis. The normal movement of the posterior leaflet should be demonstrated to exclude the diagnosis of mitral stenosis. Abnormal echoes are present behind the anterior mitral leaflet (Fig. 5.26). These speckled echoes fill the space between the mitral leaflets and are absent in systole when the tumour lies in the atrium. With a continuous scan from the left ventricle to the left atrium, the abnormal echoes should persist as the ultrasound beam passes the atrio-ventricular junction and the tumour may also be seen in the left atrium behind the aorta. The demonstration of the left atrial tumours will become even more reliable with the real-time two-dimensional scanners which are now becoming available.

Developments in echocardiography

Single element M-mode scanning which has been described on the preceeding pages, though an extremely useful technique, has several limitations. Only a selected

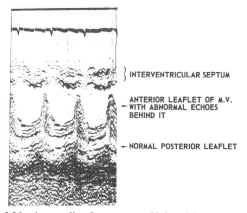

} INTERVENTRICULAR SEPTUM

ANTERIOR LEAFLET OF M.V.
← WITH ABNORMAL ECHOES
BEHIND IT

← NORMAL POSTERIOR LEAFLET

FIG. 5.26   A recording from a case of left atrial myxoma.

narrow portion of the heart can be examined at any one time and the spatial relationship of various cardiac structures can be assessed by knowing the direction of the beam of ultrasound, but with a hand-held transducer this information cannot be precise. When changing the direction of the beam one cannot be sure that the same part is not being examined twice, or conversely, that one has not missed an important part of the cardiac anatomy.

Attempts have been made, therefore, to obtain two-dimensional cross-sections of the cardiac outline. Bom *et al.* (1971), have developed a multi-element system using 20 transducers firing, virtually, simultaneously. The effect is to provide real-time angiogram-like pictures of the heart which can be viewed on a video-recorder. The results obtained by using this equipment appear promising, particularly in outlining the anatomical abnormalities in congenital heart disease (Roelandt *et al.*, 1974).

Other methods of obtaining real-time two-dimensional images are also becoming available. Mechanically-driven transducers have been used to provide a two-dimensional picture (Griffith and Henry, 1974). The newer instruments will provide supplementary information to that given by the established echocardiography machines. The present generation of M-mode scanners are not likely to be displaced completely as they will still be used for accurate measurements of valvular movement and chamber size.

Congenital heart disease

In new born infants, the examination can be performed using higher frequencies of ultrasound thus improving the resolution of structures lying close together. A 3·5 mHz focussed transducer with 5 mm diameter is usually suitable with appropriate change of the operating frequency of the machine. Infants and children often require sedation before the examination as movement during the examination makes the recording and interpretation of continuous scans difficult.

Using the standard M-mode technique the anatomical relationship of the cardiac chambers and the great vessels can be assessed. The cardiac chambers can be accurately measured. The demonstration of the interventricular septum and its relationship to the aorta is particularly important (Goldberg *et al.*, 1975). Real-time two-dimensional scanning will greatly facilitate the demonstration of the anatomical abnormalities in congenital heart disease.

Contrast echocardiography

Ultrasound can be used to show the blood-flow pattern within the heart by injecting 'contrast' in a peripheral vein. Gramiak *et al.* (1969) first used the method, by injecting 1 per cent indocyanine green through a cardiac catheter, to confirm the echographic demonstration of the aortic root. Valdez-Cruz *et al.* (1976) showed that 2–3 ml of 5 per cent dextrose mixed with patient's own blood can be injected in a peripheral vein to produce satisfactory results. Rapid injection of fluid into the venous system produces 'cavitation' and these cavities or bubbles when carried to the heart act as reflectors of ultrasound. The resulting echoes are of low amplitude so the instrument should be set at high gain and low reject.

The transducer is directed towards the aortic area (position 1, Fig. 5.3) for detection of shunts at the atrial level. In a patient with no intracardiac shunting, injection of dextrose in a peripheral vein produces echoes within the cavity of the right ventricle which clear after 3–4 cycles. When a right to left atrial shunt is present, echoes appear in the left atrium and the aortic root soon after the injection. A change of position of the transducer to the mitral area (position 2, Fig. 5.3) will show echoes appearing between the mitral cusps as the bubbles pass from the left atrium to the left ventricle.

When a ventricular right to left shunt is present, cavitation echoes are seen anterior to the mitral valve and within the aortic root but the left atrium will remain free of echoes (Valdez-Cruz *et al.*, 1976).

Seward *et al.* (1977) have shown that the diagnosis of a common ventricle can be reliably made by using the contrast echography method. In a common ventricle and two atrio-ventricular valves, the cloud of echoes appears in the tricuspid valve orifice during diastole and the space in front of the mitral valve also fills with echoes during the same cycle. The rest of the chamber then fills without outlining the septum. When a common ventricle is present with a single atrio-ventricular valve the echoes appear behind the single valve and then fill the rest of the chamber.

Contrast echocardiography is a safe and reliable method which has extended the use of ultrasound to non-invasive demonstration of intracardiac blood flow patterns.

(*References to this chapter are given on page 75.*)

6. Radiological Equipment. Contrast Media

The quality of any radiodiagnostic investigation depends on satisfactory radiological equipment. For angiocardiographic diagnosis, this equipment is expensive and requires expert technical staff for its installation, its performance and for its maintenance. The selection of this radiographic equipment is a major consideration in the establishment of a modern diagnostic cardiac unit and should be selected after mutual consultation between cardiologist, cardiac surgeon and radiologist. A unilateral decision without consultation will inevitably lead to dissatisfaction with the quality, range and versatility of the radiological investigations which can be satisfactorily performed.

One of the main difficulties encountered in making these decisions is due to the rapid technical advances being made in this field of diagnosis. A delay of several months may be desirable to assess a recently designed piece of equipment and to compare it with a model previously available and of known performance. At some stage, however, a final and agreed selection of equipment must be made. It is regrettable that because of administrative, planning, financial and building delays, this decision will have to be made many months or often several years before the equipment will be utilized for clinical investigations.

A detailed discussion of radiological equipment is outside the scope of this book, but some guiding principles may help to put the cardiologist 'in the picture' (Fig. 6.1).

There are perhaps 4 or 5 manufacturers who produce sophisticated radiological equipment for angiographic procedures. It is advisable to permit one manufacturer to supply and install the entire installation rather than employ several suppliers. It is very important to check that adequate service and maintenance facilities are available locally, for the best designed equipment becomes useless if it is inadequately installed and maintained.

Unfortunately, local service facilities for this very sophisticated equipment may leave much to be desired. A modern bi-plane angiocardiographic installation (bi-plane fluoroscopy, cine and photofluorography) costs in the region of £250,000–£300,000 at 1976 U.K. prices. 'Down-time'—i.e. the time when equipment is not functioning—is therefore very expensive indeed.

Before deciding on the equipment, the cardiologist, surgeon and radiologist must carefully consider the work-load, age of the patients and trends of clinical practice. Equipment which is ideal for coronary angiography (in adults) will not be optimal for the investigation of children with congenital heart disease. As both types of investigation must often be undertaken on the same equipment, compromises in equipment choice may well be necessary.

Before actually confirming the order for the equipment, the cardiologist and the radiologist should visit a centre using the same equipment under clinical conditions. They should witness and preferably participate in a

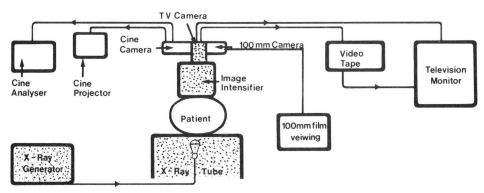

FIG. 6.1 Schematic line drawing of a typical cine angiocardiographic and photofluorographic layout.

diagnostic investigation. An installation that looks admirable in a glossy, coloured, promotional brochure or on an exhibition stand may prove to have significant limitations under actual service conditions for the exact type of work which it is desired to practise.

Fluoroscopy and radiography

An image intensifier is essential for fluoroscopy during cardiac catheter manipulation, in order to reduce patient and staff irradiation and to permit room illumination adequate for the technical procedures. An image intensifier can be used without closed-circuit television, but without this aid, fluoroscopy becomes tedious and tiring as the operator is not able to move freely, for he must view through a narrow angle mirror or periscope.

It is essential therefore that the image intensifier be linked by camera to a closed-circuit television system for a cardiac investigation suite.

Image intensifier

Size. The size of the image intensifier field is very important. The small field intensifiers provide better definition than larger ones and are considerably cheaper and easier to manipulate. For detailed visualization, e.g. of the coronary arteries, a small intensifier such as 6 in (or 7 in) may be preferred, but this size intensifier is generally considered to be too small for cardiac catheterization of adult patients. A very useful compromise is to use a 9 in (23 cm) intensifier which has an added facility to produce electronic magnification to provide a 5 in mode. A similar sized intensifier produced by another manufacturer has a 10 in/6 in mode but it must be appreciated that the area of the patient visualized is a circle of diameter of about 75 per cent of the quoted figures.

Most cardiac installations employ a 9 in/5 in (or 10 in/ 6 in) image intensifier, but a few years ago the larger 12 in/8 in intensifier was widely used. The considerable bulk, cost and poorer definition dictated a swing to the smaller 9 in/5 in intensifier, but modern technology suggests that within the next few years more satisfactory larger intensifiers may be developed. It is doubtful however, whether they will be utilized for cardiac catheterization.

A major technical improvement occurred in 1972 when caesium iodide was developed for the input phosphor screen. This new generation of intensifiers produces a higher efficiency of X-ray quantum detection, giving a much higher 'brightness' gain. This permits the use of a smaller focal spot, shorter exposure times and smaller lens apertures, all of which improve considerably the quality and definition of the radiographic image. In addition, the new intensifiers have an inherently higher resolution over the entire field so that miniature radio-graphs or photofluorograms (70 or 100 mm) can now be obtained with a quality and resolution comparable to a full-sized radiograph, but utilizing only a fraction of the exposure.

This major gain in image quality of miniature radiographs is responsible for the marked recent trend to utilize these cheaper miniature films requiring less radiation in place of the full-sized radiographs. The capital and installation cost of the miniature cameras may, however, be considerably greater, for an image intensifier is necessary for each miniature camera, thus two of each pieces of equipment are needed for bi-plane work.

A further gain in image quality is obtained by using the magnification mode (5 in) of the 9 in intensifier—there is an inevitable increase in radiation requirement ($\times 3$), but the gain in definition is very considerable—from 35 to 45 line pairs/cm and is essential for coronary angiography.

Position. In most installations, the image intensifier is placed *above* the patient who lies supine on the catheterization table: the X-ray tube is below the table. This arrangement causes less radiation scatter to the operator and enables the intensifier to be brought closer to the heart, so improving image quality. Manipulation and accessibility of cine and/or miniature cameras are much easier with the intensifier above the patient. Disadvantages of this system are that another X-ray tube will be needed if full-sized (35 cm²) radiographs are taken on a film changer, e.g. Schonander or Puck, and the access to the patient is rather more difficult with the bulky intensifier placed above the patient.

In another type of installation, the intensifier is placed *below* the catheterization table. This permits improved access to the patient and enables the same X-ray tube to be used for fluoroscopy and the A.P. film-changer. The disadvantages are that the operator may expose his hands in the direct X-ray beam (proximal to attenuation by the patient's body), the operator receives more scattered radiation (particularly to the eyes), and access to the cameras is more difficult as they are now placed below the table.

Both installations should be carefully considered, but the present consensus favours the image intensifier *above* the table for cardiac catheterization.

A recent development has been to mount the intensifier and the X-ray tube on opposing arms of large C or U which may be rotated about the patient in a transverse plane at right angles to the length of the catheterization table. In both of these U and C arm machines, the intensifier tube can be mounted above or below the table; it can also be rotated to an extreme oblique position on either side of the patient. The U arm has some advantages over the C arm; both are very satisfactory for coronary angiography (*q.v.*) but will probably not replace the traditional 'fixed' installation for bi-plane angiocardiography.

X-ray tube

The X-ray tube must have a high output, for the demands of angiocardiography, particularly in the adult, are very demanding. If cine angiography or miniature photo-fluorograms are being used, then a small focal spot (e.g. 0·6 mm²) is essential for good quality. In order to dissipate the heat resulting from small focal spot utilization, the anode of the X-ray tube rotates at about 9000 revs. per minute compared to the standard 3000 r.p.m. These high-speed rotation tubes require a special high speed stator and are expensive, but they are essential for good quality photofluorography or cine angiography.

In order to obtain maximal radiographic contrast, the kilovoltage must be reduced to the optimum value (e.g. 70 KVp) utilizing a high milli-amperage in order to obtain the required radiation energy. This requirement for low KVp and high mA necessitates X-ray tubes of high power capacity up to and exceeding 100 kW. At high-power utilization, the anode heat production increases and improved tube cooling may be achieved by cooling fans or circulating water. Newer tubes are being developed with a carbon anode mass or other material of high heat capacity.

Expert advice from the manufacturers is essential in the choice of X-ray tubes and generators.

Generators

The generator converts electrical energy supplied by the mains into a form suitable to energize the X-ray tube to produce X-rays. This process is unfortunately very inefficient for less than 1 per cent of energy supplied is converted to X-rays and less than 0·2 per cent of the energy actually reaches the X-ray film. The system is like a very expensive electric fire, for 99 per cent of the energy supplied is converted to heat.

Four-valve (single-phase, two-pulse) generators are adequate for cine angiography up to about 30 frames/s but this small capacity cannot be recommended for a modern cardio-radiological suite.

A generator of higher capacity—three phase, 6 or 12 pulse generator produces an almost constant potential and has the great advantage of reducing patient dose, increasing radiation output permitting low kV, high mA, small focal spot, low exposure time techniques. Such a generator is highly recommended for serial changer work, high speed (up to 200 frames/s.) cine and photofluorography with miniature 70 or 100-mm films.

Electronic switching permits rapid pulsing of the generator synchronous with film arrest in the cine camera gate.

For bi-plane angiocardiography, two separate genera-tors are preferable, one for AP and the other for lateral plane. A less expensive alternative is to use an extended single high-power generator which can energize two tubes synchronously or asynchronously, but the same kV must be used on both tubes, although the mA can be adjusted to allow for the increased penetration required for the lateral projection. For a major cardiac installation, it is however recommended that two generators with independent kV selection be installed.

Newly introduced generators are becoming very sophisticated, including a preliminary test exposure during which the absorption characteristics of the patient are measured and the lowest kV, maximum mA within the permitted tube loading are computerized. Measurement, calculation and setting of all these parameters takes place within a fraction of a second and the optimal factors are varied during a cine run, for example during panning or introduction of contrast medium.

It is essential to discuss in detail with the manufacturers, the type of clinical work for which the equipment is being installed. The generator and X-ray tube must be co-ordinated to ensure that the generator output suits the tube requirements.

Television cameras

Three different types of television camera (or tube) are available—the Vidicon, Plumbicon and Orthicon. Most manufacturers recommend the Plumbicon camera which has the advantage of low-image retentivity and therefore no movement lag when either the patient or the X-ray tube is moved.

Considerable advances have been made recently in the technology of television cameras. The Orthicon which was previously widely recommended for cardiac fluoroscopy, is a more complicated and more expensive tube than the Plumbicon, the performance of which has been recently considerably improved to such a degree that it has largely superceded the Orthicon. The Vidicon is small, reliable, simple, less expensive and has a good noise-to-signal ratio, but suffers from image retentivity and is not usually recommended for major cardiac installations.

Television viewing

The televised image is viewed on a monitor similar to, but built to a more exacting specification than the domestic monitor. It is often advisable to use two monitors on adjustable rotatable (pan and tilt) platforms, preferably ceiling mounted at strategic points in the catheter room.

Video-tape

Video-tape recording is an essential facility when cine angiocardiography is being used. It permits immediate play-back of the cine recording so that a diagnosis is usually possible within seconds of making the injection of contrast medium. The adequacy of the injection rate, centring of the fluoroscopic screen, the field of the patient visualized, as well as the diagnostic assessment of cardiac function can all be viewed on the video-tape replay.

Recent developments in video-tape technology have included greatly improved quality of 'still' frames, and much more reliable performance of the equipment.

A major technological improvement is about to emerge in the development of Video-Disc recorders, which enables a major reduction of radiation exposure and yet captures high resolution images for either immediate play-back or retention. This equipment is still very expensive, but there is every prospect that it will soon become available for clinical practice and may well replace the orthodox Video-Tape.

Cine-camera

The camera is mounted to photograph the output phosphor of the image intensifier tube. 35- or 16-mm cameras may be used but most authorities now prefer the larger format which provides greater detail. Medium- and high-speed cameras up to 200 frames/s are available. The high-speed cameras are very expensive and in fact the highest speeds are rarely used except in special research projects. The usual cine-speeds for coronary angiography and angiocardiography are 36–80 frames/s.

All modern cameras are equipped with contacts for *pulsing*, which causes generation of X-rays only when the shutter of the camera is fully open. During film transport, no X-rays are generated. Pulsing is essential for modern cine-cardiac radiography for it considerably reduces patient irradiation and permits pre-determined very short exposures (1–10 ms) which suppress movement blurring. A typical exposure time is 3–5 ms per frame: this requires a high powered, three-phase generator capable of high-speed electronic switching with a high-speed rotating X-ray tube.

Bi-plane radiography

For investigation of congenital heart disease, bi-plane radiography is a very useful facility: many consider it essential.

The two planes are almost always at right angles, usually AP and lateral. The two radiographic exposures may be taken at exactly the same instant—'*synchronously*' (tic-tic), permitting three dimensional visualization at that particular instant. This is desirable but the two simultaneous exposures may cause cross-fogging, so degrading the image quality.

In order to avoid cross-fogging, the two radiographic exposures can be arranged to be exactly '*asynchronous*', so that they alternate (tic-tac) and never occur at the same instant.

Asynchronous (tic-tac) is essential for bi-plane cine-recording and is advisable for bi-plane film-changer radiography.

Bi-plane radiography (either cine or film changer) is not advisable for coronary angiography where the maximum detail produced by a well-collimated beam and field is essential.

Cine film, processing and viewing

Many combinations of cine film and developer are available, and only by trial and error with consideration of patient dosage and image quality will the inevitable compromise be reached.

Some radiologists prefer fast film e.g. HPS, HP3, 4X, Cineflure, Kodak RAR with a fine grain developer, but others prefer a slower film (e.g. Plus X, Double X).

Cine-processing may be by hand on spool reels, on specially designed motorized cine-processing units, or through conventional full-size roller processors. For an active cardiac investigation unit, it is recommended that a specifically designed, motorized cine-processing unit be considered, for this will help to maintain high quality processing, and process the cine film at a much faster speed than is possible with hand processing. Some cine films however cannot be processed on some motorized processing units.

The cine film is viewed on an analysing projector which is available in 35- and 16-mm format. When analysing the cine-film, it is essential to run the film backwards and forwards repeatedly, and at variable speed. This is particularly important when analysing a cine coronary arteriogram, where it may be very difficult to identify each major branch as they move very rapidly and frequently criss-cross each other during the cardiac cycle.

A recently introduced 35 mm analysing projector has a greater illuminating power and may be viewed by several people, but most machines permit only 4 or 5 persons to study the film at one time.

For demonstration to a larger audience, it is often preferable to reduce the 35-mm film to 16 mm (by a commercial processing company), and then to project the 16 mm copy through a 16 mm projector. 35 mm projection to a large audience requires special facilities and licences.

Catheterization table

A specifically designed patient table for cardiac catheterization is essential for a major cardiac radiological installation. Modern tables are considerably more advanced than their predecessors. Recent developments include an adjustable table height which permits a comfortable catheterization position whatever the height of the operator or the size of the patient. The table may be cantilevered from one end, or have a clear tunnel

D

underneath; in either case, the film changer can be wheeled or motorized into position under the patient without having to move the patient which may displace the catheter.

The catheterization table must have a free-floating top, permitting easy movement in both longitudinal and transverse direction. This freedom of float of the table top is essential for satisfactory panning if the X-ray tube is fixed. Panning is often necessary during selective coronary arteriography using the 5-in mode of intensifier. There must be easily applied and effective brakes, preferably foot-controlled. The controls of the table must be readily accessible so that the catheterizing doctor may control the various movements whilst maintaining operating sterility.

One significant limitation of even modern catheter tables is the limited degree (15–20°) of tilt permitted. Head-down tilt may be required for resuscitation: foot-down tilt may be required during catheterization of a patient in cardiac failure, particularly from mitral or aortic valve disease. A few cardiologists (including ourselves) have utilized a conventional tilting table for catheterizing these patients in a tilted head-up position, say 30° to the horizontal. The patient may be considerably more comfortable, but these tables do not have a floating table-top facility which makes 'panning' very difficult, and the patient has to be moved a considerable distance up and down the table to utilize the film changer.

Rotating cradle

Selective coronary arteriography demands multiple projections in varying degrees of obliquity. It is difficult for the patient to be rotated without mechanical assistance. Without such assistance, the time taken to achieve the desired obliquity prolongs the catheterization study; the catheter tip may be dislodged out of, or pushed deep into, the coronary artery during the movement of the patient. These factors add very considerably to the anxieties experienced during the study, and may add an element of danger.

One approach to counter these difficulties is to employ a curved cradle which is placed lengthwise on the table. The patient is placed (or strapped) into the cradle which can then be rotated by a motorized control which is manipulated by the operator. The patient can be very easily and quickly rotated into any desired degree of obliquity; the patient remains in the centre of the X-ray beam. The axis of rotation varies so that there is always the minimum distance between the patient and the table top, and between the patient and the film. A rotating cradle is a major advantage, considerably reducing the time required for multiple oblique projections and reducing patient discomfort and operator anxiety.

The cradle does, however, have disadvantages—the patient, although fixed in the cradle, rotates relative to the table top, the catheter and monitoring equipment: this movement may dislodge the catheter. In the lateral projection the patient may feel unsafe. Because of these limitations, the rotatable tube and intensifier have been developed on a large installation which has two opposing arms, forming either the letter 'C' or 'U'.

C or U arm apparatus

The basic idea is keep the patient in a *fixed* position and to rotate the X-ray tube and the image intensifier around him in a transverse plane. The principle is the same as in the Lisholm-type skull table which has been in regular use for 40 years for skull radiography.

The X-ray tube and the image intensifier are mounted opposite each other on the end of the two arms of a C or U frame: the radius of the C or U is about 100 cm. The C or U is pivoted on a horizontal shaft, about which the two arms rotate in an axis at right angles to the longitudinal axis of the table top and the patient. A typical degree of rotation is 120° so that any degree of obliquity, including lateral projections may be obtained.

The great advantage of a C or U arm is that the patient does not move throughout the catheterization procedure so that there is much less likelihood of catheter displacement and less discomfort to the patient. The examination is quickly performed even though many oblique projections are taken, so that the catheter lies within the coronary artery for the shortest possible time.

The U arm is a significant improvement on the C arm. It can be linked with a horizontal X-ray tube and image intensifier for bi-plane angiography. The U-arm apparatus is most advantageous when multiple oblique projections are required as in selective coronary angiography for which purpose it has been specifically developed. The U arm is probably not advisable if only bi-plane full-sized film angiography is to be employed.

In coronary angiography it has recently been demonstrated that a cranio-caudal tilt of the tube and intensifier will demonstrate atheromatous lesions of the main coronary arteries (particularly the left main stem) which might be completely hidden (because of foreshortening) without this tilt. It is estimated that about 10 per cent of significant stenoses may be missed without this projection. In order to obtain this cranio-caudal tilt, the table may be swung in an arc round a vertical axis through the 'chest area': in conjunction with the U arm, simultaneous oblique and cranio-caudal angulation may then be achieved.

A more recent development is to modify the arms of the U, by construction of a parallelogram support for both the tube and the intensifier. The arms of the U are rotated to give the usual oblique projection in the transverse axis of the patient: the parallelogram is then tilted to procure the required cranio-caudal tilt. The patient remains supine on the table top and is not moved throughout the procedure. This parallelogram U-apparatus is at present being evaluated, but preliminary results suggest that it may be the most satisfactory available at present for coronary angiography.

Angiocardiographic films

Radiographs taken during angiocardiography may be full-sized or miniature.

Full-sized radiographs are individual films cut to size, usually 14 in × 14 in (35 × 35 cm) or 12 in × 10 in (30 × 24 cm), loaded carefully into a cassette which holds 30 films. The cassette is inserted into a film changer (e.g. AOT Schönander) and the films may be exposed at rates varying from 6/s to one film every 5 s, pre-determined by a program selected by the investigator. Three different rates of filming may be employed during one series of exposures, and a variable delay may be interposed before the final phase.

An alternative method is to use continuous roll film in a film changer which permits 12 exposures per s (Elema), but this model is now discontinued.

Full-sized radiographs after exposure are processed in a roller processor, usually with a 90-s cycle and the cut films are best viewed on an automated illuminated viewing machine which can hold up to 200 films at one loading.

Full-size film changers may be used either single or bi-plane at right angles, preferably asynchronously exposed.

The advantages of full-size radiographs for angiocardiography include a relatively small capital outlay and maximal clarity of definition which permits excellent quality miniature slides for projection and photographic illustrations.

Disadvantages include greater running costs due to the scarcity and expense of the silver of the films and higher radiation dosage per exposure. The use of new rare-earth intensifying screens with up to 4 or even 8 times the speed of conventional screens will soon become standard practice and will greatly reduce radiation exposure, probably to less than that required for photofluorograms.

A major disadvantage of both full sized films and photofluorography is that the dynamics of cardiac action are not portrayed. Exposures in full systole and diastole may not be obtained or recognised, small shunts and regurgitant streams may not be detected. Extra systoles cannot be recognised. For these advantages, full dynamic recording of the cardiac action is necessary, either on cine film or video-tape.

Photofluorograms are miniature films usually 70, 100 or 105 mm which are exposed in special cameras which photograph the output phosphor of the image intensifier. Our unit was one of the first to pioneer this technique (Hynes, Verel and Bates, 1970) for both congenital and acquired heart disease.

The new generation image intensifiers using caesium iodide phosphors and the new miniature camera with the larger format of 100- or 105-mm film have produced a major gain in photographic detail and image quality. Photofluorograms taken on modern equipment are comparable in quality to full-size films, enabling 45 line pairs/mm to be resolved. These miniature films may be processed through conventional roller processors or special developing machines. The films may be viewed by naked eye, aided if necessary by a hand lens. Special projecting illuminators have not been very successful and are very expensive; no doubt other projectors will be developed.

Photofluography may be used either monoplane or bi-plane, exposing asynchronously.

Advantages of photofluorograms include much reduced film costs and reduced patient radiation (but this advantage may not remain now that rare-earth screens are used in full-size film changers). Photofluorogram film loading and unloading are easier and storage space requirement for films is tremendously reduced.

Disadvantages of photofluorograms include the high cost of initial installation particularly when bi-plane photofluorography is required, for this will entail purchase of a second image intensifier and television camera. The new 100 mm camera has proved rather unreliable at full speed, but this technical problem will no doubt be solved.

Cine-filming has been included in a previous section.

Design of installation

The present trend in angiocardiography favours the continued development and utilization of photofluorography using 100- or 105-mm film as a probable replacement for full-size film changers. This trend will be particularly strong when two image intensifiers are installed for bi-plane fluoroscopy and possible bi-plane cine recording. This type of installation is advised for the study of congenital heart disease particularly in children.

For study of acquired heart disease, one image intensifier, assisted by single plane cine and photofluorography may be considered adequate.

For abdominal angiography, one image intensifier and a full-size film changer is satisfactory.

For selective coronary arteriography, a U-arm (possibly with parallelogram cranio-caudal tilt facilities), a single (small) image intensifier, cine and photofluorography is probably the best installation.

As most radiological installations need to be used for several different purposes, every new radiological facility must be very carefully considered and planned, with full regard to the pathological conditions and the age group of patients which it is desired to investigate.

Pressure pumps

Selective angiocardiography requires a pressure pump in order to inject the contrast medium sufficiently rapidly through a high resistance catheter. A rate of delivery of 30 to 40 ml/s is necessary in adult patients, particularly if there is a large left-to-right shunt.

Suitable pumps are available of different complexity and widely differing price range. The most simple pump (e.g. Talley pump) is powered by compressed air, has no electrical contact for remote control or for energizing the X-ray machine, and no heated water bath. The electric contact micro-switches may, however, be easily added to provide remote control of the X-rays.

A more sophisticated pump (e.g. Gidlund pump) has a compressed air power source, and electrical contacts for remote control with a variable preset delay for energizing the X-rays. There is a water bath maintained electrically at preset temperature.

Even more sophisticated pumps are the Viamonte-Hobbs, Medrad and Contrac pumps, which are driven by electric motor and have a complex feedback mechanism to monitor and to regulate the rate of delivery of the contrast medium. A desired delivery rate is preset on a dial and the pump compensates automatically for all of the many factors which control delivery rate, e.g. bore and length of the catheter, resistance of taps and connectors, viscosity of the contrast medium, etc.

These pumps, unlike those previously mentioned, will deliver multiple injections from one syringe loading; this is a great help particularly for cine radiography. These pumps are electrically coupled to the X-ray apparatus and are under remote control. They have a mechaninism for heating the contrast medium within the syringe.

A Cordis (1975) pump has a similar electric motor mechanism but no feedback mechanism. It has an inbuilt computer which computes the required injection pressure after the variables, e.g. catheter length and bore have been dialled. This is not as satisfactory as the fully automated Viamonte-Hobbs, Contrac or Medrad pumps, as the dialled information often does not accurately indicate the true resistance of the circuit. These electric motor pumps can be coupled to an E.C.G. and arranged to fire at a precise point in successive cardiac cycles, e.g. in diastole in 3 or 4 successive cycles.

The selection of pump will depend largely on the finances available, for any of the varieties mentioned will produce an adequate delivery rate of contrast medium. The facilities of the more complicated pumps are useful and desirable. The most complex pumps require expert maintenance for reliable use and this should be ensured before the pump is purchased. The sterilizing and the durability of the syringes must also be very carefully considered for some are plastic and cannot withstand high-temperature autoclaving. A very useful facility is the use of disposable pre-sterilized syringes on some of the electric pumps.

The injection pressures required vary between the different types of pump as they have differing mechanical advantages. Pressure readings taken from the dial cannot therefore be transposed from one pump to another variety of pump. With the Gidlund pump, a pressure of 5 to 6 kg/cm^2 is usually adequate, but a graph should be constructed for each pump, using different lengths and bores of catheters, with timing of the injections at different pressures. The rate of flow is largely determined by the catheter internal bore which is therefore of the greatest importance. The largest bore catheter possible should usually be employed when a high delivery rate is required.

Contrast medium

All modern intravascular contrast media are salts of substituted tri-iodinated benzoic acids. Three of these acids are in current use: diatrizoic acid (Hypaque, Urografin), iothalamic acid (Conray) and metrizoic acid (Triosil, Isopaque). These three acids have approximately the same toxicity.

Contrast medium salts consist of the acid anion and a cation which is usually sodium or methylglucamine. The sodium salts of iothalamic or metrizoic acid are very soluble, providing up to 100 per cent w/v solutions. Sodium diatrizoate is soluble only to 55 per cent w/v. Sodium salt solutions are much less viscous than the solutions of the corresponding methylglucamine salts with the same iodine concentration, permitting a higher delivery rate of iodine, on which the quality of the angiogram largely depends.

Unfortunately, recent evidence indicates that high concentrations of sodium ions are more toxic to cerebral and to myocardial tissue than equivalent concentrations of methylglucamine ions. Solutions of methylglucamine salts which provide the necessary iodine concentration are however too viscous for general angiocardiographic use. A compromise is therefore generally accepted, employing a solution of mixed sodium and methylglucamine salts which has a viscosity and toxicity intermediate between those of the pure salt solutions. Table 6.1 lists the intravascular contrast media in general current use in the United Kingdom.

Particular care must be exercised in the choice of contrast media for coronary angiography. Contrast media with either too low or too high a sodium ion concentration are likely to cause ventricular fibrillation. The optimum sodium concentration is about 140 mEq/ml. Urografin 76, CardioConray and Hypaque 65 are all widely used, but the former has had a much more extensive safety record. We have found Triosil 370 to be very satisfactory (Verel, Ward and Aman, 1975).

For maximal iodine flow rate, solutions of the sodium

TABLE 6.1

Contrast media for angiography: angiocardiography: intravenous urography

Registered Name	Generic Name		Iodine content mg/ml	Viscosity at 37°C Hz
CONRAY 280**	Meglumine iothalamate	60% w/v	280	4
CONRAY 325	Sodium iothalamate	54% w/v	325	2·7
CONRAY 420†	Sodium iothalamate	70% w/v	420	5·4
Cardio-CONRAY†	Meglumine iothalamate ⎱ Sodium iothalamate ⎰	52% w/v 26% w/v	400	8·6
HYPAQUE 45%*	Sodium diatrizoate	45% w/v	270	2·1
HYPAQUE 65%†	Meglumine diatrizoate ⎱ Sodium diatrizoate ⎰	50% w/v 25% w/v	390	8·4
HYPAQUE 85%	Meglumine diatrizoate ⎱ Sodium diatrizoate ⎰	56·67% w/v 28·33% w/v	440	12·2
TRIOSIL '45'* New Formula	Sodium metrizoate (with added Ca & Mg)	45% w/v	260	2
TRIOSIL '60'† New Formula	Sodium metrizoate (with added Ca & Mg)	60% w/v	350	3·3
TRIOSIL '75'† New Formula	Sodium metrizoate (with added Ca & Mg)	75% w/v	440	6·4
UROGRAFIN 60%**	Meglumine diatrizoate ⎱ Sodium diatrizoate ⎰	52% w/v 8% w/v	290	4·3
UROGRAFIN 76%†	Meglumine diatrizoate ⎱ Sodium diatrizoate ⎰	66% w/v 10% w/v	370	8·5
ANGIOGRAFIN	Meglumine diatrizoate	65% w/v	306	5·1
UROVISON	Meglumine diatrizoate ⎱ Sodium diatrizoate ⎰	18% w/v 40% w/v	325	3·3

* Cerebral and other peripheral angiography—Iodine content about 280 mg per ml.
† Angiocardiography and aortography—Iodine content 370 to 440 mg per ml.
  Intravenous urography—Iodine content 260 to 420 mg per ml.
** Preferable for cerebral angiography because of low sodium content.

salts may be preferred. There is evidence to suggest that the toxicity of these sodium salt solutions is reduced by substituting a small proportion of the sodium ions by calcium and magnesium ions—as in Triosil (new balanced formula). For most angiocardiographic purposes, however, the sodium-methylglucamine mixtures provide an adequate iodine flow rate with an effective pump, and are appreciably less toxic than the sodium (or balanced sodium) solutions.

The *catheter internal bore* is a more important factor in achieving an adequate flow rate than the viscosity of the contrast medium. Further details of contrast medium toxicity and the haemo-dynamic responses to angiocardiographic injections are given by one of the authors (R.G.G.) in *Modern Trends in Diagnostic Radiology*, Series IV, 1969.

The *concentrations of* contrast medium solutions used for selective angiocardiography generally provide an iodine content between 370 and 440 mg iodine per ml. If low injection pressures are being employed (e.g. hand injections), a higher iodine injection rate may be achieved by using a low viscosity, low iodine content medium such as Hypaque 45.

The *rate of injection* of iodine is a critical factor in producing high quality angiocardiograms: the greater the iodine injection rate, the better the angiographic contrast. The flow pattern of fluid through a catheter may be either laminar, turbulent or a combination of both. If the flow is laminar, then Poiseuille's Law is valid and the delivery rate is inversely proportional to the viscosity of the fluid. When the injection pressure rises, the flow pattern may become turbulent. Poiseuille's law is then no longer valid, and viscosity of the injected fluid becomes considerably less important (Krovetz *et al.*, 1966). In the majority of injections for selective angiocardiography, the flow is either entirely turbulent or a mixture of both turbulent and laminar patterns. A contrast medium of moderate viscosity and high iodine content (i.e. a sodium-methylglucamine mixture) is therefore generally preferable to the more toxic, low viscosity, concentrated sodium solutions which however permit a slightly greater rate of iodine delivery (Grainger, 1968).

In this Cardiac Unit, Hypaque 85 was used until 1963 when the Conray range (iothalamate) was introduced. Angio Conray 480 and later Conray 420 were then used for all angiocardiograms until 1966 when the toxicity of the sodium ion was recognized (pp. 107, 121, 145). Since then, Cardio-Conray (a 2:1 methylglucamine: sodium mixture) has been used for the great majority of angiocardiograms without noticeable deterioration in pictorial quality (Grainger, 1969).

Modern angiocardiography is based on the remarkable fact that 20 to 30 g of iodine per sec can be injected into the heart or major vessels without serious discomfort to the patient. These large injections do however produce transient haemodynamic responses which may, on rare occasions, give rise to concern (Grainger, 1969). Angiographic injections into the left-heart chambers or ascending aorta cause transient but marked peripheral vasodilatation, slight hypotension, and a moderate increase in cardiac output. Injections into the right-heart chambers or pulmonary artery may cause similar responses, but may also cause pulmonary hypertension due to an increase in pulmonary vascular resistance probably due to erythrocyte aggregation.

Pulmonary oedema, cerebral oedema and a dangerously low cardiac output are very rare but very serious reactions (chapter 17). Ten to fifteen minutes should be allowed between successive large injections of contrast medium as the haemodynamic responses will usually have subsided within a few minutes.

The volume of each angiocardiographic injection usually ranges between 30 to 60 ml in the adult. The large volumes are preferred in large adults, left to right shunts, and hyperdynamic circulations. In infants and children, a volume of 1 to 1·5 ml per kg body weight is usually given for each injection. These injections may be repeated and up to three or even four injections may be required to complete the investigation, but there is a hazard of overloading the body with contrast medium which may cause dangerous cerebral and pulmonary oedema, or severe cardiac dysfunction (chapter 17). A volume of contrast medium totalling more than 4 ml per kg body weight should rarely be exceeded during the complete investigation. Particular care with regard to contrast medium dosage must be observed in small children and neonates who are particularly sensitive to changes in osmolarity of the blood.

All water-soluble contrast media are concentrated solutions of salts of strong iodinated acids. These salts dissociate completely in solution and therefore the concentrated solutions used for angiocardiography have a very high osmolarity—up to 9 times that of blood. The introduction of a large volume of such high osmolar solution causes significant changes both in the blood and the circulatory system. Erythrocytes become smaller, crenated and form aggregates or rouleaux when they are bathed by a hyperosmolar solution which also

causes a considerable increase in blood volume. Peripheral vasodilatation, consequent hypotension, impaired myocardial contractility, increased capillary permeability, cellular dehydration result from exposure to hyperosmolar solutions.

An important recent development has been the synthesis of a non-ionic contrast medium, solutions of which have a much reduced osmolarity. Such a product is metrizamide which is a substituted amide of metrizoic acid; a solution of metrizamide containing 280 mg iodine per ml has an osmolarity of 0·456 osmols/kg, compared with an osmolarity of 1·46 osmols of meglumine metrizoate 280 mg iodine per ml which is a typical current contrast medium. Blood has an osmolarity of 0·301 osmols/kg.

Animal experiments suggest that non-ionic contrast media have much less clincal toxicity, particularly for coronary arteriography and they may well be introduced clinically for this purpose. Further development is however required, for metrizamide cannot be autoclave-sterilized in solution and it is very expensive. It has however been extensively used for clinical myelography, for which purpose it has proved very successful.

References

FISCHER, H. W. & CORNELL, S. H. (1965). The toxicity of the sodium and methylglucamine salts of diatrizoate, iothalamate and metrizoate. *Radiology* **85**, 1013.

GENSINI, G. G. & DI GIORGI, S. (1964). Myocardial toxicity of contrast agents in angiography. *Radiology* **82**, 24.

GRAINGER, R. G. (1968). Cardio-Conray—a new contrast medium formulation for angiocardiography and aortography. *Br. J. Radiol.* **41**, 674.

GRAINGER, R. G. (1969). Contrast media in *Modern Trends in Radiology*, Series IV. London: Butterworth.

HYNES, D. H., VEREL, D. & BATES, P. (1971). Value of 70 mm photofluorography in cardiac investigation. *Br. J. Radiol.* **44**, 434–440.

KROVETZ, L. J., FAIRCHILD, B. T., HARDIS, S. & MITCHELL, B. (1966). An analysis of factors determining delivery rates of liquids through cardiac catheters. *Radiology* **86**, 123.

LUDWIG, J. W. (1975). Supplementary X-ray beam projection in coronary arteriography. *Medicamundi* 59–71 (Philips) Vol. **20** No. 2.

OVITT, T., RIZK, G., FRECH, R. S., CRAMER, R. & AMPLATZ, K. (1972). E.C.G. Changes in Selective Coronary Arteriography: The Importance of Ions. *Radiology* **104**, 705.

PAULIN, S. & ADAMS, D. F. (1971). Increased ventricular fibrillation during coronary arteriography with a new contrast medium preparation. *Radiology* **101**, 45.

SNYDER, C. F., FORMANEK, A. & FRECH, R. S. (1971). The role of sodium in promoting ventricular arrhythmia during selective coronary arteriography. *Amer. J. Roentgen.* **113**, 567.

VEREL, D., WARD, C. & AMAN, M. (1975). Comparison of Triosil 370 with Urografin 76 and Hypaque 65 for coronary arteriography. *Br. Heart J.* **37**, 1049–1052.

7. Introduction to Angiocardiography. General Principles

Angiocardiography is the technique of visualization by radiography of contrast medium which has been injected into the circulation. The contrast medium may be injected into a peripheral vein or into a vena cava, but this method is generally not very satisfactory. The medium does not arrive at the heart as a discrete well-defined bolus and it therefore becomes diluted by the blood returning to the heart. It may be difficult to identify the sequence of chamber filling and the detailed anatomy of the individual chambers. One opacified chamber may obscure another chamber, for example, the opacified right atrial appendage completely obscures the pulmonary valve area in the lateral projection.

Selective angiocardiography

Because of these defects, the technique of *Selective Angiocardiography* has been developed. In this method the contrast medium is delivered through a catheter into a selected heart chamber. The contrast medium is injected by pump at high pressure so that the entire bolus is delivered in about 2–4 seconds. Radiographs, either rapid full-sized or miniature films or cine-recordings, are taken during and immediately after the injection.

Selective angiocardiography is the only radiological method which will be discussed in this text.

Angiocardiography is *not* an investigation which can be undertaken or assessed as an isolated technical procedure. It is a very important and integral part of the catheter investigation of cardiac anatomy and function. This concept cannot be too strongly emphasized, for mistakes in both manipulative technique and diagnostic interpretation become inevitable if angiocardiography is considered in isolation, or if it is undertaken by personnel inadequately informed of basic cardiological principles.

Selective angiocardiography provides information of the morphology of the heart and great vessels which cannot be obtained by any other method.

The anatomy of the different cardiac chambers can be depicted in three dimensions by means of bi-plane angiocardiography. The injection of contrast medium should be made either into the chamber which it is desired to visualize, or into the chamber immediately proximal to it. All four cardiac chambers and all the vessels entering or leaving the heart may be entered by catheter and therefore they may all be demonstrated radiologically by a selective angiocardiographic injection. The techniques necessary to

provide this anatomical information are described and discussed in subsequent chapters.

Selective angiocardiography also yields information of the *haemodynamic situation* and of the circulatory mechanics. In this context, close correlation with *oximetry* and *pressure mensuration* is essential. The three different techniques are merely different facets of the same catheter investigation and they provide a composite picture of the cardiac anatomy, function and haemodynamics which cannot be given by any single method in isolation.

Quantitative assessment of the stroke volume and end-systolic volume, ejection fraction of any of the heart chambers may be made by mensuration and calculation from bi-plane cine-angiocardiographic films. This is quite a complicated technical exercise and is probably only justified in a research project or in a few selected problems. Mensuration from ultrasonic recordings may provide this information more effectively.

Because angiocardiography entails the production of several (or many) radiographs taken in rapid succession, it provides evidence of the *sequence of filling* of the different heart chambers. For example, in complete uncorrected transposition of the great vessels, venous blood passes from the right atrium to the right ventricle and thence into the aorta for distribution to the systemic organs. In the same condition, oxygenated blood passes from the pulmonary veins through the left atrium and the left ventricle to the pulmonary arteries for a further (and useless) passage through the lungs. This abnormal sequence of chamber filling will be demonstrated by careful study of the series of films obtained during angiocardiography.

In the above example, continued life would be impossible without means for the blood in the two circulations to mix. There *must* be both a left to right and a right to left shunt of equal volume. These *abnormal shunts* may be at atrial, ventricular or ductal level and may be identified by selective angiocardiography.

Because all the four cardiac chambers and all the major vessels entering or leaving the heart can be entered by catheter, it is possible to assess angiographically the efficiency of any (or all) of the *four heart valves*.

Cine-angiocardiography is much preferred for these valve studies for it provides a more comprehensive picture of the cardiac cycle and particularly of fleeting incompetence, than does full-sized film angiocardiography in which radiographs may be taken at speeds no greater than 12 per s and often no greater than 6 per s.

In general, when anatomical detail is the prime requisite as in complex congenital cardiac malformations, full-sized film or photofluorographic angiocardiography is preferred; when valve incompetence or shunting of blood is being investigated, cine studies yield more valuable information.

Valve assessment

Any of the four cardiac valves may be normal or abnormal. The abnormality may be either congenital or acquired: the valve may be stenosed or incompetent, absent or displaced. Any of these possibilities may be investigated by the selective angiographic technique.

VALVE STENOSIS

The optimal site for angiocardiographic injection is into the chamber proximal (in the haemodynamic sense) to the suspected valve so that the blood passing through that valve will be opacified by the injected contrast medium with the minimum of dilution.

There are four basic angiographic signs of valve stenosis:

1. *Impaired mobility or separability of the valve leaflets.* In congenital stenosis of the semilunar aortic and pulmonary valves, the three cusps are adherent at the commissures but they are often otherwise quite mobile. In ventricular systole, therefore, the three valve cusps form a diaphragm which is 'blown' into the base of the aorta or pulmonary artery where it forms a thin diaphragmatic dome, convexity directed towards the artery. This evidence of semilunar valve stenosis is depicted on the angiocardiogram as a thin dark convex line, projecting into the base of the artery, and demarcated on both aspects by the opacified blood (Figs. 57A, 57C, 58B).

The mobility of the valve cusps can be assessed by comparative study of serial films, particular attention being paid to the positions adopted in ventricular systole and diastole (Figs. 57A–D). This is better evaluated on cine-angiography.

The cusps of a stenotic valve are often *thickened,* a feature recognizable on the angiocardiogram (Fig. 57). Valve *calcification* is a very frequent feature of mitral and aortic valve stenosis and can be readily recognised on cine recordings exposed immediately before the injection of contrast medium.

Stenosis of the atrio-ventricular valves does not usually provide such clear cut evidence of valve doming. Stenosis of the mitral valve is very frequent and its angiocardiographic assessment has so far proved rather disappointing, but in the right anterior oblique projection the mitral leaflets are usually seen in profile and doming and thickening of the valve may sometimes be demonstrated on cine studies.

2. *The jet of contrast medium* (and therefore of blood) which is pumped through a stenotic valve is narrower in cross-section than that pumped through a normal valve. The dimensions of the jet can be measured by ruler or dividers as it enters the receiving chamber. In the case of a normal valve, the jet appears to be as wide as the valve ring, but in valve stenosis it may be reduced to a few mm diameter (Figs. 57A and 58). The jet is often irregular in cross-section and therefore its area is difficult to measure accurately.

3. *Post-stenotic dilatation* is a frequent feature which can be recognized on the angiocardiogram. It is not seen in the ventricles when there is stenosis of the mitral or tricuspid valve, but is best seen in the aorta and pulmonary artery with stenosis of the semilunar valves. The receiving artery dilates, often eccentrically, with the maximal expansion at the site of impact of the jet which is being forced through the stenotic valve. Thus in the presence of pulmonary valve stenosis, the dilatation is usually most evident on the upper anterior wall of the pulmonary artery a few centimetres above its origin, where the vessel curves horizontally towards its bifurcation (Figs. 57 and 58).

4. *Hypertrophy of the proximal chamber* is necessary to propel blood through the stenotic valve. In the case of semilunar valve stenosis, this feature can be recognized angiocardiographically by an increase in the trabeculation and wall thickness of the ventricle. The muscle hypertrophy involves the outflow as well as the inflow tract of the ventricle: in the right ventricle this may be demonstrated by a marked narrowing of the subvalvar region during ventricular systole in patients with severe pulmonary valve stenosis (Figs. 57C, 58B).

These angiocardiographic features are best demonstrated by means of *positive* radiological contrast by injecting the medium *proximal* to the valve, i.e. visualizing the jet as a stream of contrast medium, and the valve dome as a radiolucent convex line defined on both aspects by opaque contrast medium. These latter two features may however, also be demonstrated rather less effectively, by injecting the contrast medium into the *receiving* chamber. The jet is then seen as a *radiolucent* jet being pumped into opaque contrast medium. The dome of the stenotic valve is seen as a *radiolucent* convexity projecting into the base of the *opacified* artery (Figs. 57D, 85A and 86A).

VALVE INCOMPETENCE

This is best demonstrated angiocardiographically by injecting contrast medium into the chamber on the *distal* side of the valve and then evaluating any opacification which may occur in the chamber proximal to the valve. Thus in suspected aortic valve incompetence, the injection of contrast medium is made into the ascending aorta: valve incompetence will cause opacification of the left ventricle (Fig. 86B). Cine-angiography is greatly preferable as this opacification may be incomplete and fleeting and quite invisible on large angiogram films.

The ventricle ejecting blood through the incompetent valve is often enlarged, depending on the severity of incompetence and the consequent increase of stroke volume. This enlargement will only be demonstrated angiocardiographically if the incompetent stream is sufficiently large as to opacify the entire ventricle.

There is generally enlargement of the chamber or artery, both on the proximal and the distal aspects of the incompetent valve due to increased stroke volume (Fig. 110).

Shunts

LEFT TO RIGHT FLOW

Intra-cardiac shunts of blood are usually due to congenital defects in the septa of the heart. They transmit a flow of blood which is *always* directed from the left heart chamber to the right heart chamber, provided that the septal defect is the *only* abnormality. Thus an uncomplicated atrial septal defect will transmit a shunt of blood from the left to the right atrium; a ventricular septal defect will transmit a shunt from left to right ventricle. An uncomplicated patent ductus arteriosus will transmit a shunt from aorta to pulmonary artery.

For angiocardiographic demonstration of these defects, the injection of contrast medium should preferably be made into the chamber *from* which the shunt emerges. The serial radiographs will then demonstrate opacification of the chamber receiving the shunt. In atrial septal defect therefore, it is advisable to inject the contrast medium into the *left* atrium and to detect the shunt arriving into the right atrium (Fig. 44).

If it is not possible to place the catheter tip in the chamber from which the shunt emerges, then the diagnosis may often be established by opacifying the left heart chambers from a pulmonary artery injection. This injection of contrast medium into the pulmonary artery will result, after 3 to 5 s, in opacification of the left atrium, followed rapidly by opacification of left ventricle and aorta. If there is a left to right shunt, then a right heart chamber will become opacified during left heart visualization.

Opacification of the right atrium (from A.S.D.) is best recognized in the A.P. projection: opacification of the right ventricle (from V.S.D.) is best seen in the lateral or L.A.O. radiographs: opacification of the pulmonary artery (from P.D.A.) is best assessed on the A.P. films. It is important to recognize the *most proximal* opacified right heart chamber, for this receives the shunt of contrast medium and identifies the site of the most proximal defect.

It must be emphasized that this 'follow through' technique will not detect the distal shunt if more than one shunt is present (pp. 136, 163).

Shunt detection is best demonstrated by cine-angiocardiography, the dynamics of which permit detection of very small shunts. For many years however, before adequate cine was available to us, large film format examinations proved very useful in shunt demonstration.

RIGHT TO LEFT FLOW

This direction of flow may occur when an *obstruction* in the right heart is present, distal to the *septal defect*. The septal defect may be at atrial, ventricular or ductal level; the obstruction may be at the outflow of the right atrium, right ventricle or in the pulmonary artery or arterioles (e.g. Eisenmenger Reaction). The obstruction must be *distal* to the abnormal communication and must be sufficiently severe to cause the pulmonary vascular pressures to equal or exceed those in the corresponding left chambers.

If these criteria are satisfied, then de-oxygenated blood will be passed from the right heart chambers into the left, without previous passage through the lungs: this will result in central cyanosis. For purposes of angiocardiography, the contrast medium must be injected into the right heart, preferably into the chamber from which the shunt emerges, e.g. into the right ventricle in Fallot's tetralogy. If this is not possible, then the contrast medium should be injected into the chamber immediately proximal to that from which the shunt emerges (e.g. into the right atrium in Fallot's tetralogy). This latter injection site may not be very satisfactory and every effort must be made to place the angiocardiographic injection into the right ventricle.

Whenever central cyanosis is present in congenital heart disease, there must be at least two abnormalities (1) a right to left shunt and (2) an obstructive lesion in the right side of the circulation distal to the site of the shunt. Angiocardiographic diagnosis is incomplete unless these two essential features are identified. The only important exceptions are in uncorrected transposition of the great vessels (in which venous blood passes directly from the right ventricle to the aorta without an obstructive lesion being present), total anomalous pulmonary venous drainage and a common chamber (atrium, A.-V. canal or ventricle) when mixing of arterial and venous blood occurs without an obstructing lesion.

In every patient with cyanotic congenital heart disease, at least two malformations are present (in transposition there must be a septal defect or P.D.A. in addition to the transposed great vessels). It is the objective of the cardiac catheterization including angiocardiography to detect these multiple abnormalities and to demonstrate the disturbed haemodynamics resulting therefrom.

Because of the complicated nature of the defects in cyanotic congenital heart disease, bi-plane full-sized angiocardiography has been preferable to cine-recording as it provided greater anatomical detail.

Modern bi-plane cine equipment provides much greater information about the dynamics of the circulation, and when used in conjunction with miniature films (70 or 100 mm), it provides a more satisfactory angiocardiographic study than full-sized angiocardiography alone. The capital cost is significantly greater but the film cost is much less.

Principal right heart obstructions (non-valvar)

VENTRICULAR

The great majority of obstructive lesions in the heart are at valve level. Stenosis, congenital or acquired, may affect any of the four heart valves and the principles of their angiographic demonstration have already been discussed (p. 64).

Obstructive lesions may also occur at sites other than valves. Stenosis of the outflow of the right ventricle involving the subvalvar region (or infundibulum) is by far the most frequent of these lesions and is often seen in congenital heart disease particularly of the cyanotic type.

Pulmonary infundibular stenosis may be dynamic and muscular, or fixed and fibrotic. The former type has already been mentioned (p. 64 and Fig. 57c) and usually results from an embarrassing muscular hypertrophy of the right ventricle which has developed in order to overcome pulmonary valvar stenosis. The degree of obstruction varies enormously with the muscular activity of the ventricle particularly in association with V.S.D. The infundibulum may be of full normal calibre in ventricular diastole but may be so reduced as to cause almost complete obstruction in ventricular systole (Figs. 57B and C). In order to demonstrate the dynamic nature of this variable systolic obstruction, radiographs should be taken rapidly during the angiography—either 5 or 6 per s on full-sized or miniature (70 or 100 mm) films or preferably by cine-recording.

The lateral projection is the most valuable as the right ventricular outflow is not obscured in this view by bony or soft tissue opacities. The A.P. projection is considerably less valuable as the area in question is very frequently seen almost end-on and not tangentially. The catheter tip should be placed low in the right ventricle towards its apex and the injection of contrast medium should opacify the entire right ventricular cavity. If the catheter tip is sited in the right ventricular outflow, it may irritate the muscle to spasm, and cause a spurious muscular obstruction which will confuse the angiographic interpretation.

The fixed fibrotic type of pulmonary infundibular obstruction is most frequently found in Fallot's tetralogy (Fig. 63) and is due to a marked fibrotic thickening of the outflow tract which becomes reduced to a very narrow track, often irregular in both direction and calibre. The narrowing of the outflow persists throughout ventricular systole and diastole unlike the variable stenosis of muscular hypertrophy. Fibrotic obstruction of the right ventricular outflow is commonly combined with pulmonary valvar stenosis particularly in Fallot's tetralogy, but isolated subvalvar obstruction may occur (Fig. 60).

The angiocardiographic technique is the same as for the demonstration of mobile muscular infundibular obstruction. It is important to appreciate however, that the fibrotic variety of infundibular obstruction is almost always associated with ventricular septal defects, most frequently of the Fallot type.

Progressive obstruction of the outflow of the right ventricle may develop during the first few years in a child with a V.S.D. and an initial left to right shunt. During these few years, the shunt may be either R→L or L→R; it is important to inject contrast medium into the left ventricle if a shunt has not been previously demonstrated on a right ventricular injection. Unless this is done, a V.S.D. may be missed and an isolated right infundibular stenosis could be incorrectly inferred if only a right ventricular injection is made.

PULMONARY ARTERY

Obstruction of the pulmonary artery may be caused by progressive pulmonary arteriolar obstruction (Eisenmenger Reaction), by thromboembolic disease, or by strictures involving the pulmonary arterial wall.

The *Eisenmenger Reaction* is an important concept in congenital heart disease. It is the name commonly applied to a condition in which the peripheral pulmonary arteriolar resistance increases to such a degree that the pulmonary arterial pressure rises to equal or to exceed the aortic pressure. When this occurs, any shunt between the two sides of the circulation will become bidirectional, or right to left with resultant central cyanosis.

The criteria for the development of the Eisenmenger Reaction are not well understood but it is generally believed that a large left to right shunt at any level may eventually so damage the pulmonary arteriolar bed that progressive obstructive changes develop within it. If the shunt is at atrial level (and pressure), the Eisenmenger Reaction occurs infrequently and is usually deferred to the third or fourth decade. If the shunt occurs at ventricular pressure (V.S.D. or P.D.A.), the Eisenmenger Reaction occurs more frequently and earlier. Indeed, it is already well established in many infants with V.S.D. or P.D.A. who are investigated within the first few days or weeks of birth for intractable cyanotic heart failure.

The circulation through the peripheral pulmonary arterial tree of the foetus is very small because the foetal lungs are non-functional. The haemodynamic state of the foetus is similar to that of the Eisenmenger Reaction with high pulmonary arteriolar resistance, a pulmonary arterial pressure that exceeds aortic pressure and a right to left shunt through the patent ductus (and foramen ovale).

It is essential to appreciate this concept if the cardiac

catheterization and angiocardiography are to be adequately planned and conducted. The presence of the Eisenmenger Reaction is detected by finding a pulmonary artery pressure equal to or greater than aortic pressure. The angiographic appearances of the pulmonary arterial tree in the Eisenmenger Reaction are often diagnostic as the peripheral pulmonary arteries are tortuous and taper abruptly to become smaller than normal. The main pulmonary arteries are enlarged and there is therefore a considerable discrepancy in size between the dilated central and mid pulmonary arteries and their narrow, pruned tortuous peripheral branches (Fig. 67).

These changes can be well demonstrated on antero-posterior full-sized or miniature (70 or 100 mm) angiograms with the contrast medium injected directly into the main pulmonary artery or right ventricle. The site of the right to left shunt may be demonstrated and therefore bi-plane films are advisable. If the right to left shunt is not identified by the first injection, it probably indicates that the septal defect is situated proximal to the injection site. The proximal right heart chambers are then explored by the catheter and possibly by a further angiocardiographic injection.

One of the main risks of angiocardiography is that deterioration may occur in patients with the Eisenmenger Reaction. It is likely that the contrast medium reduces pulmonary blood flow (probably by causing erythrocyte aggregation) and increases the already high pulmonary peripheral arterial resistance (pp. 61 and 145). Because of this, right sided angiocardiography is not recommended as a routine procedure in patients in whom a very high pulmonary arterial pressure is found at catheterization.

Coronary angiography

Coronary angiograms may be satisfactorily recorded either on cine or full-size films or miniature photofluorograms (70, 100 or 105 mm). Cine does not provide as good detail on each frame as do the other modes (and therefore cine frames are not ideal for photographic reproduction). Cine has the great advantage of providing dynamic studies of the rapidly moving coronary arterial branches as they criss-cross each other, and loop and twist during the cardiac cycle. It is also much easier to obtain multiple projections for each coronary artery when one is recording on cine rather than on full-size films.

The great majority of investigators therefore prefer cine-recording for selective coronary angiography, but may supplement the cine with either full-size radiographs or miniature photofluorograms.

It is important to use the magnification mode of the image intensifier in order to obtain greater detail: this will probably involve panning by moving the floating table top. The procedure should be completed as rapidly as possible with the catheter in the coronary artery for the minimum duration, and this objective is best achieved

either with a U-arm or a motorized rotating cradle (Chapter 6).

In all angiographic procedures, the contrast medium may sink to the dependent aspect of the vessel or chamber to form a 'layer', so that a vertical X-ray beam may not accurately depict the lumen of the vessel. This problem can be reduced by using a horizontal beam which will demonstrate the 'face' between the opacified and the unopacified blood within the vessel.

Myocardial function

It is essential to obtain dynamic studies provided by either cine-angiocardiography or video-tape in order to assess myocardial contractility. Films exposed at slower speeds such as the 6 or 12 per s full-size or photofluorograms are quite inadequate for this purpose.

It is important to include the whole of the ventricular chamber on the cine-recording. If the chamber is enlarged or if the intensifier is small (5 or 6 in), then 'panning' may well be required. The most frequently utilized projection for left ventricular cine-angiography is the right anterior oblique, but an additional cranio-caudal tilt may be advisable in order to reduce the fore-shortening of the left ventricle, particularly when the heart is horizontally positioned as in the sthenic individual. Two or more views may well be necessary.

With good quality cine-recording and the use of additional projections, it is possible to identify abnormalities of myocardial contractility, either generalized, resulting in a poor ejection fraction and a large end-systolic volume, or localized with zones of dyskinesia or paradoxical pulsation. Confident distinction of these latter may be very difficult.

Full-size or miniature radiographs taken at slow frequency (6 or 12 per s) do *not* permit dynamic assessment of myocardial function and it is not possible to identify full systole or diastole with the confidence that can be achieved with the dynamic recording of cine. Extrasystoles are difficult or impossible to identify by radiology unless cine recording or video-tape is available.

Summary

It is evident that in order to conduct a satisfactory angiocardiographic examination, the operator must have a sound appreciation of haemodynamic principles and of the specific situation in the particular patient being investigated. He must plan the catheterization so as to obtain the maximum information from all the different techniques at his disposal—oximetry, pressure mensuration, dye dilution, contrast medium angiocardiography. All these methods are complementary, each supplementing the others in order to build a comprehensive picture of the cardiac anatomy and haemodynamics. Each technique achieves a varying degree of importance depending on the particular clinical problem being investigated—the objective is to blend together and integrate these different technical methods to produce maximal information.

In some patients, the initial (e.g. right) cardiac catheterization may have to be supplemented by a second (e.g. left) catheterization, either performed at the same or a subsequent session. The two catheterization procedures are then planned and co-ordinated to be complementary one to the other, so that a detailed picture of the cardiac anatomy and function is secured.

No two cardiac investigation units are identical in equipment, personnel, experience or the patients whom it is necessary to investigate. Each unit will develop some diagnostic techniques more than other methods: the more practised techniques become more reliable and productive. The investigation methods described here are based on personal experience of about 10,000 selective angiocardiograms and 15,000 cardiac catheterizations performed at the Sheffield Cardio-Vascular Centre. In this centre, bi-plane large film selective angiocardiography has proved extremely reliable for congenital heart disease and has been developed to a greater extent than some of the other methods. In the last few years however, there has been a major development in radiological equipment for cine-angiography and miniature (70 or 100 mm) record-ing. There is no doubt that cine is the method of choice for demonstrating valve incompetence and shunts, and the dynamics of myocardial contraction. Miniature film recording together with cine-angiocardiography will probably largely replace the full-size format. This prediction is being taken into account in the new equipment being installed in our laboratory.

The most satisfactory method of evaluating the differing methods of various cardiac investigation units is to visit them, and preferably to work in them. Only by prolonged direct observation at several diagnostic centres, will it be possible to assess the values of the different techniques and equipment with specific reference to the group of patients being referred to one's own department.

References

EDWARDS, J. E., CAREY, L. S., NEUFELD, H. N. & LESTER, R. G. (1965). *Congenital Heart Disease*, Philadelphia & London: Saunders, Vol. II.

GASUL, B. M., ARCILLA, R. A. & LEV, M. (1966). *Heart Disease in Children*. Philadelphia & Montreal: Lippincott.

KJELLBERG, S. R., MANNHEIMER, E. , RUDHE, U. & JONSSON, B. *Diagnosis of Congenital Heart Disease*, 2nd ed. Chicago: Year Book, 1959.

ROWE, R. D., VLAD, P. & KEITH, J. D. (1956). *Selective angiocardiography in infancy and children, Radiology* **66,** 344.

8. Cardiac Catheters

Cardiac catheterization as a commonly practised diagnostic technique dates from about 1945, although it was in use for a few years before that as a physiological method. The early catheters were standard ureteric catheters, measured traditionally in French gauge. This method of measurement has persisted, being still in use today. The United States Catheter Corporation (U.S.C.I.) has introduced a colour code for the sizes up to 8F. This gives the operator a rapid method of identifying catheters. French gauge is converted to millimetres (O.D.) by dividing by three, so the catheters and their sizes are:

French gauge	Colour of band	Size mm (O.D.)
4	red	1·3
5	silver	1·7
6	green	2·0
7	yellow	2·3
8	blue	2·7
9	none or black	3·0
10	none	3·3
11	none	3·6
12	none	4·0

Other methods of measurement are applied to certain products. The thin walled tubing made by Kifa-Odman in Sweden is made in four sizes distinguished by colouring the plastic from which the various sizes are made. These are described on page 73. Many other types of plastic tubing are described in millimetres for internal diameter (I.D.) and external diameter (O.D.—'O' for overall or outside).

Stainless steel tubing is often described in a numbered gauge, usually S.W.G. or standard wire gauge; sometimes, however, the gauge used is a different needle gauge. A slotted steel plate giving the gauges is obtainable but a better guide is a micrometer. In most cases the needles are supplied for a particular purpose and should be carefully reserved for this. Confusion is worse confounded by the (engineering) practice of giving the diameters of wires in thousandths of inches, or as decimals of an inch. Thus, the Ross needle is measured in inches for length, and in needle gauge for its external diameter. The catheter through which it is passed is measured in centimetres for length and French gauge for diameter. The Seldinger wire passed through the needle is measured in centimetres for length, but in inches for diameter, e.g. 0·035 indicates a wire of 35 thousandths ('thou') diameter. Most wire incidentally is slightly oval in section, a truly circular section being a rare phenomenon.

The tubing from which catheters are made may be radio-opaque or radio-transparent. Most fabricated catheters are radio-opaque to a varying extent, and are supplied with a metal hub which has a Luer-lok female fitting so that it can be securely attached to a Luer male nozzle. A variety of fittings are available for making connections to plastic tubing, and taps, junctions etc. are produced in metal and plastic by a number of manufacturers. In all of these, the size of the hole drilled through the fitting tends to be smaller than the catheter bore, so in diagnostic work the number of junctions should be kept to a minimum particularly in angiography when constrictions due to junctions reduce the rate of injection.

The following catheters are useful for particular purposes in venous catheterization.

Cournand catheter

This is the original ureteric type catheter with the addition of a bend of about 45° placed some 5 cm from the tip. It is used for routine work and for wedge pressure measurement. In many cases the balloon catheter provides an easier way of getting a reliable wedge measurement (Batson et al., 1972). It is easily seen on fluoroscopy as the wall is thick and radio-opaque. Its main disadvantage is that it is not suitable for angiography (p. 70). Many Cournand catheters are made with an inner surface which is a woven tube of plastic filament. This has many crevices and makes a clean injection of tracer substances difficult if the tracer is washed in. If tracer techniques are in regular use, the teflon type of Cournand catheter is the most suitable, but it is a little more difficult to control than those made with a woven lining, as a rotation applied at the operator's end of the catheter may be absorbed in the flexible wall. In other words, it transmits torque less efficiently. The 125 cm length in sizes 6F to 8F is most generally useful. Most manufacturers provide catheters with a steel mesh incorporated in the wall. These have excellent torque but their narrow bore makes a rapid injection through them difficult.

Alternatives to the Cournand catheter are the *Goodale-*

Lubin and the *Lehman* catheters. The Goodale-Lubin catheter has two lateral holes close to the open tip which makes its use in wedge pressure measurement unreliable, although it is less easily blocked by the endocardium. The Lehman catheter has a nicely curved end but is thin walled making it difficult to see during fluoroscopy, and is easy to kink. These catheters have not been used in this unit since an initial trial some years ago.

Catheters for selective angiography

Selective angiography demands a catheter which will not recoil, particularly when the right heart is being investigated. In the right heart, only those injections of contrast medium made into the right atrium are free of the tendency for the catheter to spring back from the injection site to the chamber proximal to that which the injection is intended to delineate. This recoil tendency is less when injections are made into the left heart by way of the aorta or by left atrial puncture. No catheter is entirely free of a risk of movement when a pressure injection is made through it, but a catheter with a blocked end and open side holes is much more satisfactory than an open ended one. Movement in a blocked end catheter in which there are side holes close to the tip is due mainly to the pressure of the injection causing the catheter to straighten. In a wide bore, open ended catheter there is a violent recoil and a real risk of perforating the heart. The Lehman and Goodale-Lubin catheters are therefore not suitable for pressurized selective injections of contrast media.

A series of blocked end catheters is available. Although most were developed originally for arteriography before the Seldinger technique became widely practised, today they are used almost exclusively for *right* heart angiography. The most convenient is the *Eppendorf* which is made with a radio-opaque plug at the distal end. This plug is easily visible on fluoroscopy and offsets the poor visibility of the catheter wall which is necessarily thin in order to allow as wide a bore as possible for contrast medium injections. It is, however, currently available only in sizes 6F to 8F. These are not large enough for work in adult patients. The most generally useful catheter is the *N.I.H. catheter*, sizes available (1976) being 5F to 10F. This catheter is about two-thirds the price of the Eppendorf catheter. In this unit, the N.I.H. catheter is used routinely for all venous catheterizations in patients suffering from congenital heart disease. In adults, catheters 100 cm long are used. In children 80 cm is a better length. Cordis catheters are cheaper, but of narrower bore than the corresponding U.S.C.I. catheters, giving a slower injection rate.

The pig-tail catheter, although primarily intended for ventriculography is sometimes useful for reaching difficult sites from which angiography is required.

Percutaneous catheterization of the right side of the heart is mainly used in the investigation of rheumatic heart disease. The measurement of right heart pressures and the estimation of cardiac output supplement the information which is obtained by transseptal catheterization of the left atrium and ventricle undertaken at the same investigation through the same venous puncture. For this purpose the *Gensini* percutaneous catheter is useful if it is necessary to reach the pulmonary artery. It may be used for angiography in adults but needs a tip occluder. The multiple side holes make it unsuitable for wedge pressure measurement (but this measurement is unnecessary if the left atrial puncture succeeds). Percutaneous introducers for blocked end catheters are available (e.g. those made by Vigon).

For transseptal catheterization, the *Brockenborough* teflon catheter is used, both adult and child sizes being in regular use. The high cost of these simple catheters is to some extent offset by their long life. As a satisfactory catheter can be made for about a fraction of the cost of the commercial article, however, many centres fabricate these catheters which are essentially similar to those used for aortography and left heart studies (p. 73).

Platinum electrode catheters are used for tracer techniques with hydrogen or ascorbic acid, and are convenient instruments for recording the intracardiac electrocardiogram. They are narrow bore catheters of the Cournand type, with the addition of one or more platinum rings which encircle the tip of the catheter, additional rings being placed 10 cm, or 6 and 16 cm proximal to the tip in the two and three electrode types respectively. They are *not* suitable for angiocardiography because of their narrow bore. Percutaneous insertion is possible with the *Brancato* type of platinum electrode catheter, but these catheters are used primarily in shunt detection on the right side of the heart, where the need for a large bore catheter with a blocked end for angiography usually involves a surgical cut down. The percutaneous electrode catheter, therefore, has a very limited usefulness.

Balloon catheters, until recently, were primarily used for research. For this purpose the Dotter-Lukas triple lumen catheter is the most versatile. It is of 9F size with a balloon which can be inflated, situated between two orifices. It has therefore three lumens, one to each hole and one to the balloon. The balloon should always be inflated with a low viscosity radio-opaque liquid, and if blown up in a blood vessel (e.g. the pulmonary artery) it should not be advanced or withdrawn before being completely deflated. The manipulation in an artery of a partly inflated balloon may cause the distal tip to become invaginated into the latex sheet of the balloon. If this happens, it is difficult to persuade the balloon to empty.

A very useful balloon catheter with a double lumen designed to float through the right side of the heart to the pulmonary artery has been devised. This is the Swan-Ganz catheter, made by the Edwards company. Similar catheters are now made by several manufacturers. One lumen provides inflation of the balloon, the other pressure recording. Its use is described on page 93.

A therapeutic balloon catheter technique is also in general use. The *Rashkind* septostomy balloon catheter is used to create an atrial septal defect in infants suffering from transposition of the great vessels. The double lumen type is the easiest to use as the distal orifice can be used to confirm the site of the catheter in the left atrium by blood sampling and pressure measurement. Its diameter of 6·5F, however, makes it a big catheter for an ill, premature infant (p. 77 and Fig. 19).

Coronary arteriography may be undertaken by a variety of catheters. Radio-opaque catheters are essential. In general it is easier to make use of catheters specifically designed for the investigation. The most widely used are the Sones catheter (U.S.C.I.) or the Judkins catheter (Cordis). Both are suitable for percutaneous insertion over a guide wire. We have found the Judkins catheter easier to use (Chapter 13). The Bourassa catheters (Vygon) are not unlike the Judkins type.

Selective arteriography is being increasingly practised to demonstrate individual vessels in the abdomen, thorax, or limbs. A radio-opaque end-hole catheter is needed for this technique, and as hand injections of contrast medium are usual, recoil is not a problem. Seldinger introduction is usual. Most investigations can be done using red, green or yellow Kifa tubing giving a terminal bend to suit the operator. There is also a wide range of catheters designed for this investigation made by Cordis, Cook, Vygon and Surgimed.

Controllable tip catheters of several makes are available. We have found them of limited usefulness, possibly because of insufficient practice. The chief disadvantage has been a tendency for the catheter to become displaced when the controlling guide wire is drawn back. They are also expensive to operate. Some colleagues, however, find them invaluable especially in catheterizing infants with complex congenital anomalies.

Finally, there is the intracardiac pressure head and phonocardiograph. This consists of a very small transducer mounted on the extremity of the catheter. It is capable, with suitable electrical filtering, of recording both sound and pressure waves. The catheter is provided with a lumen so that blood samples can be taken. It is possible to record sounds generated within the heart and determine their origin. The pressure records are free of artefacts which may distort recordings made in the conventional way with a transducer connected to the end of a liquid filled catheter. The catheter is not suitable for angiocardiography. It provides, however, the best method of pressure measurement when the rate of change in pressure (dp/dt) is determined.

Care of catheters

Cardiac catheters are a potential cause of infection to the patients investigated. In addition, the bore of many types of catheter is a mesh of woven filaments in which particles of clotted blood and plasma may adhere so that foreign protein reactions may occur. Their cost may preclude single use. Cleaning is therefore very important: storage is a matter of widely differing practice.

Cleaning must begin as soon as the catheter is removed at the end of an investigation. It should immediately be washed out with 20 to 40 ml tap water. Ten per cent hydrogen peroxide is then run through the catheter for one hour, followed by tap water for 24 hours. Distilled water is then run through for one hour and the catheter is then allowed to drain vertically for some hours. Since adopting this cleansing routine, reactions due to foreign protein in the catheter have been rare.

Catheters in regular use are sterilized after cleaning by autoclaving in paper packs which permit sterilization of the catheter straight, not coiled. The catheters may be enclosed in a length of slit rubber tubing which preserves their shape and protects them from damage in the C.S.S.D. where they are at risk when softened by heat.

Catheters in occasional use are stored in air, either hanging straight in bundles or packed coiled in polythene bags in boxes. When a catheterization is planned, the catheters likely to be needed are placed in hibitane solution or some suitable liquid disinfectant, each catheter being filled by syringe as it is inserted to make sure that the lumen fills completely. Plastic container tubes about 1·3 m long and 6 cm bore, closed with a rubber bung, are suitable for this immersion, which should last 30 minutes. An unexpectedly needed catheter can be immersed for 5 minutes in an alcoholic solution of hibitane. Catheters stored in liquid for more than a few hours get too soft. Sterilization with formaldehyde makes the catheter wall brittle and dangerously liable to crack. Autoclaving or gas sterilization are possible but require a large and expensive stock of catheters; it is difficult to sterilize by these methods except by coiling the catheters up. A catheter which has been stored in a coil can be peculiarly difficult to manipulate, particularly when introduced from the leg. It must be recognized, however, that the liquid sterilization recommended here is not as safe as heat sterilization by the autoclave. It is safe only in combination with the thorough cleaning technique and storage in a room in a clean area remote from contact with the wards or other sources of cross infection.

Connections and taps for the tubing and catheters used in cardiac investigation should have the qualities of those used to draw off beer—all holes drilled for the passage of fluid should have the same diameter as the tubing, the taps and junctions should not leak, and the taps should have a long working life. Unfortunately, to provide a leak-tight joint in a tap on tubing having a bore of 2 mm (the inside diameter of thin wall 9F tubing) requires large surfaces, and such a tap would be bulkier than most operators would tolerate. Fortunately, the bore is not critical for pressure measurement where the actual movement of fluid is minute, so the problem is one which primarily affects angiocardiography where the rate of injection is of first importance. The only practicable solution is to use as few junctions as possible in angiocardiography, for example, connecting the catheter directly to the injection apparatus whenever possible, and by drilling out all connectors and taps used to as large a bore as possible, consistent with their continued function. Most connectors and simple taps can be enlarged to 2 mm bore without rendering them inefficient. No 3-way tap known to the author can be treated in this fashion, but this is not important as 3-way taps are not needed in the connections for angiocardiography.

Equipment for the Seldinger technique

Needles of several types are available for the Seldinger technique. The original needle is made in two sizes, a 205 size fitting a guide wire of diameter 0·045 in (1·14 mm) and 160 fitting a wire 0·035 in (0·89 mm). The large needle and wire are rarely necessary and for arterial work should be avoided if possible as complications are more common when they are used. The smaller needle that fits a 0·035 in wire is preferable for angiography, and all sizes of catheter can be tapered to fit this diameter wire. Vessels which are surrounded by much scarring as, for example, that resulting from previous venotomy or arteriotomy are an important exception. In these, the thinner guide wire may be too flexible to enable a catheter to be pushed through into the vessel. Here the 0·045-in needle and wire are preferable.

The original *Seldinger needle* consists of an outer thin walled blunt cannula fitting closely over an inner needle which is in turn plugged with a stilette. It is essential that the cannula fits the needle snugly with a minimum of 'shoulder' where the cannula ends on the needle. Sharpening these needles (when blunt) is a skilled job as the bevel must not be ground down to lie within the cannula. If this happens the cannula must be shortened. This is work for a skilled instrument maker, and where this service is not available, a simpler needle may be used. Such a needle is the *Sutton needle* which is simply a sharp needle (without cannula) with a bore just large enough to accommodate the wire. A similar needle with a stylet is preferable. In using needles with no stylet,

there is some risk of cutting a core of tissue and so plugging the needle if the cutting point is inexpertly ground. We prefer the Seldinger needle for most purposes, as it is easier to thread the cannula up the vessel.

The *Cournand needle* resembles the Seldinger needle but the outer cannula has a blunt bevel at its tip which follows the bevel of the sharp inner needle. The cannula is therefore a blunt atraumatic needle. This is easier to introduce into the vessel than the Seldinger needle but more difficult to sharpen satisfactorily. For small vessels in children and infants, the paediatric Cournand needle is the most satisfactory, using a 0·024-in guide wire.

Other types of needle are available. A disposable *polythene cannula* with an inner needle may be used. Many types are available, for example those of Portex (Plextrocan), Braun, (Braunula), Vygon (Arterioflex) or Bardic (Angiocath). The Portex is the softest and is readily threaded up a vein once the needle is withdrawn. The Guest needle (Avon) is particularly suited to the arm. The Vigon cannula is supplied in a sterile pack with a 5F pacing catheter and is very useful for emergency pacing but the cannula, although plastic, has a hard sharp edge and can perforate thin veins. All are thicker than a metal cannula and more difficult to insert.

Guide wires were originally guitar strings, and the usual type are made on the machinery used to make strings for steel stringed guitars. They consist of a central core of straight wire, around which is wound a finely coiled spring. The tip of the coil is sealed with solder and the core usually terminates 5 cm from the end of the coil at one end, leaving a soft flexible tip, but at the other end it is continued into the solder and so anchored. In another type of guide wire the core protrudes from the coil at the operator end and can be moved to and fro inside it, so varying the length of the flexible tip at the other end. The surface of these guide wires is a series of arcs formed by the successive coils of wire of circular section. By using a coil of flattened wire for the winding, the surface is formed by flat sections and a smoother wire is formed. The guide wires may be coated by a very thin film of teflon which considerably reduces friction with the catheter. This is very useful when using polyurethane catheters which tend to bind on to the wire. The coating tends to be slightly uneven and increases the diameter of the wire to 0·036 in. or even more. This may be too large for some introducing cannulae. It is particularly important to check the wire by passing it through the cannula before attempting a Seldinger introduction

The diameter of the guide wires and cannulae is a source of a minor confusion. Three methods of expressing the sizes are in common use. In Britain and North America the diameter is usually given in thousandths of inches ('thou'). In Europe millimetres are normally used. A third nomenclature is the 'P.E.' number. This refers to a practice, now abandoned, of drawing out different sizes of polyethylene tubing to different tip diameters. The number identified the external diameter of the plastic tube, not the guide wire size. Guide wires over 0·035 in are now rarely used and all P.E. tubing is usually drawn to a tip which fits the 0·035 in wire. This results in the apparently paradoxical situation that polythene catheters of sizes P.E. 160, P.E. 205, P.E. 240 and P.E. 280 all fit the 'P.E. 160' wire. The sizes are tabulated below:

DIAMETER OF WIRE

mm	in	P.E. No.
0·610	0·024	60
0·889	0·035	160
1·194	0·047	205
1·321	0·052	240

In choosing guide wires, the primary considerations are their rigidity, malleability and smoothness. Only extensive practice with different types will give the practitioner the 'feel' of the various models (much as experience gives the feel of a fishing rod). The rigidity is primarily a function of the *core* wire, particularly its diameter and hardness. It is also related to the initial tension of the spring which determines the softness of the tip of the wire where the core is absent. If a guide wire will not tolerate an acute bending to less than a right angle and subsequent straightening, it is not sufficiently malleable to be safely used for any manoeuvre more complex than the simple introduction of a catheter. The flat wound wires are smoother and therefore more easily passed down long catheters. They were originally developed for passage through the Ross needle which is 24 in (62 cm) long. Guide wires with a sliding core and a J-shaped tip are very useful for negotiating tortuous vessels. The wire is introduced straight, the centre wire is withdrawn a few centimetres in order to form the J, and the smooth, non-traumatic curve of the J becomes the leading segment and will traverse most tortuous vessels.

One danger in using a coiled spring wire is that the coil may fracture, usually 5 cm from the tip—where the central core terminates. This accident results in the end of the coil being left in the punctured vessel. Most wires are now constructed with a second (safety) fine wire running within the entire length of the coil and soldered to both of its ends.

An alternative to the spring coil wire is one in which the *steel core* is covered with a *plastic sheath*. Again there is a terminal flexible 5 cm tip with no core. These wires are very flexible and are very useful for negotiating particularly tortuous arteries or 'difficult' aortic valves. If a catheter introduced on a spring guide cannot be manoeuvred past a tortuosity, it may be possible to negotiate it by replacing the spring guide wire by a flimsy plastic one. The catheter should be withdrawn a few centimetres, the plastic-covered guide wire inserted with the flimsy end first and gentle manipulation may pass the section which has proved impassable by catheter or the original wire. Plastic-coated wires without a coil spring are not suitable for introducing a catheter through tougher than usual skin because they are not sufficiently rigid. Another possible disadvantage is that a sliver of plastic may be scraped off by the needle and be left in the subcutaneous tissue or artery. Coiled spring safety-wires with adjustable core and J-tip will usually negotiate even very tortuous vessels.

For an adult of normal size, a 120 cm guide wire and a 100 cm catheter are suitable for a left ventricular catheterization or a right sided investigation intended to reach the pulmonary artery from the groin. If wedge pressures are to be measured, a longer catheter of 120 cm is needed in an adult to be sure of reaching the pulmonary capillaries. Longer wires (up to 200 cm) are then needed and they are useful for changing catheters (p. 81). The guide wires made with a flat wire coil are particularly suitable for this purpose.

With careful cleaning it is possible to use guide wires several times. The risks of accident, however, are such that single use is recommended. An official directive to this effect has been issued.

Catheters for Seldinger technique

The original *Kifa-Odman* radio-opaque catheters were manufactured in three sizes—red (internal diameter = 1·2 mm; external diameter = 2·2 mm), green (internal diameter = 1·2 mm: external diameter = 2·6 mm); yellow (internal diameter = 1·55 mm: external diameter = 2·8 mm). A few years later a grey, radio-opaque catheter (internal diameter = 1·8 mm: external diameter = 2·8 mm) was introduced. For cardiac catheterization in the adult, the grey Kifa-Odman catheter is the most satisfactory as it permits a greater rate of contrast medium injection. The grey catheter, however, is less controllable than the yellow catheter which has a thicker wall (but the same O.D.) and has therefore more torque and can be more easily rotated within the vessels. A yellow Kifa-Odman catheter may therefore be preferred in some situations because of this increased control. The grey Kifa-Odman catheter is of satisfactory design and its easy visibility during fluoroscopy is very helpful, but in the author's (R. G. G.) experience, femoral artery thrombosis has been more frequent with these catheters than with a non radio-opaque polythene catheter of comparable size. This is probably because of the rougher outer surface of the Kifa-Odman catheter.

Non radio-opaque polythene tubing can be used for cardiac catheterization and we prefer sizes P.E. 280 (I.D. = 2·0 mm: O.D. = 3·0 mm) or P.E. 240 (I.D. = 1·67 mm: O.D. = 2·42 mm) for the adult, and sizes 205 (I.D. = 1·57 mm: O.D. = 2·08 mm) and 160 (I.D. = 1·14 mm; O.D. = 1·57 mm) for small children. This type of polythene catheter is cheap and is discarded after use.

All sizes are easily tapered to the 160 guide wire (0·035 in) and side holes are readily made by a sharp borer. The smooth outer wall reduces to a minimum the arterial trauma and the risk of arterial thrombosis after the catheterization. The main disadvantage of the non radio-opaque polythene catheters is that they are not visible on the fluoroscopy screen and in order to see the catheter and screen it into position, it must be filled with contrast medium. In the course of complete left ventricular and aortic assessment, several catheter adjustments are necessary and an additional 30 ml of contrast medium may be required merely to visualize the polythene catheter. Modern contrast media have such low toxicity, however, that this extra volume does not constitute an additional hazard.

A particularly useful catheter for left ventriculography is the pig-tail catheter in which the terminal curve is a small circle of tapered catheter, proximal to which are staggered side holes. These catheters have wire braid stiffening their walls. They should be used in conjunction with teflon coated guide wires. As the tip of these catheters is soft, their introduction into the artery should be preceded by the use of a dilator (e.g. a short piece of teflon or Kifa tubing slid along the guide wire).

At the time of writing, we prefer polythene 280 or Judkins (Cordis) polyurethane pig-tail catheters for routine left ventriculography in the adult. A major advantage of the polythene catheters is that they are more flexible and less rigid at the tip than the radio-opaque catheters. The tip of a polythene catheter is less likely to penetrate the endothelium of the left ventricle. Intramural injection of contrast medium is almost unknown with these soft flexible catheters.

Teflon radio-opaque tubing may be used for making left heart catheters and a useful gauge is the U.S.C.I. 7315 8F. This tube has a larger internal diameter than the previously mentioned catheters but it is not as radio-opaque as the grey Kifa-Odman catheter and it is more expensive, more difficult to prepare and especially to taper, more easily kinked and more rigidly tipped (and therefore more hazardous) than the Kifa-Odman or polythene catheters.

All of the above catheters may be purchased as tubing which is cut to the required length and then fashioned into catheters. As mentioned above, the catheters used are almost invariably tapered to fit closely around the 160 (0·035 in) guide wire. The different types of catheter tubing are 'worked' with differing degrees of ease—the most difficult being Teflon. In each case, the taper is prepared by heating the tubing over a spirit lamp to a critical temperature at which softening occurs; the catheter is then carefully pulled out over the previously inserted guide wire. The catheter is then cut by a sharp razor blade at the point where it snugly meets the guide wire. Four side holes are bored by a sharp boring tool (Kifa) within 2 cm of the tip of the catheter, at staggered points on the circumference to prevent weakening the catheter. The syringe end of the catheter is then flanged with a heated tool (Kifa) so that it is firmly held in the appropriately sized catheter tap holder.

The catheters are packed singly into polythene envelopes. The packages are then sterilized by gamma irradiation. A batch of 100 catheters are prepared, packed and sent to a commercial unit for gamma irradiation sterilization, the cost of which is negligible. Individual catheters can be sterilized by immersion in hibitane in spirit, care being taken to fill the lumen of the catheter by syringe. The polythene and Kifa-Odman catheters are used once and then discarded.

Many catheters are manufactured commercially, complete with end hole, side holes, pre-formed curves and a flared end for the connector. A very wide range of such catheters, generally prepared from dacron, teflon, polyurethane or polyethylene is available from specialist medical suppliers. These catheters are expensive. The manufacturers recommend their use for one procedure only.

Soft radiolucent polythene catheters (complete with flange, taper, holes and preformed curve) have become available—prepacked in gamma-ray sterilized envelopes. These catheters are less expensive and therefore readily disposable. They have proved of considerable value in saving time previously spent in making catheters in the X-ray department. Careful quality control is quite essential and must be maintained whether the catheters are prepared commercially or in the department.

The introduction of a catheter over a guide wire is facilitated by preliminary dilatation of the track with a short length of rigid catheter tubing—the *dilator*.

Closed-end catheters may be introduced percutaneously through a *sleeve introducer* (e.g. Vygon) pages 80 and 101. Recent introducers incorporate a valve allowing use of different size catheters.

Connections and Taps

It is essential to make certain that satisfactory and sterile taps, connectors and connecting tubing are readily available to secure connection of the catheter to the injecting pump or pressure transducer.

The connection link must not impose an additional resistance to the injection circuit and therefore large bore polythene (or nylon) tubing is used. All connections should be tested for leaks before being coupled to the catheter—a weak or leaking connection may 'blow' when subjected to the high pressure injection from a pump. This may result in useless radiographic exposure to the patient and waste of perhaps 40 films. All connections should be Luer-Lok. Some taps and connections are delivered with too small a lumen, which imposes an unnecessary constriction on the injection system. All such connections must be carefully examined to prevent this; if necessary they should be exchanged or re-bored by an expert instrument repairer.

References

BATSON, G. A., CHANDRASEKHAR, K. P., PAYAS, Y. & RICKARDS, D. F. (1972). Comparison of pulmonary wedge pressure by the flow directed Swan-Ganz catheter. *Cardiovasc. Res.* **6**, 748.

RASHKIND, W. J. & MILLER, W. W. (1966). Creation of an atrial septal defect without thoracotomy. *J. Am. Med. Ass.* **196**, 991.

Catalogue of catheters supplied by many manufacturers.

References to Chapter 5: Echocardiography

BOM, N., LANCER, C. T., HONKOOP, J. & HUGENHOLTZ, P. G. (1971). Ultrasonic viewer for cross-sectional analysis of moving cardiac structures. *Bio-medical Engineering* **6**, 500.

BROWN, O. R., HARRISON, D. C. & POPP, R. (1974). An improved method for echographic detection of left atrial enlargement. *Circulation* **50**, 58.

EDLER, I. & HERTZ, C. H. (1954). Use of ultrasonic reflectoscope for the continuous recording of movements of heart walls. *Kung. Fysiograf. Sallsk. Lund. Fordhandl.* **24**, 40.

FEIGENBAUM, H., WALDHAUSEN, J. A. & HYDE, L. P. (1965). Ultrasound diagnosis of pericardial effusion. *J. Am. Med. Ass.* **191**, 107.

FEIGENBAUM, H. (1975). Echocardiographic examination of the left ventricle. *Circulation* **51**, 1–7.

FEIGENBAUM, H. (1976). *Echocardiography.* Philadelphia: Lea & Febiger.

FEIZI, O., SYMONS, C. & YACOUB, M. (1974). Echocardiography of the aortic valve. *Br. Heart J.* **36**, 341–351.

FORTUIN, N. J., HOOD, W. P. SHERMAN, M. E. & CRAIG, E. (1971). Determinations of left ventricular volumes by ultrasound. *Circulation* **44**, 575.

GIBSON, D. G. (1971). Measurement of left ventricular volumes in man by echocardiography—comparison with biplane angiographs. *Br. Heart J.* **33**, 614.

GOLDBERG, S. J., ALLEN, H. D. & SAHN, D. J. (1975). *Paediatric and Adolescent Echocardiography,* Chicago Year Book Publishers.

GRAMIAK, R., SHAH, P. M. & KRAMER, D. H. (1969). Ultrasound cardiography: contrast studies in anatomy and function. *Radiology* **92**, 939.

GRAMIAK, R. & SHAH, P. M. (1971). Cardiac ultrasonography. A review of current applications. *Rad. Clin. N. Am.* **9**, 469.

GRIFFITH, J. M. & HENRY, W. L. (1974). A sector-scanner for real-time two dimensional echocardiography. *Circulation* **49**, 1147.

LINHART, J. W., MINTZ, G. S., SEGAL, B. L., KAWAI, N. & KOTLER, M. N. (1975). Left ventricular volume measurement by echocardiography. Fact or fiction? *Am. J. Cardiol.* **36**, 114.

LUDBROOKE, P., KARLINER, J. S., PETERSON, K., LEOPOLD, G. & O'ROURKE, R. A. (1973). Comparison of ultrasound and cineangiographic measurements of left ventricular performance in patients with and without wall motion abnormalities. *Br. Heart J.* **35**, 1026.

MURPHY, K. F., KOTLER, M. N., REICHIK, N. & PERLOFF, J. K. (1975). Ultrasound in the diagnosis of congenital heart disease. *Am. Heart J.* **89**, 638–656.

NICHOL, P. M., GILBERT, B. W. & KISSLO, J. A. (1977). Two-dimensional echocardiographic assessment of mitral stenosis. *Circulation* **55**, 120.

POPP, R. L. & HARRISON, D. C. (1970). Ultrasonic cardiac echography for determining stroke volume and valvular regurgitation. *Circulation* **41**, 493.

QUINONES, M. A., GAZSCH, W. H. & ALEXANDER, J. H. (1974). Echocardiographic assessment of left ventricular function. *Circulation* **50**, 42.

ROELANDT, J., KLOSTER, F. E., TEN CATE, F. J., VAN DORP, W. G., HONKOOP, J., BOM, N. & HURGENHOLTZ, P. G. (1974). Multi-dimensional echocardiography: An appraisal of its clinical usefulness. *Br. Heart J.* **36**, 29–43.

SEWARD, J. B., TAJIK, A. J., HAGLER, D. J. & RITTER, D. G. (1977). Contrast echocardiography in single or common ventricle. *Circulation* **55**, 513.

SIMON, A. L., ROSS, J. & GAULT, J. H. (1967). Angiographic anatomy of the left ventricle and mitral valve in I.H.S.S. *Circulation* **36**, 852.

STEFADOUROS, M. A. & WITHAM, A. C. (1975). Systolic time intervals by echocardiography. *Circulation* **51**, 114.

VALDEZ-CRUZ, L. M., PIERONI, D. R., ROLAND, J. A. & VARGHESE, P. J. (1976). Echocardiographic detection of intracardiac right to left shunts following peripheral vein injections. *Circulation* **55**, 558.

WEYMAN, A. E., DILLON, J. C., FEIGENBAUM, H. & CHANG, S. (1974). Echocardiographic patterns of pulmonary valve motion in valvular pulmonary stenosis. *Am. J. Cardiol.* **34**, 644–651.

WRAY, T. M. (1975). The variable echocardiographic features in aortic valve endocarditis. *Circulation* **52**, 658.

9. Insertion of Cardiac Catheters

Cardiac catheters may be inserted into veins or arteries either by dissecting out the vessel and incising it, or by passing a suitable catheter over a guide wire which has been led into the vessel through a hollow needle. In this chapter the methods of venous dissection are first described, followed by an account of the percutaneous (Seldinger) technique.

Dissection techniques

EXPOSURE OF VEINS

Having chosen the appropriate site for introducing the catheter into the venous system, the skin is inspected.

Upper limb

In the upper limb the *medial cubital vein* is the easiest to use if it is large enough, for it provides the only reasonably good chance of a blind entry into the thorax. The cephalic vein, although frequently larger than the medial cubital, has an unpleasant habit of thinning out near the shoulder and the catheter may stick at this site, or difficulty may be experienced in negotiating the catheter under the clavicle and into the thoracic cavity. If the antecubital vein is too small or is represented by a leash of venules, it may be necessary to try further up.

The brachial vein is approachable at almost any point in its length. The operator should feel for the pulsation of the brachial artery and then make an incision parallel to the artery and overlying it. If the tissues are gently split with a pair of haemostats, the brachial bundle will soon appear and the vein may be selected for catheterization. A larger vein is available in the *axilla* but is rarely required for catheterization. The arm should be abducted, rotated so that the hand lies palm upwards with the forearm parallel with the patient's head. The anterior axillary fold is palpated and the pulsation of the axillary artery identified. An incision is made over the pulsation and blunt dissection performed until the vein is isolated between temporary ligatures. For special purposes the *external jugular vein* may be used but it is generally not desirable as a site of entry for catheterization, partly for cosmetic reasons and partly because there is a slight risk of air entering the vein.

Lower limb

The *long saphenous vein* is best approached by the following technique. The pubic tubercle is first identified

and a point vertically below this in the thigh is noted (if the thigh is slightly externally rotated, the vein will be found on a line joining the pubic tubercle and internal femoral condyle). The distance below the ilio-inguinal ligament depends, to some extent upon the size of the patient; in an average adult it is 5 cm, in an infant as little as $1\frac{1}{2}$ to 2 cm. An incision is made at this point parallel to the inguinal ligament and blunt dissection should reveal the large saphenous vein deep to this point.

The *femoral vein* in infants is approached by a very similar incision made about 0·5 cm below the inguinal ligament. In puny infants under 3 kg an incision in the line of the vein made across the inguinal ligament is easier. In dissecting for the femoral vein, it is usual to find the long saphenous vein near the surface and occasionally it is large enough, even in a 3 kg infant, for a No. 5 or No. 6 catheter. If it is too small, it should be gently retracted. The dissection is carried down until the femoral bundle is exposed and the vessels lying in it are cleared by blunt dissection with the tips of a pair of curved haemostats. It should be noted that in this site the femoral artery is normally the more superficial vessel. The femoral vein lies behind the femoral artery and it is the author's (D.V.) practice to put a loop of plain catgut around the artery, in order gently to retract it, and then to place a double loop of plain catgut round the femoral vein. The lower loop is tied lightly with a single overhand knot and used to support the vein during the insertion of a catheter. If there is a clear indication of a valve (this is common), the vein should be incised just below this and a No. 6 catheter passed up. In occasional puny infants weighing under 3 kg, even a No. 5 catheter can only be introduced with some difficulty, but it is usually possible to perform any diagnostic manipulation including selective angiocardiography through this vein. At the end of this investigation, the vein should be repaired. This can usually be done using a figure-8 stitch to approximate the edges of the hole. If this fails, the upper ligature is lightly tied over the catheter and round the vein, the blood lost is replaced by packed cells and the catheter is withdrawn. The single knot is tied lightly. The femoral vein is thus left with a double ligature above and below the incision, and providing absorbable catgut is used for this procedure, it has been our experience that there are no sequelae. (In infants with a good layer of fat the femoral vein may be left without ligation providing the subcutaneous tissues are carefully approximated by sutures.) The foot of the investigated infant is usually somewhat blue for a day or two but re-catheterization later will reveal that patency of this vein is restored very quickly and no lasting disability occurs. It is possible at the same time to catheterize the femoral artery. If the arterial repair should fail, the vessel may be ligated at this point without danger to the infant's leg. The femoral vein technique described here has only been used on puny infants weighing under 4 kg.

The Rashkind catheter (for the creation of an atrial septal defect in infants suffering from transposition of the great vessels) is often too large to pass into the femoral vein of a small infant when the vein has been exposed in the way described in the preceding paragraph. When transposition seems likely in an infant weighing 4 kg or less, the following exposure is preferable. A vertical incision is made under local anaesthesia in the line of the pulsation of the femoral artery and directly over it. The cut should be about 2 cm long with about 0·75 cm above the inguinal ligament and the remainder of the incision extending into the thigh. The femoral canal is exposed by blunt dissection and the femoral artery identified. The femoral vein is at this level found lying medial to the artery. A double loop of plain catgut is passed under the vein after gently mobilizing it. The ends of the lower loop are passed through a small length of fine plastic tubing and snared to prevent bleeding. A short longitudinal incision is made in the femoral vein and a No. 6 angiographic catheter inserted to enable the diagnosis of transposition to be established. The angiographic catheter is withdrawn and the Rashkind catheter is then inserted. Should either catheter fail to occlude the femoral vein, the upper catgut loop is used to snare the vein over the catheter to stop the leak. At the end of the catheterization, the incision in the vein is repaired with fine 00000 thread on an atraumatic needle by sewing it up transversely. The repair is tested by releasing the upper snare. If leaking is insignificant, the skin is sutured using vertical mattress stitches and light pressure applied if necessary. Veins are much more difficult to repair than arteries as their walls are much thinner, but leaks are easily controlled by external pressure. At this level, ligation of the femoral vein should be avoided as persistent oedema may occur. This approach to the femoral vein should not be undertaken unless there is a clear suggestion from clinical evidence that transposition is present, because the repair is difficult and the incision, which crosses the fascial planes, is unsightly.

Umbilical vein

A further method of venous access, which is occasionally of great value, is the umbilical vein. This can be used in new-born infants up to the 5th or 6th day of life in favourable cases. It is most easily approached by wiping away the withered umbilical stalk and cleaning the scar until the umbilical vein becomes apparent. The umbilical vein should first be explored with a 5F soft polyvinyl umbilical catheter of the type used for exchange transfusions. Having reached the right atrium with this catheter, a right atrial angiocardiogram can be performed. If further investigation is needed, a No. 6 catheter can usually be inserted without difficulty and with a little manipulation the right atrium can be reached. Occasionally, the vein lumen narrows, presumably owing to the physiological thrombosis, and the catheter will only pass for a short distance. In such cases it is best not to try to force the catheter up, since it then usually passes through the vein wall into the peritoneal cavity, where its mobility can be extremely confusing during fluoroscopy. Many satisfactory cardiac catheterizations have been performed through the umbilical vein in small infants.

INSERTION OF CATHETER

Having selected a suitable vein and exposed it, the next problem is the insertion of the catheter. A small V-shaped nick is made in the vein wall with a pair of fine pointed scissors. This can be made to be a reasonably tight fit round the catheter in patients with a large vein, or may have to involve a large part of the circumference of the vein in small infants. It is important not to extend the incision round to include 50 per cent or more of the circumference of the vein, lest the vein wall be so weakened that the vein tears in two during catheterization. In very small veins it is safer to make a short longitudinal incision which does not significantly weaken the vein wall. The hole in the vein being made, the insertion of the catheter may proceed. A wide variety of tools is available for this manoeuvre. A fine pointed pair of curved ophthalmic forceps is commonly used. The points are inserted into the lumen of the vein, gently opened by inserting scissor points between the jaws of the forceps, and pressed laterally to stretch the vein wall. The catheter is then inserted between the tips of the forceps which are subsequently withdrawn. In another technique the vein is lifted by a small hook inserted into the incision in the vein so that the incision is stretched out longitudinally, and the catheter tip inserted gently into this slit.

Another method is the use of a pointed piece of stainless steel tubing (e.g. a needle) ground off so that only half the circumference remains; a suitably trimmed piece of plastic tubing of similar shape may be used. The tube is thus converted to a channel section and is given a blunt point. The vein is picked up by inserting the pointed end of the channel section with the concavity downwards into the lumen through the incision in the vein wall. The catheter is then slipped into the concavity of the channel section and enters the vein easily. It is necessary to have a series of these channel sections made from different gauge tubing to suit the varying sizes of the cardiac catheter.

Arterial cut-down

The exposure of arteries is usually easier than that of veins as the arterial pulsation is a good guide to the site of the vessel. On the rare occasions when a Seldinger approach is inappropriate (usually in infants), the artery is exposed and a catgut loop placed round the vessel to control it should difficulties arise. The insertion technique depends on the size of the artery.

In puny infants a 19 gauge needle is used to prick the artery below the controlling loop and a 0·035-in flat wound guide wire is inserted through the prick hole retrogradely towards the heart. A Portex polythene catheter of suitable length with a moulded plastic hub is then inserted over the guide wire, using a size as large as the artery will comfortably accommodate. This catheter is given a terminal bend in hot water to facilitate manipulation. 30-in catheters should be obtained and cut to an appropriate length before insertion. For angiocardiography, the plastic hub should be shortened to fit tightly into a Luer-Lok adaptor. Alternatively a 4F Lehman catheter (U.S.C.I. Cat 5470) is particularly useful in small infants. Its main limitation is the long leader which makes aortography in the ascending aorta difficult. Before angiographic injection, the catheter outside the patient should be fixed by a sand bag to prevent it whipping back. On removing the catheter, the bleeding is controlled with the cat-gut loop while the adventitia over the puncture is approximated by a single stitch of 00000 silk on an atraumatic needle.

Should a larger artery be opened, e.g. for the insertion of a Sones catheter, the vessel wall should be incised *longitudinally* with a fine pointed scalpel, making the incision as short as possible. The catheter is inserted as described in the preceding section. The incision in the artery is sewn up by making stitches with 00000 silk on atraumatic needles into the adventitia and media. They should not extend to the lumen or intima. When the incision is a small one, a figure of 8 stitch will close it satisfactorily: with larger incisions, a series of stitches in the line of the artery convert the longitudinal incision into a transverse suture line. The repaired artery usually bleeds slightly after the sutures are tied, but this responds to light pressure. Arteries should *not* be incised transversely as the repair tends to occlude the lumen of the vessel.

Percutaneous insertion of cardiac catheters

Percutaneous arterial catheterization is considerably less traumatic both to the artery and the surrounding tissues than is an open exposure of the artery. We therefore prefer the closed percutaneous technique whenever it is practicable. The cut down technique is reserved for very small infants.

The most practical technique for the percutaneous insertion of cardiac catheters is that described by Seldinger (1953). The method consists essentially in the passage of a flexible guide wire into the vessel, and the threading of a catheter over the wire which is then withdrawn from the vessel. The method is applicable to both arteries and to veins. Its main disadvantage is that the catheters necessarily have an end hole so that there may be a recoil when they are used for the high pressure injections of angiocardiography. This tendency is reduced to acceptable proportions by making the end hole small in relation to the larger side holes. Alternatively, a terminal metal occluding device retained by a fine wire may be used to block the end hole (Straube tip occluder, U.S.C.C. Cat. No. 9535-9645). The veins usually chosen for the Seldinger technique are the femoral and the antecubital. The most convenient arteries are the femoral and the axillary. The brachial artery is very liable to spasm and is best avoided.

The technique requires a certain modicum of manual dexterity and instruments which are in good order and carefully assembled. It is essential to check the condition and the fit of the catheter on the guide wire and the integrity of the wire before the procedure is commenced. Manual dexterity cannot compensate for badly prepared or maintained equipment.

A description of the needles, guide wires and catheters used in the Seldinger technique is presented in Chapter 8, page 69.

Curving the catheter

Before the patient is towelled up for catheterization, the tapered tip of the selected sterile catheter is curved by immersion into a bowl of very hot sterile water and the curve is fixed by immediate immersion into sterile cold water. The type of curvature induced is important, for an incorrectly curved catheter may not be successful. Usually for arch aortography and left ventriculography, the terminal 4 to 6 cm of catheter is formed into an arc approaching a half the circumference of a circle of about 4 cm diameter. The younger the patient, the nearer the curve should approach the semi-circle, for in young patients an inadequately curved catheter will tend to pass from the descending aorta into the left subclavian artery. In children a complete semicircle curve is prepared of reduced diameter depending on the size of the patient. It is important to avoid side holes on the convexity of these bends, as in changing the catheter (p. 81), it is possible to pass the second guide wire through a hole so placed. If this happens, the wire may catch in the hole and damage either the wire or catheter. This accident may rarely require surgery to remove the catheter or wire.

Terminal curves of different shapes are often successful in traversing the aortic valve when the 'standard' semicircle tip has failed. Some operators prefer a J shaped catheter curve, S bend or a complete circle. It may be helpful to have several short sterile copper wires pre-curved to the desired shapes so that they may be inserted into the cardiac end of the catheter before immersion into the hot water for moulding.

An increasing range of preformed catheters of varying material, bore, wall thickness, terminal curvature, pre-packed and sterile is available from several manufacturers. Increasing use is being made of these preformed catheters.

SELDINGER TECHNIQUE

The technique is almost always performed under local anaesthesia, using 5 to 10 ml of 1 or 2 per cent procaine or lignocaine to infiltrate the skin and around the vessel at the site selected for puncture. The puncture site in the skin is enlarged with a scalpel point and a track bored out towards the chosen vessel with a closed fine pointed haemostat to facilitate later manipulation of the catheter.

The selected needle is then introduced along the track which has been made and the vessel is punctured. In the case of a venepuncture, it is usually not possible to feel the needle enter the vein, but in the upper limb the puncture can usually be seen. In the lower limb the *femoral vein* is found 5 to 8 mm medial to the pulsation of the femoral artery just below the inguinal ligament. The puncture is facilitated if the thigh is rotated externally in slight abduction as in this position the femoral vessels are straightened.

Very sharp needles are necessary for easy *arterial puncture*. A fine point with a short bevel gives the most satisfactory results. The arterial wall has a tough, rubbery consistency and a blunt needle will push an artery out of its way instead of pricking its surface and then entering it. An oblique puncture of the arterial wall is more easily controlled than one made vertically (Verel & Rickards, 1973).

In the *upper limb* the artery should be fixed with the fingers of one hand and the needle introduced at an angle of about 20°. The pulsation of the artery may be felt, transmitted along the needle, and it may then be possible to push a simple needle into the lumen, lower the hub, and thread it up the vessel. The desirability of a short bevel is here apparent. If the needle has a long point, the tip may 'pick up' the intima on the far side of the vessel so that the artery is transfixed. With a Seldinger or Cournand needle, this technique of puncturing only the superficial wall of the artery rarely succeeds. The artery can be deliberately transfixed, the stylet and needle withdrawn, and the cannula carefully drawn back, until a pulsatile jet of blood indicates that the tip of the cannula lies in the arterial lumen. The cannula is then threaded up the artery.

For the *femoral artery*, the point of entry should be 1 to 3 cm below the fold of the skin corresponding to the inguinal ligament. Here again with the needle it is usually possible to identify the pulsation or the resistance of the arterial wall. With the Seldinger or Cournand needles, the artery may be entered either after transfixing it as described above, or, in favourable cases, it may be possible to enter the lumen without touching the distal wall of the artery. The authors have rarely experienced bleeding from the puncture of the posterior wall in this transfixing technique.

As soon as the blood pulsates through the cannula, the hub is depressed to lie parallel to the skin and the guide-wire is threaded up the artery.

The guide wire should only be inserted if there is a free flow of blood from the cannula or needle. A slow flow from an artery or ooze from a vein indicates that the cannula is not free in the lumen of the vessel. Commonly this is due to the end of the cannula lying against the far side of the vessel. If withdrawing it by 1 to 2 mm does not produce a good flow, blood may be coming from a puncture of the vessel but the cannula may lie outside it. The cannula should then be withdrawn, the needle and stylet re-inserted, and another puncture made. Before passing the guide wire through the cannula, the angle between the cannula and the vessel should be reduced by lowering the hub towards the skin so that the cannula lies as parallel as possible to the vessel.

The guide wire (flimsy end foremost) should be passed through the needle or cannula for not more than 20 cm, the needle or cannula carefully withdrawn, and the puncture site lightly compressed with a swab to prevent bleeding. The wire is held firmly, the cannula drawn off, and the wire wiped clean with a damp sponge.

It is most important not to use any force in introducing the guide wire through the needle as this invariably indicates an unsatisfactory puncture with the wire penetrating into the arterial wall. If the passage of the guide wire is not *very* easily achieved, the needle should be withdrawn, the artery compressed until it has ceased to bleed and a further attempt to puncture the artery should be made.

After the satisfactory insertion of the guide wire, the pre-formed catheter is threaded over the wire until it reaches the skin. The guide wire may not at this stage protrude from the hub (operator) end of the catheter. In order subsequently to withdraw the guide wire, it must always protrude through this end of the catheter. The guide wire is therefore carefully withdrawn from the vessel by gentle traction at the point of skin puncture until the end of the guide wire protrudes 2 or 3 cm from the hub end of the catheter. This is essential.

The catheter and wire assembly are then carefully and gently pushed through the skin puncture until the catheter enters well into the vessel as indicated by blood flowing freely through the catheter.

If the guide wire enters the artery easily but the catheter cannot be introduced, the usual cause is that the catheter is badly tapered and does not fit snugly on to the wire. A dilator should be passed over the wire to enlarge the track of the guide wire. Another cause of this difficulty is an unusually thick skin and subcutaneous tissues preventing the threading of the catheter into the artery (e.g. after a previous incision, etc.).

When the catheter has been successfully introduced into the vessel, the guide wire may be either completely or partially withdrawn depending on the particular technique being adopted.

The further progress and manipulation of the catheter and wire are described in the appropriate sections (Chapters 10–12).

The original Seldinger technique does not allow the introduction of catheters with occluded ends. This is possible by the use of the percutaneous catheter sleeve introducers, for example, those made by U.S.C.I. or by Vygon.

Subclavian vein catheterization

Percutaneous catheterization of the subclavian vein is a technique of considerable value when an approach to the heart from the superior vena cava is necessary and a brachial approach is not possible. The puncture may be made either above or below the clavicle. The cardinal structure is the scalenus anterior muscle which separates the subclavian artery from the vein. This is identified in the conscious patient by palpation and by asking the patient to raise and lower the head while lying supine. In supraclavicular puncture the needle is inserted just lateral to the lateral margin of the sterno-mastoid muscle, about 1·5 cm above the upper margin of the clavicle, and the point of the needle is directed backwards, downwards and medially to enter the subclavian vein where it passes over the first rib lateral to the scalenus muscle. In a subclavian puncture the needle is passed in at the junction of the medial and middle thirds of the clavicle about 2 cm below the clavicle. The needle is passed medially backwards and slightly upwards to enter the vein.

In either case a free flow of blood is obtained and a guide wire inserted. We have had surprisingly little trouble in finding the vein by this technique and have found the supraclavicular approach suitable for occasional left atrial transseptal punctures where for some reason it was not possible to approach from below. The infraclavicular approach is extremely useful for getting a permanent endocardial pace-making catheter into position using a big catheter introducer passed down the superior vena cava by a Seldinger approach. Clear descriptions of the technique are given by Loskot et al. (1965), Macauley and Wright (1970) and by Epstein and Coulshed (1971). These papers should be consulted by anyone attempting this technique.

Artery catheterization

The axillary, brachial or radial artery may be utilized for arterial catheterization and the catheter may be passed retrogradely into the aorta. These arterial approaches from the arm are generally not as satisfactory as the approach from the femoral artery, which is larger, easier to puncture, less closely related to important structures and less liable to arterial spasm and other complications.

The authors believe therefore that the *femoral* artery should be the standard catheterization approach to the left heart. Occasionally this is not practical: there may be no femoral arterial pulsation (e.g. coarctation of aorta), it may be impossible to traverse a tortuous or atheromatous iliac artery, or a shorter more direct approach may be required (e.g. some methods of coronary arteriography).

The *brachial* artery is notoriously liable to spasm after arterial catheterization, particularly with a large catheter.

The *radial* artery is difficult to catheterize percutaneously and usually requires surgical exposure and catheterization under direct vision. This may be considered necessary—as for the introduction of the Mason Sones coronary artery catheter or for counter-current aortography in small infants.

The *axillary* artery is easier to catheterize percutaneously than is the brachial or other arm arteries and it is utilized by the authors when the femoral artery approach is not practical

The technique is basically the same as for the femoral artery catheterization. The artery is punctured in the axilla at a point of easy palpation; this usually corresponds to the undersurface of the humeral head. A very high or medial puncture should be avoided as it may not be possible subsequently to apply proximal arterial compression in order to secure haemostasis.

Only the small (size 160) needle should be used, together with the 160 wire and a catheter no larger than polythene 240. The grey Kifa-Odman catheter is probably too big for safe axillary artery catheterization.

The patient is positioned with the arm abducted to a right angle. After successful arterial puncture, the guide wire is introduced carefully and threaded slowly along the axillary artery. This should be performed under screen control for the guide wire often curves upwards into the vertebral artery—this should be avoided. When the guide wire has been successfully introduced for about 10 cm, the tapered catheter is threaded onto the wire in the usual way and introduced into the axillary artery. The introduction of the catheter should be continued under fluoroscopic control in order to ensure that the catheter negotiates the subclavian artery and then turns down to enter the innominate artery (right) or aorta (left).

Not infrequently the catheter may enter the vertebral artery or (less frequently) the lateral thoracic branches of the axillary artery. A curved catheter tip and varying the position of the arm aids manipulation and the avoidance of these vessels.

It is occasionally quite difficult to encourage the catheter to curve downwards into the first part of the subclavian artery. The catheter should then be withdrawn into the third part of the subclavian artery, rotated so that the concavity of its curve faces downwards and the arm rotated and abducted to varying degrees until the correct catheter course is gained. Sometimes a thin walled catheter may be too flexible and buckles under the skin instead of threading easily into the artery. It is useful in these circumstances to stiffen the catheter with a 205 (thick) guide wire, taking care that it does not protrude into the artery. Once the catheter has negotiated the first part of the subclavian artery, it is easy to traverse the innominate artery into the aortic arch.

The positioning of the catheter tip within the aorta or within the heart depends on the diagnostic problem to be investigated. For assessment of the left ventricle or of mitral incompetence, the left ventricle should be entered as described in Chapter 12. For assessment of aortic incompetence, the catheter tip should be sited in the middle of the ascending aorta for the angiographic injection of contrast medium (p. 120). For coronary artery catheterization, the individual coronary arteries may be selectively catheterized utilizing manufactured radio-opaque pre-curved, pre-tapered catheters (e.g. Mason-Sones or Judkins catheters). The latter are designed for percutaneous, Seldinger introduction and are highly efficient.

In patients with coarctation of aorta, the catheter tip should be placed in the upper part of the ascending aorta so that the aortic arch and its branches will be demonstrated. If the catheter tip is placed in the upper part of the descending aorta, the full collateral circulation may not be visualized.

Because of the possible danger of damage to the brachial nerve plexus during the axillary arterial catheterization, some investigators prefer to utilize the left axillary artery in right-handed persons. For patients with coarctation, the right axillary artery is preferred, as the left subclavian artery is often involved in the aortic deformity.

Axillary artery catheterization may be performed under local or general anaesthesia—the author prefers the latter.

After the radiological examination has been performed, the catheter is withdrawn and very considerable care is necessary to secure haemostatic control of the puncture site. The compression must be applied high in the axilla, proximal to the puncture and a haematoma must be meticulously avoided as it may involve the brachial plexus or impair the arterial lumen.

When the examination is concluded, careful examina-

tion of the arm pulses, and hand and arm movement and sensation should be made. If the examination has been performed under general anaesthesia, the clinical examination of the arm must be repeated when the patient has regained full consciousness. Examination of the hand function and arterial integrity should be repeated on the next day as delayed symptoms have occasionally been observed after axillary artery catheterization.

In recent years we have made infrequent use of axillary artery catheterization, preferring follow through studies from the pulmonary artery injection or trans-septal angiography.

Changing the catheter

A particular advantage of percutaneous Seldinger catheterization is that a catheter may be changed without further arterial puncture (Fig. 9.1). This facility should be utilized whenever it is desired to change a catheter for one of different material (e.g. Kifa-Odman, polythene, teflon, woven nylon) or for a catheter with a different terminal curve. The shape of the curve is of considerable importance in traversing an aortic valve or in selectively entering a specific artery (e.g. coronary, renal).

If a decision has been made to change the catheter, then the new catheter should be selected, mounted on its holder-tap-adaptor, and its desired curve preformed by immersion in very hot water. This new catheter, like the original one, must be tapered to fit the guide wire being used and must be at least 10 cm shorter than the wire.

The original catheter is withdrawn into the abdominal aorta and the guide wire fully reinserted, flexible end foremost, so that the wire end nearest the operator is flush with the catheter holder-tap. This will mean that 10 cm or more of the wire leader protrudes through the tapered end of the catheter and lies freely in the aortic lumen.

The catheter guide wire assembly is then slowly withdrawn until the tapered tip of the catheter emerges from the skin puncture. The guide wire is then held firmly so that no more of it is withdrawn, and a finger is placed firmly over the skin pucture to prevent bleeding. The catheter is then carefully withdrawn over the guide wire by the assistant, and placed on the trolley. The exposed guide wire is wiped clean with a wet sponge.

The new catheter is then threaded over the original guide wire and introduced into the artery in the usual way. The guide wire can then be withdrawn leaving the new catheter in the aorta.

Another method which we have often found useful employs a 200 cm flat wound guide wire. This is passed through the original angiographic catheter to the tapered end of the catheter which is then withdrawn over the guide wire. The tip of the guide wire remains at the site of the tip of the original catheter. A new catheter can then be passed cautiously over the guide wire and is

E

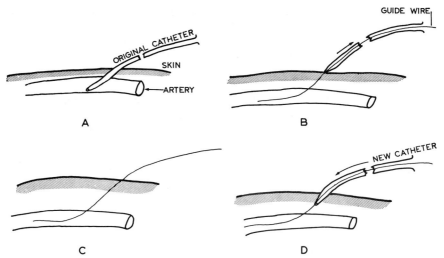

FIG. 9.1 *Changing the Catheter*. A. Withdraw the catheter so that its tip lies just within the artery. B. Thread a guide wire through the catheter. When the wire is well in the artery, withdraw the catheter through the puncture site.

C. Keeping the guide wire well inside the artery, pull the catheter off the wire. D. Thread the new catheter onto the wire and introduce it through the old puncture into the artery.

thereby guided to the desired position. This procedure is regarded by some as potentially hazardous.

A difficulty sometimes encountered in changing catheters is due to too tight a fit between the tapered end of the original catheter and the guide wire. If the fit is too snug it may be impossible to rethread the flexible end of the guide wire through the end hole of the catheter. If this occurs, the situation may sometimes be salvaged by using a new thinner (e.g. paediatric) wire for threading through the original catheter. The change of catheter may then proceed as outlined above.

It is preferable, however, not to change to a thinner guide wire for then introduction of the new catheter may be made more difficult. In order to avoid this problem, it is important to be careful in preparing the taper on the original catheter and in testing it on the guide wire to be used, before introduction into the patient. The fit between the end hole of the taper and the guide wire should be 'comfortable', i.e. it should be reasonably snug with a minimum of 'shoulder' but it should not be so tight as to prevent easy movement between the catheter and the wire. This mutual fit is an essential part of the Seldinger technique and the ideal fitting of the catheter taper to the guide wire is only achieved by practical experience—and usually after a humiliating failure.

Recently guide wires and catheters of 36 and 38 thou. have become available in addition to the original 35. This has further complicated matching up of guide wire and catheter particularly in the middle of a procedure.

Losing the guide wire up the catheter
Occasionally the operator end of the guide wire slips into the catheter during manipulation, particularly through a

tortuous artery. The usual predisposing cause is that only one or two cm of wire protruded through the hub end of the catheter at the beginning of the catheter manipulation. Once the distal end of the guide wire has slipped inside the catheter, it cannot be retrieved and the whole technique is in danger of being spoilt.

A very useful trick which may save the situation is to cut off the hub end of the catheter with a sharp razor blade. The cut is made proximal to the end of the guide wire which then protrudes from the cut end of the catheter. The guide wire is then removed from the catheter. The cut end of the catheter will be pouring forth blood and therefore cannot be flanged for use in the catheter holder. Fortunately the outer cannula of the 205 Seldinger needle makes a very close fit inside polythene 205 or 240 catheter. The 160 outer cannula makes a very good fit inside the polythene 160 catheter. Depending on the catheter being used, the appropriate cannula is inserted well into the cut end of the catheter to make a watertight junction, and the hub of the cannula is then connected to the syringe, either directly or by means of a short connecting tube. In this way the original catheter may be utilized and the investigation may be continued.

Another approach is to clamp the catheter and guide wire together at the puncture site by powerful forceps, withdraw the catheter slowly until the guide wire appears at the skin.

Control of bleeding
When the catheter is finally withdrawn from the vessel after completion of the catheterization, considerable bleeding will occur.

Venous bleeding after percutaneous catheterization is

readily controlled by light pressure over the vein. A few minutes' light pressure is all that is required. After venous catheterization by surgical cut down and exposure of the vein, bleeding tends to be more severe and more prolonged. The bleeding can usually be easily controlled by light pressure without ligature of the vein, but occasionally one or two catgut ligatures may be considered necessary. The catgut is readily absorbed and within a few weeks the vein is usually recanalized and patent. Care must be taken (whether or not the vein is ligatured) that the full thickness of subcutaneous tissues and skin be carefully stitched back superficially to the vein. We prefer to use vertical mattress sutures on all occasions for closing skin incisions. This soft tissue support is of considerable importance in limiting venous bleeding.

Arterial bleeding is always profuse after arterial catheterization but it can always be controlled by firm pressure carefully applied directly over and proximal to the puncture site. It is therefore essential that the point of arterial puncture can be reached by the fingers of the operator and brought under direct digital control. The bleeding always occurs from the puncture wound which has admitted the catheter on the superficial aspect of the artery.

The digital pressure must be quite firm and will have to be applied for several minutes. Usually the bleeding ceases within 10 to 15 min but occasionally pressure may be required for 30 min or longer. The operator must have the patience to maintain this arterial control and must not delegate it to inexperienced staff. A few seconds of uncontrolled arterial haemorrhage may result in a very large haematoma. In almost every case, pressure for 30 min will control the arterial puncture, rarely an arterial wall stitch of 00000 nylon on an atraumatic needle may be required. This has occurred only once in approximately 8000 arterial catheterizations in our clinic.

Although digital pressure on the artery should be continuous, it is advisable to allow one or two arterial pulsations to be transmitted every minute. It is advisable to permit bleeding for the first second from the proximal segment of the artery to facilitate any clot being washed out. The applied pressure must not be too heavy as the arterial lumen should not be occluded. The minimum pressure necessary to control the haemorrhage should be used. These precautions will reduce the incidence of arterial thrombosis (Chap. 17).

Causes of prolonged bleeding are hypertension, obesity, recent anti-coagulant therapy, arteriosclerosis, too large a catheter, poor technique and an inaccessible puncture site.

The patient should be carefully observed for several hours after the catheterization for, in exceptional cases, brisk bleeding may restart even after perfectly adequate initial arterial control. The same procedure of digital pressure should again be employed and is invariably successful.

It is strongly advised that the patient remain in bed for 24 hours after Seldinger femoral arterial catheterization.

References

Both, A., Gleichman, U., Loogen, F., Maurer, W. & Ressl, J. (1969). Erfahrungen bei der anwendung von mikrokathetern in der kardiologischen diagnostik. *Zeitschr. fur Kreislauf.* **58,** 1212.

Filston, H. C. & Johnson, D. G. (1971). Percutaneous venous cannulation in neonates and infants: a method for catheter insertion without 'cut-down'. *Pediatrics* **48,** 896.

Seldinger, S. I. (1953). Catheter replacement of the needle in percutaneous arteriography. *Acta radiol.* **39,** 368.

Verel, D. (1958). Percutaneous intubation of the femoral vein for transfusion. *Lancet* **1,** 716.

Verel, D. & Rickards, D. F. (1973). Effect of the site of the puncture of the femoral artery upon haemorrhage following aortic angiocardiography. *Clin. Radiol.* **24,** 62.

Subclavian Vein Catheterization

Loskot, F., Michaljanic, A. & Musil, J. (1965). Right and left heart catheterization via the subclavian veins. *Cardiologia* **46,** 114.

Macauley, M. B. & Wright, J. S. (1970). Transvenous cardiac pacing. Experience of a percutaneous supraclavicular approach. *Br. Med. J.* **4,** 207.

Epstein, E. J. & Coulshed, N. (1971). Transseptal catheterization via right subclavian vein. *Br. Heart J.* **33,** 658.

10. Right Heart Catheterization

General considerations

Any attempt to describe the technique of cardiac catheterization in words must, to a greater or lesser extent, be inadequate. It is probably correct to say that although certain manipulations of the cardiac catheter are practised by most people who perform diagnostic catheterizations, each practitioner will develop his own technique. The first decision of importance to be made is an appraisal of the likely scope of the investigation. Clearly, in a right-sided catheterization of the patient suffering from rheumatic heart disease, the measurement of pulmonary wedge pressure is going to be of considerable importance. This will inevitably mean the choice of a catheter with a single end hole, since side holes render the wedge pressure measurement even more uncertain than it normally is. If congenital heart disease is being investigated, then the size of the patient in relation to the available veins becomes of considerable importance. Thus, in a small infant, adequate selective angiography usually requires a 6F catheter, although in infants of under 3 kg a number 5F will usually do. (In such small infants a number 6F catheter may be too big for safe manipulation in a small heart and discretion demands that a No. 5 is used.) In infants of less than 3 kg weight, the femoral vein is the only easily accessible vein likely to be big enough to take an adequate catheter and the appropriate incision must be made for reaching it. In a large adult, on the other hand, an 11 or 12F catheter may be needed to get good angiocardiograms. Should the arm for some reason be selected for catheterization, unless there is a large antecubital vein, the axillary or brachial vein must be approached. Similarly, in children it may be desirable to enter the internal saphenous or brachial vein rather than the vein at the antecubital fossa in order to insert a catheter of sufficient size to permit rapid injection of contrast medium.

The possible lesion under consideration may also affect the choice of site for catheterization. If there are any grounds for suspecting an *atrial septal defect*, then the approach from the thigh holds out a much easier prospect of reaching the left atrium through the defect, since the plane of the inter-atrial septum is so placed that a catheter introduced from below will easily pass through from one side to the other, whereas a catheter introduced from above may have to be acutely bent if a high atrial septal defect is to be entered. Conversely in very large patients,

it is often easier to reach the pulmonary artery from the left arm than from any other site. Against this, however, must be placed the possibility that the catheter introduced into the left arm may not be long enough to permit an adequate wedge pressure measurement in the pulmonary capillary in a large patient. The not infrequent presence of a *left superior vena cava* is a further possible snag. When this is present, it is usually impossible to catheterize adequately from the left arm as the catheter is led down behind the heart, through the coronary sinus, into the lower part of the right atrium and, in many cases, will only pass down into the liver from this site (Fig. 5.6). It is sometimes possible successfully to complete a cardiac catheterization using a catheter passed down the left superior vena cava. In such cases there is likely to be an ostium primum defect of some considerable size which permits an undue mobility of the catheter tip in the right atrium.

Some authors writing on this topic have advocated the right arm as the easiest to use, others the left. The opinion of the writer is that the left arm is, on the whole, easier for manipulation, particularly if the catheter is fairly stiff. The right arm, not infrequently, poses considerable difficulties in negotiating the entry into the superior vena cava and in some patients the catheter has a distressing habit of wandering across to the other side or up into the neck. It is also more difficult to control when it is in the right ventricle if passed from the right arm.

Having decided on the likely scope of the investigation and on the most promising site for the approach to the heart, a vein is catheterized by one of the methods described in the section on insertion of catheters (p. 76 et seq.).

Manipulation of the catheter

EARLY HOLD-UP

Once the catheter is inserted into the vein it should be advanced towards the heart. Occasionally after an easy passage for 2 cm or less the catheter jams or further passage becomes difficult. There are several possible reasons for this. The most common is probably the failure to insert the catheter into the lumen of the vein. It is not difficult, particularly if working in an awkward site, to introduce the catheter, not into the lumen of the vessel, but into the plane between the media and the intima.

This is particularly the case if a messy incision has been made and the blood is not kept carefully wiped away. An uncommon reason for the catheter sticking is that the vein has narrowed. In one patient catheterized in Sheffield, a total of seven attempts at cardiac catheterization in different sites were made by three different investigators. All failed and in no instance did the catheter pass more than 4 cm along the vein. At surgery, the patient was found to have Fallot's tetralogy and the veins in the periphery were found to have retained their primitive plexiform character. A more common cause of a hold-up is encountered when the long saphenous vein is used. Here the catheter tends to pass up the inferior hypogastric vein and stick, instead of passing into the femoral vein. This can usually be circumvented in the following way: when the catheter is arrested it should be gently brought back about 3 cm, the saphenous vein pulled gently towards the feet and so stretched. The catheter will then usually pass readily into the femoral vein, although sometimes it is necessary to rotate the tip of the catheter.

Increasing use of percutaneous insertion of all types of catheter through the Vygon introducer into the femoral vein, has greatly reduced the problems of early hold-up. The patient with tetralogy of Fallot mentioned earlier has been easily catheterized by this technique to demonstrate her post-operative state.

Late hold-up

Not infrequently when the antecubital vein is used, there is some hold-up at shoulder level. This is usually due to the catheter passing down the lateral thoracic vein. It can be circumvented easily by withdrawing and turning the catheter tip towards the head. Once past this point, the tip should be rotated anteriorly until it points towards the feet and the catheter will usually pass down into the superior vena cava with little trouble. Occasionally a great deal of difficulty is experienced in this manoeuvre, particularly when the right arm is catheterized. This is commonly due to the bend on the end of the catheter not suiting the bend in the veins. The catheter tip lodges in the lower end of the innominate vein. It is sometimes possible to achieve the manipulation into the superior vena cava by withdrawing the catheter and either changing it or bending the tip to a different shape in hot water, fixing the bend by plunging it into cold water. If it is then rapidly inserted it is not infrequently possible to persuade it to pass an obstruction which previously was impassable. Other possible tricks are to manipulate the tip of the catheter up to the neck and form a loop at the junction of the internal jugular vein and the subclavian vein. This loop will sometimes pass down the superior vena cava and the tip will follow it (Fig. 10.1). It is sometimes of use to inject a small quantity of contrast medium to try and get some idea as to where the catheter should be going. As has been mentioned, catheterization from the

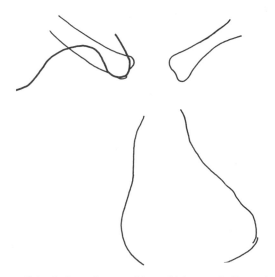

FIG. 10.1 Catheter in a position which may facilitate the passage from the right arm to the heart when the tip of the catheter is held up at the origin of the superior vena cava. The tip of the catheter is in the jugular vein with a loop at the origin of the superior vena cava. When the catheter is advanced, the loop descends into the right atrium. (This illustration is a tracing of a radiograph, as are the other illustrations in this chapter.)

left arm is often easier than the approach from the right arm. The main reason for this is that the passage from the left arm to the right side of the heart involves no reflex bends in the catheter, which is, therefore, much more easily turned when it is within the heart cavity.

The *cephalic vein* is best avoided because of the frequent difficulty in passing the catheter beyond the level of the clavicle. If, for some reason, this vein has to be used and the catheter sticks at this site, it is well worth trying the following manoeuvre. The patient's wrist is firmly gripped by the operator and the arm is brought up close to the ear. The catheter may then pass on. If not, the wrist is firmly pulled with sufficient force almost to move the patient along the table and the catheter, after a gentle withdrawal of perhaps 3 cm, is advanced. This will usually pass it beyond the kink at which it has been obstructed. The most common cause of failure of this manoeuvre is due to the pull on the arm not being sufficiently strong. It may also help to inject contrast medium and watch its course to see where the catheter is going wrong. Often it will be found to have passed the main channel and be lodged in a tributary. It is usually possible to manoeuvre it into the correct vein if the catheter is first withdrawn and a suitable bend made at the tip. The catheter is then quickly re-introduced, 3 or 4 ml contrast medium injected by hand to show the site where the catheter has previously gone astray, and the catheter manoeuvred into the axillary vein.

Manipulation in the heart

The manipulations of the catheter within the heart are largely a matter of individual preference and considerable experience. The operator must familiarize himself with the movement of the catheter tip. When this is seen only in one plane, as in the normal screening, it is difficult for the beginner to know which way the tip of the catheter is moving when it is rotated. The appreciation of whether it is turning towards or away from the operator is essential to intelligent use of the catheter. Some manoeuvres are in general use. For example, it may be difficult to enter the *right ventricle*, either because the catheterization is being performed from below and so the tricuspid orifice is difficult to reach, or because the catheter tip has become straightened in the course of its passage into the heart and it will not bend sufficiently to enable the tricuspid ring to be approached. In these circumstances, it is useful to manipulate the catheter up and down until the tip catches in the wall of the atrium and the catheter can be bent into a loop (Fig. 10.2). This U-shaped loop may be rotated until it lies in the plane of the tricuspid valve and then the catheter gradually withdrawn until the tip is seen to make a slight movement towards the left side of the heart (Fig. 10.3). This usually occurs as the tip slips through the tricuspid valve, the catheter is then rapidly advanced, and if the situation has been correctly judged, will pass immediately into the pulmonary artery. A precisely similar manoeuvre in a slightly different plane can be used to pass the catheter through an atrial septal defect. When the groin approach is used, an atrial septal defect is usually passed at the initial entry of the catheter and indeed the main difficulty in the catheterization may be avoiding this easy path to the left atrium. It can be exasperating when it appears to be impossible to enter any chamber other than the left atrium.

The manipulation of the catheter from the right ventricle into the *pulmonary artery* can be exceedingly difficult. It is most easily achieved when the catheter is passed from the left arm since there is a natural tendency for the catheter to form a wide loop which passes from

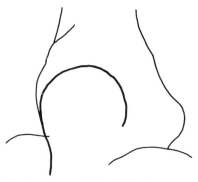

FIG. 10.3   The loop shown in Fig. 10.2 has been rotated so that the tip lies medially. As the catheter is withdrawn the loop opens and the tip of the catheter enters the right ventricle.

behind forwards through the ventricle and out into the pulmonary artery. It is less easy from the right arm where the catheter is bent into a U-shaped loop which is more difficult to rotate. It may be completely impossible in occasional cases when a catheter is passed from below, although in other cases passing the catheter from the right ventricle to the pulmonary artery by the inferior vena cava approach is a matter of great ease. Two situations are particularly unpromising. The first is most commonly encountered when the catheter is passed from above and passes out towards the apex of the ventricle. If it is seen lying horizontally along the lower border of the heart and a check shows that it is not in fact in the coronary sinus but is genuinely in the ventricular cavity, it is almost impossible to manipulate it up into the pulmonary artery (although the position is ideal for an indwelling pacemaker—Fig. 20). The only thing to do is to pull the catheter back towards the atrium rotating to see whether the tip can be persuaded to rise up to the outflow tract. It usually will not and a fresh passage of the tricuspid valve has to be attempted. Occasionally repeated manipulations fail to produce a hopeful position and the catheter should be withdrawn. It may be that it is too soft or too hard or the tip is not adequately bent. It is worth trying a new bend in the tip of the catheter, using hot water followed by cold immersion to fix it. If this does not work, another catheter may be tried. When passed from below it is more usual to find the catheter will stick halfway up the lateral border of the right ventricle and refuse to pass up to the outflow tract. The most suitable manoeuvre in these circumstances is to withdraw gently, watching the tip until it is apparent from its mobility that it is free in the cavity of the ventricle. Clockwise rotation is then applied and the tip gently advanced. With repeated withdrawals and advances and further clockwise rotations, it is usually possible to wind it up into the outflow of the right ventricle and on to the pulmonary artery. In very large and trabeculated ventricles, however, it is sometimes necessary to confess failure. If it is essen-

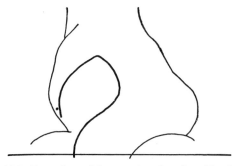

FIG. 10.2   Loop formed for entering the tricuspid valve by catching the catheter tip in a crevice in the atrial wall.

tial to know what the outflow tract is like, a small angiocardiographic injection will usually show this clearly and permit assessment of the valve. It is important to bear in mind all the time during this type of manipulation that the patient has a limited time of endurance for investigation and the study must not be unduly protracted.

Once in the pulmonary artery, it is usually a straightforward matter to obtain blood samples and wedge pressures. Occasionally, however, difficulty is experienced either because the catheter is too short to wedge satisfactorily and keep contact with the pressure head or for some other reason. It is desirable to have a number of different sized connectors to enable the catheter to be connected to the pressure head by a length of plastic tubing. Sometimes the catheter cannot be wedged because instead of the tip advancing, a loop forms in the atrium whenever more catheter is pushed up the vein through which it has been introduced. There is sometimes no remedy for this but to accept defeat (Figs. 10.4 and 10.5), and change to a balloon float catheter.

Occasionally the catheter will advance if it is rotated slightly in order to straighten it. The beginner is advised to rotate the patient (in whom this difficulty is experienced) through 90° and inspect the catheter in the lateral plane. This will usually reveal the reason for his failure to advance the catheter in the shape of an acute change of direction from posterior to anterior in the atrium. Occasionally it is possible to achieve success by stiffening the catheter with a guide wire, or changing to a stiffer catheter, or one in which the terminal bend is different, but usually the trouble is unsurmountable because of the size of the heart. A very large catheter (9F or 10F) can easily be wedged in such circumstances but such a catheter is quite unsuitable for measuring a satisfactory wedge pressure. The best it can do is to produce an indifferently damped pulmonary artery tracing

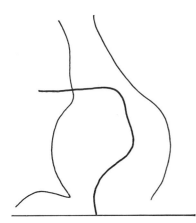

FIG. 10.4 Catheter passed from below to the pulmonary artery.

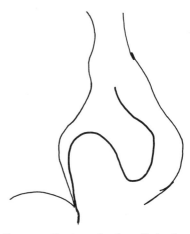

FIG. 10.5 On attempting to wedge the catheter shown in Fig. 10.4 by passing more of the catheter into the heart, a loop forms in the atrium and the tip, instead of advancing, moves back into the right ventricle.

of no value whatever. In such circumstances there may be nothing for it but to 'grasp the nettle' firmly and aim for the left atrium with a Ross needle to measure the left atrial pressure.

The *order of events* in any catheterization is to some extent dictated by chance and it is important to make use of such opportunities as present themselves. When all goes more or less according to plan, however, it is probably best to start by passing the catheter through the right atrium and out into either the superior or inferior vena cava, depending on the route by which the heart has been approached. A series of samples is then taken, one from the inferior vena cava, low down, one from the inferior vena cava near the heart, three or more from the atrium and one from the superior vena cava. These samples are passed to a technician for immediate oxygen analysis. If an indicator technique is available, it is useful to record a curve from the atrium and if there seems likely to be a shunt at this level, to repeat these curves in the superior and inferior vena cavae. For this purpose, a method which permits the recognition of a left to right shunt is most useful (e.g. that using ascorbic acid). The intra-atrial pressure is then recorded and the catheter passed to the right ventricle and pulmonary artery. Samples are obtained from both pulmonary arteries and the main pulmonary artery, the ventricle in the outflow tract and the ventricle close to the tricuspid valve. Pressure recordings are made in all sites and careful withdrawal traces obtained at the sites of the valves. In some cases, it may be desirable to record the wedge pressure and, if this is the case, a single end hole catheter must be used.

The results to date are then considered. If there is evidence suggesting the presence of arterial blood at any site, the next stage is planned. A careful search with the catheter is made for anomalous veins or septal defects in the right atrium and the problem of the best form of angiography considered. It is not infrequent in cyanosed cases to enter the aorta from the right ventricle. This would suggest that a selective right ventricular angiogram programmed to show the outflow tract of the right ventricle will be the most useful investigation. If manipulation of the catheter in the pulmonary artery has resulted in the passage into the aorta, suggesting the presence of a patent ductus, it may be reasonable to make a small injection of contrast medium into the aorta at this site, in the hope of visualizing the lesion. This is particularly important in small infants where the differentiation between patent ductus and aorto-pulmonary window is of great importance. High pressure injections should not be made into the duct. In cases where an atrial septal defect or foramen ovale has been found, a complete investigation of the heart may be obtained by sampling from the left ventricle, the left atrium, the right side of the heart and then by performing right and left-sided angiography. This type of investigation requires great experience and much knowledge of the possible anatomical abnormalities in the heart if the best use is to be made of the opportunities which chance presents. In many cases of congenital heart disease, the best results are obtained by catheterizing the patient throughout with an angiographic catheter. This has the advantage that it is possible to utilize the opportunity for angiography whenever it may arise. This is particularly the case when cinegraphy is being used in a single plane as the only method of visualizing the heart chambers. Here it is probably better to proceed little by little with fairly frequent short film records of angiocardiograms rather than to consider a considerable mass of catheter results before deciding on one or two sites for injection of contrast medium.

It will be apparent that if the best use is to be made of the apparatus and the opportunities which are presented by catheterization, the operator must have both an intimate knowledge of the limitations of his technique and a considerable appreciation of the abnormalities he may encounter. Careful judgement is needed to enable the best use to be made of any situation which may arise during cardiac catheterization, particularly since the patient's condition may limit the time available for investigation.

As the investigator's experience increases, he comes to recognize the scope of investigation possible in commonly encountered conditions. In the next few paragraphs, some of these are described. One of the fascinations of cardiac catheterization, however, is its infinite variety, and with increasing experience, the operator is able to take better advantage of the opportunities for establishing a diagnosis which chance may present.

The scope of investigation possible in patients with an *atrial septal defect* can be remarkable. It has already been mentioned that the left atrium is most easily entered from below. In a secundum defect it may only be possible to enter the left atrium and pulmonary veins from this approach. If the operator has more experience and confidence a more rewarding approach is made from the arm. Here the left arm is the one of choice and the occasional occurrence of left superior vena cava should not be regarded as a deterrent since it is of interest to the surgeon to know that this anomaly is present. [During open heart surgery for atrial septal defect, a stream of blood pours over the operating field from the coronary sinus. Continuous suction with several pumps may be necessary to keep it clear during closure of the septal defect.] When present it is usually necessary to abandon catheterization from the left arm and start again from the right. Having reached the right atrium from above, the catheter should be bent in a loop by catching its tip in the wall of the atrium. This U-shaped loop is rotated so that the tip of the catheter points postero-medially. It is then gently worked up and down the atrial septum until a lateral movement, often very slight, indicates that it has entered a septal defect; it is then usually possible to manipulate it out into a lung vein (Fig. 10.6). Samples and pressures and angiocardiography from the left atrium can all be done and with experience the left ventricle can be entered with ease and certainly by the following manoeuvre. The catheter is gently withdrawn from the pulmonary vein until the loop originally formed to pass it to the left atrium has been drawn up into the superior vena cava

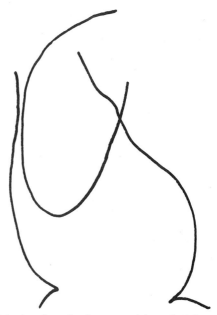

FIG. 10.6   A catheter has been passed from the left arm to the pulmonary veins of the left upper lobe by way of the right atrium, an atrial septal defect and the left atrium.

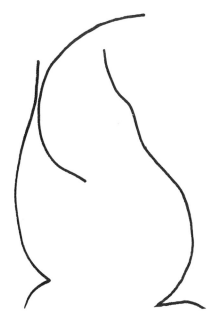

FIG. 10.7 The catheter shown in Fig. 10.6 has been drawn back until the tip lies just within the left atrium. The position suggests a high defect as the tendency for the catheter to straighten will usually result in the catheter springing out towards the lateral wall of the right atrium once the tip is no longer constrained by the lower margin of the defect. This deduction is of very little worth, however. A catheter sterilized in a coil, for example, will tend to adopt the position shown naturally.

(Fig. 10.7). The tip of the catheter is thus pulled back until it almost reaches the midline and the catheter is then rotated slightly clockwise and advanced. It will then enter the left ventricle and pass out usually to the apex (Fig. 10.8). The most common cause of failure is entry into the left atrial appendage. If this has happened, the appearance of the catheter can be very misleading. It is possible, in infants, to manipulate it clear of the heart shadow so that it appears to lie in a pulmonary vein. Occasionally there is a notable pressure difference between the left atrium and the left atrial appendage (Fig. 10.9). In the atrial appendage a considerable A wave is sometimes recorded and this may give rise to much confusion. The position can be clarified by injecting a small quantity of contrast medium by hand down the catheter. If the catheter is lodged in the atrial appendage it should be withdrawn, rotated clockwise and again advanced, when the ventricle should be entered. Once in the ventricle it is possible to perform an angiocardiogram which will exclude with certainty ventricular septal defect and patent ductus.

A further advantage of this approach is that from the left arm it is frequently possible to enter a *sinus venosus defect* or anomalous drainage of the right upper lobe. This can be further clarified by angiocardiography. It is, therefore, possible in favourable circumstances to make a

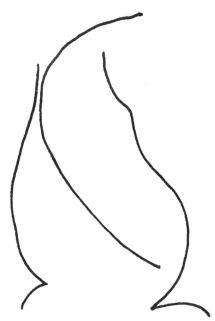

FIG. 10.8 The catheter shown in Fig. 10.7 has now been advanced to the apex of the left ventricle. This manoeuvre is usually most expeditiously achieved if some clockwise rotation is applied to the catheter as it is advanced. The reason for this is easily understood if the position in Fig. 10.6 is considered. The catheter is passing here from a relatively anterior position (the right atrium) to the pulmonary vein (lying at the back of the left atrium). Merely to draw it back and, push, after it has straightened, it in again without rotation will result in the tip of the catheter entering the lower lobe pulmonary vein or the left atrial appendage. Clockwise rotation will turn the tip anterior to the atrial appendage so that it will enter the ventricle across the aortic cusp of the mitral valve. Counter-clockwise rotation should be applied if the pulmonary veins of the left lung are to be entered. Note that the direction of rotation is the same whichever arm is catheterized, but is reversed when the leg is used. (To illustrate this point—suppose a catheter lies in the right atrium, the tip pointing posteriorly. If passed from above, a clockwise twist will turn the tip medially. If passed from below, a clockwise twist will rotate the tip laterally.)

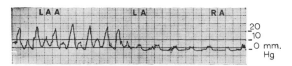

FIG. 10.9 A misleading pressure tracing, occasionally encountered in patients with a long atrial appendage. This tracing was thought to represent a drawback through a foramen ovale. In the left atrial appendage a high systolic pressure was recorded with an aortographic catheter (30/0 mmHg). Left atrial angiocardiography showed a large atrial appendage and an atrial septal defect was found at surgery. The high systole in the atrial appendage is uncommon, but can be extremely misleading.

complete examination of the heart with a venous catheter when atrial septal defect is present, the only valve not traversed by the catheter being the aortic valve and the state of affairs in this region should be clearly demonstrated by the left ventricular angiocardiogram.

An *ostium primum defect* by contrast is all too readily traversed by a catheter passed from the upper limb and may rarely be impossible to traverse from below. When it seems deceptively easy to pass from one ventricle to the other, an ostium primum defect with cleft valve should be suspected. The ease with which the chambers can be entered in this condition is well exemplified by the author's experience mentioned earlier of making a complete catheterization involving entering into all chambers of the heart following catheterization through a left superior vena cava.

Tricuspid atresia can present a most puzzling picture when it is investigated for the first time. The usual emotions associated with its encounter are an initial gratification with the ease with which it is proving possible to enter the ventricle and a growing suspicion that the route by which the ventricle is being entered is not normal. The catheter will readily pass from right to left high up through what must be an atrial septal defect to enter the left ventricle with extreme ease. It is usually correspondingly difficult or impossible to persuade it to leave the ventricle by either of the great vessels. A gradual suspicion that the right ventricle, if present, is somewhat fugitive, dawns on the operator and, usually rather late, enlightenment comes and he realizes there is no right ventricle to enter. Here the most informative manoeuvre is an angiocardiogram from the right atrium. A large bolus should be injected and rapid filming set for the early part of the injection, in contrast to most atrial injections where slow filming is usually sufficient as the atrium fills. This angiocardiogram should show the triangular wedge of tissue containing the blind right ventricle which in most cases does not fill with contrast medium (Fig. 75). Cine-angiography will usually demonstrate the condition convincingly, but is best avoided since stenosis of the pulmonary valve is not uncommon in deeply cyanosed children with this condition, and the cine film may not show it. A selective left ventricular injection with two-plane changer is usually satisfactory, but the author has had very little luck in his attempts to find its outflow tract. Tricuspid atresia is, however, an easy condition to diagnose when the electrocardiogram shows left axis deviation in a cyanosed infant.

Another condition which gives rise to much confusion is *anomalous pulmonary venous drainage* of the type in which the venous drainage of the left lung enters the coronary sinus. These patients do not have the appearance so characteristic and easy to recognize on the P.A. chest radiograph which has been termed the 'cottage loaf'. They present, as a rule, as patients with an atrial

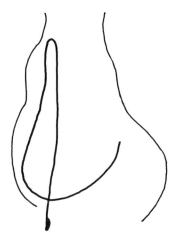

FIG. 10.10   Catheter passed up the vena azygos from below the diaphragm into the superior vena cava, and thence to the right atrium and right ventricle.

septal defect and a very large shunt. The condition should be suspected when it is found that all the intra-cardiac samples, with the exception of those from the venae cavae, are in the high 80's or low 90's percentage saturation. It is good practice to make a pulmonary artery angiocardiogram to show the lung venous drainage in every case diagnosed as atrial septal defect, although where open-heart surgery is routinely done with bypass and hypothermia, it is not a vital matter to the patients to establish the presence of such anomalous venous drainage. Should simple hypothermia be used, however, the patient's life may hang on the diagnosis.

Azygos venous drainage is another condition which is quite mystifying when first encountered. In this anomaly the inferior vena cava either does not form or does not connect with the femoral vein selected for catheterization (Figs. 10.10, 10.11 and 10.12). If the catheter is passed from below it appears to reach the heart normally and

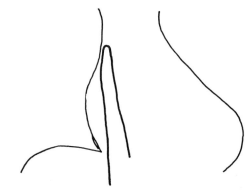

FIG. 10.11   Catheter passed up the inferior vena cava to the right atrium and thence to the superior vena cava and then down the vena azygos.

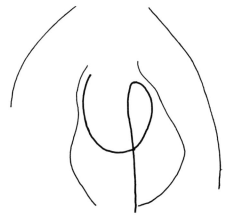

FIG. 10.12 Catheter passed up the left vena azygos to the left atrium, left ventricle and aorta in a case of anomalous venous drainage of the lower body to the left atrium.

then becomes quite refractory and will neither enter the superior vena cava nor any other chamber. The true state of affairs is revealed if the patient is rotated into the lateral position. The catheter is seen to lie *behind* the heart and if contrast medium be injected it is usually possible to persuade it to follow the vena azygos into the right atrium proper, from which it is sometimes possible to complete a satisfactory cardiac catheterization. When the subject is very small, for example an infant, this is not possible and a disappointing and inadequate investigation results. The right atrium in such patients is a strange chamber with, as a rule, separate entries for the two azygos veins and a separate drainage of the right and left hepatic veins. These, together with the coronary sinus, the superior vena cava and the four pulmonary veins may present a surgeon repairing a large atrial septal defect in such a case with a nice problem of geography. Such a patient recently repaired proved to have no less than fourteen holes in the atrial cavity in addition to an atrial septal defect sufficiently large as to constitute a common atrium. A large patch was stitched in and appears to have been successfully positioned in that the patient survived, is better and is not now cyanosed.

It is necessary always to be on the lookout for odd rarities. Such a curiosity is the entry of veins from the lower part of the body to the left atrium instead of to the right. Drainage of the inferior vena cava to the left side of the heart has been described, but we have not encountered this. We have, however, one patient in whom a left-sided vena azygos entered the left atrium and permitted catheterization from the left side of the heart while an approach from the arm gave full data from the right side of the heart (Figs. 10.12 and 10.13). Unfortunately he proved to have Eisenmenger's reaction to a septal defect so surgery has not been attempted. Another curiosity identified was a direct communication between

the pulmonary artery and left atrium. Both these cases were met by investigators early in their experience of cardiac catheterization and were successfully recognized by careful reconnaissance and the application of a routine procedure. Whenever in doubt, the pressure should be carefully recorded, a sample taken and an injection of contrast medium made.

A note on timing angiocardiograms from the right side of the heart may be made here. Injections into the cavity of the ventricle usually stimulate extrasystoles during which the onward movement of blood is much reduced. It follows that if, for example, a dye curve gives a circulation time from right ventricle to ear of seven seconds, the film programme should be run for eleven or twelve seconds if adequate follow on pictures of the left side of the heart are wanted. Even with this allowance the films may run out before the aorta is adequately filled. Ventricular extrasystoles are avoided if a slow injection (15 ml/s) is given, but poor-quality angiocardiograms may result.

Catheterization for cardiac pacing

INDICATIONS
An intracardiac electrode catheter is usually inserted in one of three circumstances:

1. To institute cardiac pacing as an emergency in a patient in whom frequent and prolonged Adams-Stokes attacks are threatening survival.

2. As a less acute procedure in a patient in whom established heart block has failed to respond to medical treatment.

3. As a precaution in a patient in whom a recent cardiac infarction seems likely to precipitate complete heart block.

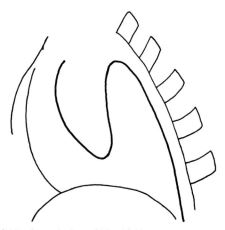

FIG. 10.13 Lateral view of Fig. 10.12.

CATHETERS

Electrode catheters consist essentially of a platinum electrode tip with a wire conducting core leading to a suitable terminal for connecting to the pace maker. The core is covered by an insulating radiopaque coating. Two main types are available.

1. *Single electrode catheters.* These have a simple platinum tip and a single conducting core leading to a single terminal. They are most commonly used with an implanted pacemaking unit which is inserted subcutaneously, usually in the axilla. A second terminal, usually only a few cm long is placed in the axilla or the metal casing of the pacemaker forms the indifferent electrode.

2. *Double electrode catheters.* These are made with one electrode at the tip and a second platinum ring electrode 1 cm from the tip. Two wires run through the catheter to a pair of terminals at the hub end of the catheter. They may be used:

(i) for permanent pacing by a suitable external unit.
(ii) for testing the effect of pacing in a patient with established heart block.
(iii) for emergency pacing.

These catheters are available in sizes 5F and 6F. The 5F size is a little more difficult to manipulate but is preferred, as the only cardiac perforation by the catheter in our experience with over 1,000 insertions occurred with a No. 6F catheter which is stiffer than the thinner 5F.

INSERTION OF THE CATHETER

The *percutaneous catheter introducer* (Vygon Desilets) is a very convenient tool for getting the catheter into the vein in an emergency. It consists of a flexible introducing catheter of 7·5F external gauge and 5F internal bore, together with a 5F inner catheter and a 0·035-in guide wire.

The 0·035-in guide wire is passed into the selected vein by the Seldinger technique. The 5F inner catheter is passed over the wire into the vein. The introducing (outer) catheter is then pushed over the 5F inner catheter until it lies in the vein. The wire and inner catheter are then removed leaving the introducing catheter in the vein. The pacemaking catheter is then inserted through the introducing catheter which is then withdrawn. The introducing catheter cannot be removed from the pacing catheter and remains on it until the pacing catheter is removed. This introducer is only suitable for emergency pacing.

The temporary pacing catheter made by Vygon (see p. 72) is used in a similar fashion. It has the advantage of being supplied ready sterilized with a plastic cannula which can be removed once the catheter is inserted. In difficult cases, however, the flexibility of the Vygon pacing catheter makes it more difficult to position satisfactorily.

SITE OF INSERTION

The site selected for inserting the catheter is partly determined by the patient's clinical condition and partly by practice in the medical unit concerned. The choice is usually between the jugular vein, the axillary vein and the antecubital vein.

Jugular vein. This may be the only visibly dilated vein in an acutely shocked patient. It is easily entered and a flexible guide wire can be passed down to the superior vena cava. The flexible catheter introducer should be passed down to this level before withdrawing the introducing catheter, as the electrode catheter is sometimes held up at the thoracic inlet.

The jugular vein may also be used for permanent pacing with an intracardiac electrode and an external pacemaker. For this purpose it is necessary to insert the catheter by cutting down. When a catheter inserted into the jugular vein is used with an implanted axillary pacemaker, the catheter hub is drawn down by a long forceps passed up from the axilla subcutaneously. Most operators bring the catheter down in front of the clavicle.

Axillary vein. For emergency pacing the axillary vein is very suitable if a wholly percutaneous technique is available (see p. 79). For permanent pacing it is a feasible approach. A coil of catheter should be left in the axilla and the catheter anchored with a stitch to fascia close to the vein and another stitch close to the pacemaker.

Antecubital vein. This is the site of choice for temporary pacing. It is easily accessible, the insertion of the catheter is usually easy, and, if permanent pacing is envisaged, the insertion at this site permits a trial of pacing without compromising the sites used for implantation of a permanent pacemaker.

It is particularly important to avoid the jugular vein if the insertion of the permanent pacemaker is not to be performed until after a day or two of trial. Mediastinal infection is a considerable risk of the jugular route.

Subclavian vein. We now use the subclavian vein for all permanent pacemaker catheter insertions. The infraclavicular approach is used, the catheter being introduced by a Vygon catheter introducer through the skin incision used to place the pacemaker coil (Lucas type) or pacemaker unit in the pectoral region (see p. 80).

PLACING THE TIP OF THE PACEMAKER CATHETER

The optimal site for the catheter tip is the apex of the right ventricle where it is held in place by being entangled in the chordae tendinae. In this site it should be possible to pace the heart with a 1 to 2 volt impulse. Getting the catheter to this site has taken an experienced operator less than 6 seconds screening time on an indifferent X-ray set. It has also occupied the same operator for more than an hour in ideal radiological conditions. Like all catheter work, the ease with which the manoeuvre can be accomplished is quite unpredictable. The catheter should lie in a smooth curve along the lower border of the right ventricle and the tip should point directly at the apex of the heart (Fig. 20). If a 3 volt impulse does not produce a satisfactory response the site should be checked by recording the electro-cardiogram from the catheter. If a right ventricular pattern is obtained the catheter should be gently manipulated until a satisfactory response is gained. Other possible positions (coronary sinus, pericardium) are apparent from the E.C.G. and the catheter is then manipulated into the right ventricle.

When a satisfactory response and position have been achieved, the catheter is taped to the skin at the incision and, if the antecubital vein has been used, the catheter is doubled back up the arm to the shoulder, being taped to the skin at frequent intervals. The pacemaking lead is passed over the head pillow and connected to the end of the catheter at shoulder level. Fixed in this position it is usually not necessary to immobilize the arm.

The *apex* of the ventricle is the only satisfactory site. The heart can be paced from the right atrium but up to 30 volts are needed and each stimulus may produce enough contraction of skeletal muscle to shake the bed. Low voltage pacing can be obtained from the outflow tract of the right ventricle but the catheter is unstable in this position and is likely to work its way up into the pulmonary artery or be pushed back to the right atrium or even into the inferior vena cava by the heart's action.

Good quality fluoroscopy is necessary for this catheter manipulation. If a policy is adopted of inserting pacemaking catheters into patients with acute myocardial infarcts and a bundle branch block pattern, a portable image intensifier is desirable. This should be kept on the Intensive Care Ward for immediate screening in cases where emergency pacing has failed. To take and develop a radiograph to decide whether the failure is due to the electrode catheter moving up the pulmonary artery, into the right atrium or into the pericardial sac, may be to delay too long.

Float catheterization

By float catheterization is meant the insertion of catheters into peripheral veins with the intention that the natural flow of blood will sweep them up to the desired site. The various techniques have a valuable if rather limited usefulness in diagnosis and therapy. Several distinct methods can be distinguished. The use of a float catheter in association with the Ross needle is described elsewhere (see p. 95).

Float catheterization for the *monitoring of pulmonary artery* pressure has been advocated in the management of acute heart failure, particularly when due to respiratory disease. When successful, it permits a valuable observation to be made in acutely ill patients with virtually no disturbance and without the need for X-ray screening to

position the catheter. Suitable catheter material is polyethelene of 0·5 mm bore, 0·75 mm O.D., or the slightly larger Cardioflex catheters manufactured by Vygon specifically for the purpose. Introduction should always be by a plastic introducing cannula since these fine walled catheters are very easily sheared off by a needle or metal cannula.

The method is to introduce the plastic cannula and needle into a suitable vein, preferably the medial cubital. Suitable plastic cannulae are the Portex Intracath, the Vygon arterioflex or the Braunula. The needle is withdrawn leaving the cannula in place. The catheter connected to a pressure transducer and filled with saline is then passed into the vein and 10 cm or more passed up. The cannula is withdrawn and remains threaded over the catheter. Light pressure is now applied to stop bleeding. Once bleeding has stopped the catheter is advanced while the pressure record is observed continuously on an oscilloscope or direct recorder. If all goes well the ventricle is entered, signalled by an obvious change in the pressure tracing and shortly afterwards entry into the pulmonary artery causes a much less obvious alteration to an arterial wave form. The operation is made much more certain if the intracardiac E.C.G. is monitored by filling the catheter with sodium bicarbonate solution and connecting the chest lead of the monitoring E.C.G. to the lumen of the catheter. This is most easily accomplished by having a metal connector for the catheter to which a suitable alligator clip is attached. The alligator clip has a socket to fit the pectoral lead. The characteristic E.C.G. pattern enables the position in the atrium to be recognized as well as the ventricle and artery.

The main disadvantages of the technique are its uncertainty (it is impossible to know what is happening if it fails) and the damping which may occur. This may be reduced by using a catheter as short as possible and avoiding long connections. The pressure transducer should be attached direct to the catheter—and having a metal nipple makes a suitable connection point for the E.C.G. alligator. Damping can also be greatly reduced in these catheters by a very slow continuous saline or bicarbonate infusion of less than 1 ml per minute made by a suitable power-driven syringe. It is essential to check before insertion that the rate of infusion is not high enough to cause a spurious rise in the pressure recorded by the transducer. Success with this technique is improbable if the heart is very large and virtually impossible if the right atrium is dilated, e.g. by rheumatic carditis.

The second technique, which we have found of great value, is the use of the *Swan-Ganz catheter*. This is a soft radio-opaque double lumen catheter. One lumen provides an end hole for pressure monitoring. The second permits the inflation of a small balloon of 2 ml capacity just proximal to the end of the catheter. The catheter is introduced by cut down or large plastic cannula into the medial cubital vein. It is passed to the superior vena cava when the balloon is inflated with 1 ml of air. It is quickly swept to the periphery of the pulmonary arterial tree monitored by the pressure and/or intracardiac electrocardiogram as described above. A reliable wedge pressure can then be obtained by inflating the balloon with a further 1 ml air which effectively blocks the pulmonary artery. The tracings are of high quality and we have found the wedge pressure measured in this way to be a more consistent reflection of the directly measured left atrial pressure than the measurement of W.P.C.P. with a Cournand catheter (Batson et al., 1971). We have had about 85 per cent success with this catheter, the failures include being held up at the thoracic inlet, failing to traverse a large atrium, or rarely, failing to pass beyond a very large ventricle. The Swan-Ganz catheter is particularly valuable for assessing very ill patients with rheumatic heart disease or investigating patients as outpatients. It is sometimes useful for pressure measurement in difficult congenital lesions (Jones & Miller, 1973).

A third float catheter technique may be described as *selective float catheterization*. There are occasions when no amount of manipulation will persuade a catheter to pass through a stenosed pulmonary valve or pulmonary artery band. If a measurement beyond the suspected narrowing is essential it is rarely possible to pass a float catheter through it from a peripheral insertion because the blood streaming up the aorta will usually take the catheter with it. In these circumstances a suitable open end catheter should be passed up to as close to the area as possible to act as a guide. A fine polythene catheter is then passed through this guiding catheter and should then be swept through into the pulmonary artery. We have found this situation arises particularly in transposition of the great vessels with pulmonary valve stenosis, or after pulmonary artery banding, or operations on the pulmonary valve or infundibulum.

Any open ended catheter with a smooth bore is suitable for use as a guide catheter but clearly, it must be possible to pass it to the required position and it must be possible to pass the float catheter through it. On varying occasions a teflon Gensini catheter, a Ross needle introducer and a length of teflon tubing have been used. The use of a Gensini catheter requires very fine polythene tubing as the end hole is 0·035 inches diameter. It is difficult to push this float tubing through a full-length catheter, particularly if the catheter contains blood. We have found that a slow infusion of saline through the float catheter while it is being passed down the guide catheter greatly facilitates its passage. As already mentioned the float catheter should be kept as short as possible. The tracings obtained are often somewhat damped, but even with a long float catheter good records are possible.

Another float technique which can be of great value is a semi-float *pacemaking catheter*, the Vygon pacing catheter. It is possible for an experienced operator to place this catheter in the right ventricle in a position suitable for artificial pacing using only the intracardiac electrocardiogram for guidance. However, most centres undertaking pacing would have suitable fluoroscopy which greatly simplifies the procedure. The flexibility of the catheter which justifies its description as 'semi-floating' makes it easy to use in most patients. However, on occasions when entry to the ventricle is difficult, its poor torque is a considerable disadvantage. It is supplied ready sterilized in a pack with an introducing needle and plastic cannula—the Vygon arterioflex. After introduction, the cannula can be completely removed as the pacemaking catheter has a constant diameter. The plastic cannula (like the Braunula) has a rather sharp end and is moulded out of hard material. It is not difficult to drive it through the vein wall after removal of the introducing needle, if it is roughly handled. This can make the percutaneous introduction of the pacing catheter, intended to save time, into a time waster when seconds may count, since the catheter is easily passed up in the subcutaneous tissues. Since there is no lumen, the only clues to the fact that the catheter is not in the lumen of the vein are the discomfort to the patient and difficulty in its passage. Both these warning signs may be very slight.

References

BATSON, G. A., CHANDRASEKHAR, K. P., PAYAS, Y. & RICKARDS, D. F. (1972). Comparison of wedge pressure measured by the flow directed Swan-Ganz catheter with direct left atrial measurement. *Cardiovasc. Res.,* **6,** 748.

SWAN, H. J. C., GANZ, W., FORRESTER, J., MARCUS, H., DIAMOND, G. & CHARETTE, D. (1970). Catheterization of the heart in man with use of a flow-directed balloon-tipped catheter. *New Eng. J. Med.* **283,** 447.

JONES, S. M. & MILLER, G. A. H. (1973). Catheterization of the pulmonary artery in transposition with Swan-Ganz flow directed catheter. *Br. Heart J.* **35,** 298.

11. Left Atrial Catheterization

The introduction of a needle or cardiac catheter into the left atrium can provide information of very great value in acquired and congenital heart disease. The main stimulus to this approach to the heart has been the investigation of mitral valve disease where the use of the wedge pressure measurement in the pulmonary capillaries proved a somewhat uncertain weapon in diagnosis. The pulmonary wedge pressure is often a reduced and damped version of the pressure in the left atrium and, all too frequently, many attempts to record wedge pressure in the human lung result only in varying degrees of damped pulmonary artery tracings (Fig. 11.1). The difficulties in obtaining a satisfactory recording of the wedge pressure are discussed in the section dealing with right-sided cardiac catheterization. Three lines of approach to the left atrium have been devised.

The simplest direct approach is by the *insertion of a needle* into the back (Bjork *et al.*, 1953). This is advanced past the vertebral bodies into the left atrium. It is a procedure not without risk, it requires a general anaesthetic and the results obtained are indifferent since the patient must be placed either on one side or prone to enable access to the back. This requires considerable manoeuvring of an unconscious patient and the procedure is not too well tolerated by ill subjects.

The second approach to the left atrium is *via the bronchoscope* (Allison & Lenden, 1955; Faquet *et al.*, 1952). In this technique a bronchoscope is passed down the trachea and a long needle is stabbed through the carina into the left atrium. This procedure is also open to the objection that the patient is either anaesthetized or, if conscious, can hardly be regarded as in a state of rest when the measurement is made. The insertion of the needle may produce considerable pain and it seems unlikely that any measurement made under these conditions can have much value.

The most commonly used technique of reaching the left atrium at present is *transseptal puncture* (Ross, 1959; Ross *et al.*, 1960). In this, a long needle is passed up the femoral vein to the right atrium and stabbed through to the left atrium, passing through the fibrous area of the inter-atrial septum. In the description which follows, the original technique of Ross will first be described and then the subsequent modifications of this discussed.

The apparatus needed for the puncture of the atrial septum includes a suitable needle. The standard model is

24-in long and is equipped at the lower end with a needle hub to which is attached a pointer indicating the direction of the curve at the other end. The end which is inserted has a bevelled point designed to pass readily up the inside of an introducing catheter. This is of size 9F for the standard needle and is approximately 1 cm shorter than the length of the needle from the tip to the beginning of the hub. This ensures that when the needle is pushed fully up the catheter only 1 cm of unguarded steel projects beyond the sheath of the catheter. It is convenient to have a plastic tube connection suitable for joining the hub of the needle to the recorder. A further piece of equipment is a long flexible fine plastic tube which will pass down the lumen of the needle and project beyond the tip for some 10 to 20 cm. The operator end of this tube should be splayed out and connected to a suitable hub so that recordings of pressure or injections can be made through it.

Under local anaesthesia the long saphenous vein is exposed in the upper part of the thigh, preferably the right. The right side of the heart may be catheterized

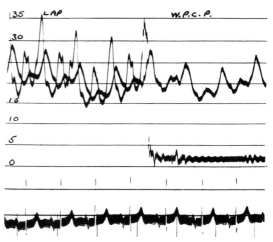

FIG. 11.1 Simultaneous recording of left atrial pressure and wedge pulmonary capillary pressure to show the usual distortion in the W.P.C.P. record. On the left both are recorded, on the right L.A.P. transducer has been switched off. The W.P.C.P. is damped compared to the L.A.P. with a lower systolic pressure. Transmission through the pulmonary capillary bed has also caused a slight time lag as well as loss of detail.

and then the left atrial puncture undertaken. The introducing catheter is first passed up the inferior vena cava into the right atrium and carefully screened so that the tip is seen to lie free in the cavity of the atrium. A Ross needle is then inserted and passed gently up until it is evident from the contour of the catheter that the needle tip has reached the right atrium. Care is taken to ensure the tip does not protrude beyond the end of the Cournand catheter by maintaining a distance of just over 1 cm between the hub of the Ross needle and the hub end of the Cournand catheter. Patients occasionally experience a little discomfort as the curved tip of the needle passes up the inferior vena cava and in some patients considerable discomfort may be experienced if the left leg is used for this procedure rather than the right. The tip of the catheter is now passed up the right atrium with the needle curve directed antero-laterally until it is judged to be well above the level of the tricuspid orifice. If the shadow of the left atrium cannot be made out by adjusting the screening current, help in this respect may be obtained from the inspection of a plain film of the chest taken before the procedure commences. The needle is now rotated until its tip is directed postero-medially. It is then possible to move the tip gently up and down the inter-atrial septum. It is usually easy to determine when the tip lodges in the foramen ovale as a very characteristic sensation of arrest occurs, often with a forcible transmitted pulsation.

The needle tip is then gently advanced from the end of the catheter and if the site has been correctly chosen, it is usually possible to feel the septum being punctured by the needle tip. The pressure tracing will commonly change its character and a sample of blood may be taken to confirm that the left side of the heart has been entered. In addition the circulation time may be measured using an ear oximeter. The shortened time from the left side of the heart also confirms the passage through the atrial septum (Fig. 11.2). It is convenient in this technique to connect the pressure recorder to the end of the Ross needle by a length of plastic tubing. The recorder may now be disconnected and the narrow plastic tubing passed up the lumen of the needle into the left atrium. This may pass through the mitral valve in favourable cases and permit measurements of the gradient across the valve. It is sometimes possible to pass through the aortic valve by this technique, but it must be remembered that every additional length of catheter of this bore makes accurate recording increasingly difficult and unless extremely sensitive gauges are used, no useful pressure tracing will result. Further information may be obtained by injecting tracer substances into the ventricle beyond the mitral valve. In mitral incompetence there is a characteristic broadening of the tracing obtained which contrasts with that found in mitral stenosis.

There are a number of hazards attached to this tech-

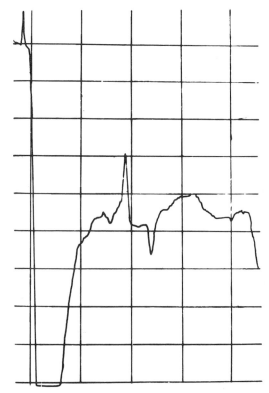

FIG. 11.2   A dye curve recorded with ear oximeter. Injection into the left atrium. Confirmation that the catheter has reached the left side of the heart is given by the appearance at the ear 2 seconds after injection. The subsequent vagaries of this tracing were unexplained. This occasional odd behaviour of dye curves lead to the trial of other indicators of intracardiac shunts.

nique. It is clearly a very blind procedure in which the identification of the left atrium depends on lodging the catheter tip in a site which is not visible on X-ray, but depends on the feel of the catheter. However, few complications have been reported by those using the Ross needle. The main hazard encountered has been the loosening of the soldered connection between the needle hub and the needle itself. This results in a misleading situation in which rotating the hub with its indicator does not produce any change in the position of the catheter. Once this phenomenon has been recognized it causes no difficulty since the needle can be withdrawn and a replacement inserted.

It is when one turns to the further developments of the Ross technique that the major hazards are encountered. An obvious advance was to pass the catheter itself into the left atrium (MacDonald and Millar, 1962). The Cournand catheter originally used would permit recording of pressure with a much less sensitive pressure gauge than is needed for the fine catheter passed through the lumen of the needle. The Cournand catheter, however, is unsuitable for angiography and selective angiography from the left side of the heart is an attractive prospect, allowing accurate diagnosis to be made in a variety of conditions.

Brockenborough et al. (1962) described a technique for left atrial catheterization which has been widely used but which has been associated with a higher incidence of complications than the simple Ross puncture. It has, however, many advantages; in particular, it is suitable for percutaneous insertion of the catheter and for left heart angiocardiography. Two needles are employed, both somewhat longer than the Ross needle. One is a straight blunt-tipped needle used for introducing the catheter as far as the right atrium, the other a curved-tip puncture needle whose terminal 1·5 cm consists of fine gauge tubing. Both needles are made of tubing of slightly small gauge than the Ross needle, with thinner walls. They are, therefore, much more flexible.

The Brockenborough technique employs specially made catheters which are radio-opaque and terminate in an end hole with multiple side holes. The tip of the catheter is kept on a wire former when not in use so that when this is removed the catheter assumes a curve of about three-quarters of a circle. The diameters of these circles range from 2 to 6 cm and are intended to facilitate the passage of the catheter through the mitral valve; the smaller diameters in normal atria, the larger ones in dilated atria. The straight introducing needle is about 1 cm shorter than the catheter; the fine tip of the curved puncture needle protrudes about 1 cm beyond the end of the catheter.

The method of insertion is as follows. A Seldinger wire is first inserted by the usual percutaneous technique into the right femoral vein. The Brockenborough catheter is passed over it on the straight introducer and advanced to the right atrium. The straight introducer is then withdrawn, the puncture needle inserted into the catheter and a puncture of the inter-atrial septum performed as in the Ross technique.

The fine gauge tip of the Brockenborough needle permits a very much smaller puncture of the left side of the heart than is possible with the Ross needle. Despite this apparent advantage, the Brockenborough needle has been a much more difficult instrument to work with than the Ross needle. The main hazard with the needle is its greater flexibility. This results in a number of unpleasant characteristics. The most dangerous is the failure of the needle tip to rotate despite the rotation of the hub. Thus, it may be that the needle with its catheter lodges in an anterior position in the right atrium. It is possible then to turn the needle hub to the correct postero-medial position and then to move the needle up and down the atrial wall in an apparently satisfactory fashion, until it catches in what appears to be the correct place. On advancing the needle tip, if it has lodged in some crevice in the anterior

part of the atrium, the aorta may be directly punctured with the needle. This accident has been reported by a number of investigators. In a similar fashion the needle may lodge posteriorly and may provide a somewhat unexpected method of diagnosing a pericardial effusion. There are verbal accounts of samples being obtained from the lung alveoli and from other structures outside the heart.

Another hazard of this technique is due to the nature of the catheter used. In order to permit the rapid injection of contrast medium, a plastic catheter with multiple lateral holes near the open tip is normally used for the insertion of the needle. The plastic wall of this catheter is readily perforated by the tip of the Brockenborough needle which is in any case sufficiently small to leave the catheter by way of one of the side holes near its end. It is thus possible to pass the needle up the lumen of the catheter to the right atrium where the needle makes a false passage through the side of the catheter wall. Good screening conditions are necessary to appreciate that this has happened, particularly if the patient is large. Clearly, attempts to pass the catheter through to the left atrium after this accident has occurred are dangerous.

The hazard of a false passage is considerably reduced by a modification of the technique suggested by Cope (1963). In this a fine flexible stainless steel guide wire is passed through the Brockenborough needle and projects beyond its tip for about a centimetre. The wire required for this purpose should be springy but somewhat soft, and its end should be rounded. If a suitable wire has been obtained, it should be passed until it protrudes through the needle. Frequent passes of the catheter with the wire in position should be attempted to make sure it is working satisfactorily before the catheter is inserted.

The attempt to puncture the atrial septum may sometimes be frustrated by the flexibility of the Brockenborough needle. On advancing the needle to puncture the septum, it sometimes happens that the curve near the end of the needle increases its convexity and the needle, instead of passing through to the left atrium, jumps up the inter-atrial septum. If this happens, it may be necessary to withdraw the needle and insert another with a less acutely curved end. Having punctured the septum and confirmed the position in the left atrium by the pressure tracing and either blood sampling or dye curve, the catheter and needle are advanced and, if all goes well, pass through into the left atrium. To achieve this smoothly the catheter end hole must fit the needle tip closely. Once within the left atrium the needle is withdrawn and pressures and dye curves recorded and angiocardiograms made.

The considerable risks and uncertainties of the Brockenborough technique has limited the use made of the method (Ardrouny et al., 1963; Libanoff and Silver,

1965). A modification which has proved more reliable and safe makes use of a Seldinger wire and the Ross needle (Verel, 1967). It has been used by a succession of registrars and post-graduate students without mishap, and may, therefore, turn out to be of general usefulness, and not merely one of the numerous techniques which are workable only in the hands of an unusually skillful few. The atrial septum is first punctured by the Ross needle, using the largest size available (16 gauge). For this purpose the point of the needle is directed either directly backwards or turned 10° to the patient's left rather than at 45° as recommended by Ross. A Seldinger wire wound from flattened stainless steel wire 0·035 in diameter and 180 or 200 cm long is then passed through until it lies well out in the lung field in a pulmonary vein (Verel, 1966) (Fig. 11.3). The Ross needle and introducer are then withdrawn, the wire wiped clean, and a Brockenborough left atrial catheter on a curved, blunt introducing needle passed over the wire into the left atrium. The Seldinger wire and the Brockenborough introducing needle are then withdrawn, leaving the catheter in the left atrium.

Once in the left atrium, it has usually proved possible to manipulate the catheter into the left ventricle, either by direct passage at the first attempt, but more usually after a period of manoeuvring. Useful tricks for this purpose are the redirection of the catheter with the curved introducing needle and the reinsertion of the Seldinger wire. The usual cause of failure to enter the ventricle is the large size of the left atrial appendage which tends to lie directly in the path of the catheter tip. If the introducing needle is reinserted until its curve is within the left atrium, it can be used to direct the catheter anterior to the appendage (it may be more correct to say anteromedial). The catheter is then advanced into the ventricle

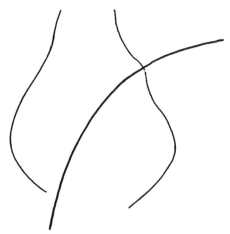

FIG. 11.3   Seldinger wire passed through puncture in the interatrial septum to the left atrium and then into a pulmonary vein.

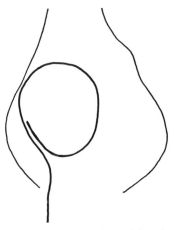

FIG. 11.4   Seldinger wire coiled up in the left atrium.

and the needle again withdrawn. If this fails it is often possible to get in with the wire. This is inserted with the catheter drawn well back towards the septum and a loop formed in the left atrium (Fig. 11.4). This is gradually withdrawn and the tip of the wire watched until a slight lateral movement shows that it is entering the mitral orifice; it will usually then advance to the apex of the left ventricle. The catheter is then pushed along the wire into the ventricle. Catheters are readily changed using the wire as a guide. Yet another manoeuvre is sometimes helpful in cases of difficulty: a springy obturator used to occlude the end of a Gensini catheter is bent at its tip to a curve of about 4 cm diameter and three-quarters of a circle; this can be inserted to the tip of the Brockenborough catheter and will not infrequently result in a curve which easily enters the left ventricle (Ross, 1966).

Transseptal puncture of the left atrium by any of the foregoing methods is still a potentially hazardous procedure. Much of the risk of this manoeuvre is due to the use of the needle which may be misdirected. Aldridge (1964) has described successful penetration of the foramen ovale by a stiffened catheter, and with practise this technique can be used successfully in over 90 per cent of cases. The following routine is at present regarded as the safest for transseptal catheterization.

A blunt Brockenborough introducing needle (U.S.C.C. Catalogue No. 9152) is bent at its tip for some 6 cm to a smooth curve of about 10 cm radius thus resembling a Ross needle with no point. A smooth 180 cm guide wire of 0·035-in diameter is passed to the right atrium via a needle puncture in the femoral vein. The Brockenborough catheter (U.S.C.I. Catalogue No. 7720-7735) is passed over the wire to the right atrium and the wire is then withdrawn. The bent introducing needle is now passed to the right atrium, if it sticks at any point it can usually be advanced by drawing the catheter and needle back 3 cm or so and then advancing the needle 3 cm.

Both catheter and needle are then advanced together. The difficult area is usually traversed in this way and the needle may be advanced.

The catheter is now passed up the atrium with the curve directed antero-laterally until it is at the upper extremity of the right atrium. The tip is rotated to a postero-medial position 15° to 30° from a true posterior direction and drawn down the atrial septum. It is usually possible to both feel the tip jump into the foramen ovale and also to see the slight medial movement on the X-ray screen. The catheter and introducer should lodge firmly if they are now advanced. The hub of the introducer is now rotated gently to turn the tip of the catheter from a true lateral to a true posterior position while the catheter tip is watched on the screen. A gentle to and fro rotation is continued and in over 90 per cent of cases this is followed, after a few twists, by a sudden or slow advance of the catheter through to the left atrium. This may be easily felt as a definite loss of resistance, or may be appreciated only by the change in the position of the catheter tip and the character of the tracing. The site of the catheter is confirmed in the usual way by injecting contrast or tracer and by blood sampling for oximetry.

The failures of this blunt dissection are usually due to failure of the catheter to lodge in the foramen ovale. This may happen in subjects with a normal left atrium (e.g. with aortic stenosis) in whom the foramen is flat and not easily picked up by the rather blunt catheter. Occasionally it happens in a subject with a dilated left atrium that the catheter rebounds up the septum each time pressure is exerted on it. Another cause of failure is to mistake the tricuspid orifice for the foramen ovale. Usually the catheter will not lodge securely in this site.

The higher position of the foramen in a normal atrium compared with the mitralized heart may cause confusion and the site to be missed. When the foramen ovale cannot be found, it is usually instructive to watch a pulmonary artery angiocardiogram on the television screen to see where the left atrium is. In patients with aortic stenosis the foramen ovale is usually much higher than it is in mitral stenosis.

Finally, caution is necessary in this blunt dissection. An incorrectly placed catheter can be pushed into the pericardial space with little difficulty. If blunt dissection fails, the Brockenborough catheter should be withdrawn after passing a guide wire to the atrium. The Ross introducer is then passed in over the wire, assisted, if necessary, by a polythene sheath over the wire. A Ross needle puncture is then performed. The position of the needle in the left atrium is confirmed by sampling and tracer curve. The guide wire 180 cm long and 0·035-in diameter is passed through the Ross needle into the left atrium until its tip is seen to lie well out in the lung field. The Ross needle is then cautiously withdrawn and the Brockenborough catheter on its bent introducer is passed up over the guide wire and through to the left atrium.

In rare cases the passage of a needle to the right atrium is a cause of considerable discomfort, and the introducing catheter is tightly gripped at the pelvic brim. This greatly reduces mobility of the catheter and makes the technique uncertain and dangerous. A complaint of discomfort from the patient, with a reduction in catheter and needle mobility is best treated by abandoning the investigation. The paper of Ross (1966) discussing the pros and cons of this technique should be read by all embarking on this investigation. Nevertheless, the relative ease and certainty of this approach to the left ventricle have led to its adoption for the assessment of aortic stenosis as the method of choice (Verel and Taylor, 1967). A combined left atrial catheterization and retrograde aortic approach to the left ventricle will, in most cases, permit the measurement of pressure in the left atrium, ventricle and aorta, together with angiocardiographic visualization of the entire left side of the heart. In this way a complete anatomical and functional assessment of the left side of the heart can be obtained.

The foregoing account describes the diagnostic catheterization of the left atrium and any pressure measurement or angiocardiogram needed for diagnosis can be made thereby. For research purposes it may be desirable to introduce a phonocardiographic catheter into the left atrium by transseptal puncture. The phonocardiographic catheter has a blocked up end and will therefore not pass along a guide wire. Forman et al. (1962) have found an ingenious solution to this difficulty. They pass a Ross needle and introducer, suitably shaped at the end, with an outer tube of thin-walled teflon into the left atrium. The needle and introducer are then withdrawn leaving a thin-walled tube leading into the atrium. The phonographic catheter can be introduced through this. Those interested will find the paper describing the technique gives an admirable account of the method.

The detailed references given for this section are, indirectly, an index of the difficulty of the technique. The unique information which it yields, however, makes its perfection a matter of great importance. Those who, like the author, have suffered many disappointments and frustrations in attempting transseptal puncture will find the very clear account of the technique by Soulié and his co-authors (1961) helpful. When the left atrium appears to have defeated the investigator, their simple statement should be recalled 'in effect, the right side of the auricular septum in man looks downwards, forwards and to the right, that is to say, roughly at the orifice of the inferior vena cava'.

The left atrium may be punctured by passing a shortened Brockenborough catheter to the right atrium by a right subclavian vein puncture made above the clavicle (see p. 80). A shortened introducing needle is then passed into the catheter and a suitable site on the left atrium found for puncturing the inter-atrial septum. We have used this technique occasionally when an approach from below was impossible because of pelvic vein thrombosis or other technical reason. It is also much easier to pass the catheter through a tight mitral stenosis from above. However, we have not adopted it as routine because the manipulation in the neck is alarming to the patient and the position is an awkward one if the patient has to be catheterized tilted head up at 30° to avoid pulmonary oedema. The descriptions by Loskot *et al.* (1965) and by Epstein and Coulshed (1971) should be consulted.

References

ALDRIDGE, H. E. (1964). Transseptal left heart catheterization without needle puncture of the inter-atrial septum. *Am. J. Cardiol.* **13**, 239.

ALLISON, P. R. & LENDEN, R. J. (1955). Bronchoscopic approach for measuring pressures in the left auricle, pulmonary artery and aorta. *Lancet*, **2**, 9.

ARDROUNY, Z. A., SUTHERLAND, D. W., GRISWOLD, H. E. & RITZMAN, L. W. (1963). Complications with transseptal left heart catheterization. *Am. Heart J.* **65**, 327.

BJORK, V. O., MALSTROM, G. & UGGLA, L. G. (1953). Left auricular pressure measurement in man. *Ann. Surg.* **138**, 718.

BROCKENBOROUGH, E. C., BRAUNWALD, E. & ROSS, J., Jr. (1962). Transseptal left heart catheterization, review of 450 studies and description of improved technique. *Circulation*, **25**, 15.

COPE, C. (1963). Transseptal left heart catheterization. Details of technique. *Circulation*, **27**, 758.

EPSTEIN, E. J. & COULSHED, N. (1971). Transseptal catheterization via the right subclavian vein. *Br. Heart J.* **33**, 658.

FAQUET, J., LEMOINE, J. M., ALHOMME, P. & LEFEBRE, J. (1952). La mesure de la pression auriculaire gauche par la voie transbronchique. *Archs. Mal. Couer*, **45**, 741.

FORMAN, J., LAURENS, P. & SERVELLE, M. (1962). Le cathétérisme des cavités gauches au micromanomètre par la voie transseptale. *Archs Mal. Coeur*, **55**, 601.

LIBANOFF, A. J. & SILVER, A. W. (1965). Complications of transseptal left heart catheterization. *Am. J. Cardiol.* **16**, 390.

LOSKOT, F., MICHALJANIC, A. & MUSIL, J. (1965). Left and right heart catheterization via the subclavian veins. *Cardiologia*, **46**, 114.

MACDONALD, J. S. & MILLER, B. L. (1962). Selective transseptal angiocardiography of the left side of the heart. *Clin. Radiol.* **13**, 195.

ROSS, J. (1959). Catheterization of the left heart through the inter-atrial septum: A new technique and its experimental evaluation. *Surg. Forum*, **9**, 297.

ROSS, J. (1966). Considerations regarding the technique for transseptal left heart catheterization. *Circulation*, **34**, 391.

ROSS, J., BAUNWALD, E. & MORROW, A. G. (1960). Left heart catheterization by the transseptal route. A description of the technique and its application. *Circulation*, **22**, 927.

SOULIÉ, P., SERVELLE, M., FORMAN, J., OSTY, J., BALEDENT, P. & EAGLE, C. C. P. (1961). Le cathétérisme des cavités gauches par la voie transseptale. *Archs. Mal. Coeur*, **54**, 481.

VEREL, D. (1966). An improved Seldinger wire. *Lancet*, **1**, 1107.

VEREL, D. (1967). Catheterization of the left atrium by Ross needle and Seldinger wire techniques. *Br. Heart J.* **29**, 380.

VEREL, D. & TAYLOR, D. G. (1967). Assessment of aortic valve gradient by left ventricular puncture and simultaneous transseptal catheterization. *Br. Heart J.* **29**, 633.

12. Left Ventricular Catheterization

The most satisfactory catheter approach to the left ventricle is by retrograde catheterization of a peripheral artery, followed by the passage of the catheter through the aortic valve into the left ventricle. Because of the ease of puncture and the low incidence of complications, the *femoral artery* is the most satisfactory routine point of entry into the arterial system.

If the femoral artery approach is found impossible, e.g. because of tortuous iliac arteries or aortic coarctation, other approaches to the left ventricle may be used. These include retrograde catheterization of the *axillary artery*, *transseptal* puncture from the right to the left atrium, and rarely, by direct *percutaneous left* ventricular wall puncture. If there be a patent foramen ovale, an atrial or a ventricular septal defect, the left heart chambers can often be entered by a catheter introduced from the peripheral veins into the right heart chambers.

The femoral artery may be catheterized either by a closed percutaneous puncture using the Seldinger technique or, rarely, by surgical exposure of the artery with direct-vision arteriotomy or puncture. The latter technique may be necessary in children under 1 or 2 years but with experience, Seldinger catheterization may be successfully performed even in neonates.

If the Seldinger approach is used, the catheter must have an end hole to thread onto the guide wire. If it is desired to introduce a catheter without an end hole, e.g. N.I.H. catheter, this can be accomplished by means of a *percutaneous catheter introducer*, e.g. Vygon desilet. This is a very useful adjunct: a very thin plastic sleeve is introduced into the femoral (or brachial) artery (or vein) via a modified Seldinger guide-wire technique, the catheter is then passed through the sleeve into the artery or vein. The catheter can be exchanged for another catheter if desired, through the plastic sleeve without the use of the guide wire. In this way, catheters without end holes can be satisfactorily introduced into the right or left side of the heart, by a very satisfactory percutaneous technique.

The Seldinger catheterization of the femoral artery is the standard approach for a catheter with an end hole, and is used by the great majority of investigators in all patients above the age of 2 or 3 years. The technique used by the authors has been discussed in detail (p. 79).

Retrograde catheterization of the left ventricle

Once the catheter is successfully introduced into the femoral artery, the tip of the guide wire may be withdrawn a few cm until it lies within the catheter. This can be checked by fluoroscopy or by measurement of the protruding length of wire. Blood will pour from the catheter at this stage and the tap cannot be closed because of the guide wire. A very useful technique is to pass the free operator's end of the wire into a piece of wide-bore polythene or nylon connecting tubing which links the catheter to a hand syringe which can perfuse the catheter with saline or contrast medium. This technique results in a bloodless procedure, apart from a few drops of blood lost before the guide wire has been introduced into the needle.

In the great majority of patients, the catheter guide wire assembly can be threaded without difficulty through the iliac arteries into the aorta. In elderly patients, the iliac arteries may be very tortuous and it may be difficult or impossible to negotiate the convolutions. No force should ever be used; the catheter should be gently advanced under fluoroscopic control, injecting a few ml of contrast medium to visualize the course of the artery. If the catheter cannot be threaded through the iliac artery, the catheter should be withdrawn a few cm, the original wire withdrawn and replaced by a *J-wire* with an adjustable centre core wire. The J-guide wire is a most valuable implement and with skill, it can be induced to traverse very tortuous vessels. The manipulation of the J-wire is discussed on p. 73. An alternative is to use a pig-tail catheter, the curved floppy end of which is very useful to negotiate a tortuous vessel as it does not penetrate into the arterial wall as does a straight catheter or guide wire.

Occasionally the guide and catheter will pass into the circumflex iliac artery (Fig. 17): after about 8 cm of catheter has entered the artery it becomes arrested and fluoroscopy will demonstrate that it has passed sharply laterally above the inguinal ligament. The catheter is then withdrawn under fluoroscopic control until the catheter and guide wire lie almost at the puncture site, the catheter is rotated, directed medially and may then be induced to enter the external iliac artery and reach the common iliac artery and aorta. Quite often, this manoeuvre is unsuccessful and the catheter and guide must then be withdrawn and a completely new femoral artery puncture performed. Before the catheter is withdrawn, it is well worthwhile trying a J-tipped guide wire, the curve of the J often inducing the guide wire to take the main stream direction up the external iliac artery.

If at any stage in the catheter manipulation, blood does not flow through the catheter when the syringe is disconnected, this is a strong indication of an unsuccessful catheterization and usually means that the catheter is passing into the arterial wall. The catheter is then withdrawn until a brisk blood flow is resumed and a further attempt made to thread the catheter or guide wire up the arterial lumen. Usually this will be unsuccessful and the catheter will have to be withdrawn again to obtain a brisk blood flow. A J-shaped guide wire should then be introduced into the catheter and an attempt is made to pass the flexible J tip through the tortuous vessel. If this is achieved, it is usually possible to thread the catheter over the guide wire.

It is unusual for trauma to the intima to cause clinically significant arterial damage, provided that care is exercised throughout the procedure.

Once the aortic bifurcation has been reached, there is rarely difficulty in passing the catheter up to the aortic arch. Exceptions are in aortic coarctation or severe atheromatous obstruction of the aorta which may occasionally be quite impossible to traverse.

In many patients, particularly under 40 years of age, the catheter-guide wire assembly will tend to pass directly into the left subclavian and vertebral artery rather than curve round the aortic arch. When this occurs, the guide wire is withdrawn so that its tip lies well within the catheter which will then assume its preformed curve. The curved catheter can then usually be threaded with ease round the aortic arch into the ascending aorta. Occasionally the catheter tip will enter the innominate artery; this will be readily seen on the screen and the catheter is then withdrawn into the aortic arch, rotated, advanced and usually enters the ascending aorta without difficulty.

If these manipulations are unsuccessful and the catheter cannot be passed round the aortic arch but repeatedly enters the major arch branches, then the curve of the catheter is not tight enough. The original catheter is then withdrawn, *leaving the guide wire in the iliac artery*. The same or a new catheter with a more sharply curved end or a pig-tail shape is threaded over the guide wire and will usually negotiate the aortic arch.

When the ascending aorta is gained, the E.C.G. monitor should be checked and the tracing should be constantly observed for any change in wave form or dysrhythmia. These may occur if a coronary artery is unwittingly entered or if the left ventricular outflow is entered and irritated.

The catheter tip is carefully passed down the ascending aorta to the aortic valve. In many cases, the catheter tip will continue retrogradely unimpeded through the valve into the left ventricle. This can be seen at fluoroscopy and

is usually heralded by two or three ventricular extrasystoles as the left ventricular outflow is always sensitive to the presence of the catheter.

In soft cases, the catheter will not traverse the aortic valve so readily. The guide wire is then withdrawn a few centimetres to allow the catheter to assume its full preformed curve. The catheter (if non radio-opaque) is kept filled with contrast medium in order to permit continuous fluoroscopy. The catheter is then advanced a little further, its tip will reach the aortic valve, be deflected and the convexity of the terminal curve of the catheter will then come to lie against the aortic aspect of the aortic valve cusps. Further gentle advancement will usually enable the curved presenting part of the catheter to traverse the valve and enter the left ventricle. If this does not occur, the catheter is withdrawn a little and again presented to the valve. This procedure can be repeated several times in a few seconds and in most cases, the catheter will eventually pass through the valve. For this technique, the extreme pliability of the non radio-opaque polythene catheter is a considerable advantage.

If this technique is not successful, the catheter is withdrawn into the middle of the ascending aorta, the guide wire threaded through the catheter tip until about 8 cm of the flexible end of the wire protrudes. The catheter guide wire assembly is cautiously advanced up to the aortic valve and played upon its surface. Often the wire finds the lumen of the valve and enters the left ventricle. The guide wire must not protrude for more than one minute (p. 130).

During these attempts to traverse the aortic valve, the catheter can be rotated either clockwise or anti-clockwise as it is advanced, but with polythene or Kifa-Odman catheters, one has little control of rotation of the tip of the catheter due to the low torque of the tubing.

If the aortic valve is not negotiated after 5 or 10 minutes of attempts as outlined above, the catheter should be withdrawn and replaced by a catheter with a different shaped terminal curve. Another type of catheter may be tried e.g. a pig-tail polyurethane type (e.g. Cordis).

The attempts to traverse the aortic valve are then repeated with the new catheter.

With a normal aortic valve, the left ventricle can be entered by the above technique in about 95 per cent of patients. With aortic valve stenosis or a grossly deformed incompetent valve, the success rate is considerably less.

Many operators prefer to start with a manufactured (expensive) pig-tail catheter, as it is usually easy to traverse the aortic valve and lies well in the left ventricle, making sub-intimal injection and recoil very unlikely.

It is important to avoid, wherever possible, withdrawing the protruding guide wire through the tapered end of the catheter in the left ventricle, ascending aorta or aortic arch. This is because platelets and red cells

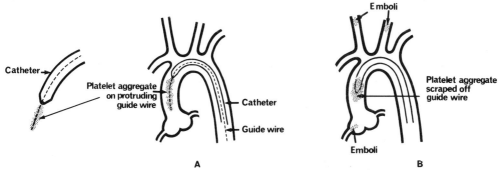

A   **B**

FIG. 12.1 Thrombo-embolic complications of Seldinger Technique.

A. The guide wire protrudes through the catheter, and platelets aggregate on the surface of the guide wire. This is shown in the close-up drawing on the left.

B. When the guide wire is withdrawn through the catheter,

the tapered tip of the catheter scrapes the platelets off the guide wire to produce a dangerous unsupported aggregation of platelets at the tip of the catheter. Fragments may be broken off and may lodge in a critical artery such as a coronary or cerebral artery causing a major clinical complication.

aggregate on the protruding length of guide wire and become scraped off as the guide wire is withdrawn through the tapered catheter tip. This may result in a blood aggregate being left on the tip of the catheter, and the clot may break off and embolize into a vital artery such as a coronary or cerebral artery. This complication may arise during ascending aortography, left ventriculography as selective coronary or cerebral arteriography. The problem is illustrated in Figure 12.1. The important point is that, whenever possible, the guide wire should never be allowed to protrude through the catheter in the left ventricle, ascending aorta or aortic arch. On a few occasions however, it is necessary to allow the guide wire to protrude through the catheter for a few seconds in order to achieve the desired catheter position.

Difficulties may arise during the above procedure of aortic valve approach.

The catheter may curve back on itself at the aortic aspect of the valve and further advancement may result in the lengthening of the tapered limb of the catheter curve (Fig. 12.2) so that the catheter tip re-enters the aortic arch whilst the catheter curve is still at valve level. Further catheter advancement will result in the tip entering the head and neck arteries or it may even pass round the aortic arch to reach the descending aorta.

In this state, the convexity of the catheter curve lies against the aortic valve and it is not unusual for the operator to be able to pass this convexity into the left ventricle. If the returning limb of the catheter tip is short, sufficient of the catheter may be introduced into the left ventricle to permit the catheter tip to enter this chamber and achieve a position suitable for injection of contrast medium. It is not uncommon however for the curved loop of catheter to enter the left ventricle, but the tip of the catheter to remain in the aorta, perhaps caught at the origin of the innominate artery (Fig. 12.2B).

Further introduction of the catheter merely lengthens the catheter loop, the catheter tip with its holes remaining in the aorta. This is a frustrating situation but it does indicate that the aortic valve is capable of being traversed. The catheter should then be withdrawn into the descending aorta and straightened as discussed (pp. 104 and 121, Fig. 14.4). It should then be re-advanced and again presented to the aortic valve. If this procedure fails, then the

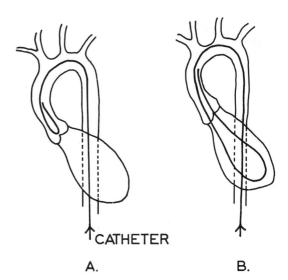

A.   **B.**

FIG. 12.2 *A Problem in Left Ventriculography*

A. The catheter tip is coiled back on itself, just above the aortic valve. This is a good position for traversing the valve.

B. Sometimes and unfortunately, the bend of the loop traverses the aortic valve, leaving the tip of the catheter (with its delivery apertures) remaining in the aorta. The angiographic injection cannot be delivered into the left ventricle. The long loop must be withdrawn into the aorta and straightened as shown in Fig. 14.4.

catheter should be changed for one of a different terminal curve preferably a more rigid catheter of the pig-tail type.

This excessive curving of the catheter usually occurs when the guide wire has been withdrawn far into a soft polythene catheter, or when the guide wire has been completely withdrawn and the valve has been 'played' with an unsupported catheter. Another cause is an incorrectly preformed (soft) catheter curve. To deal with this, the coiled catheter is bodily withdrawn into the descending aorta; this measure will often straighten the catheter which can then be re-introduced into the ascending aorta. If the catheter does not uncoil itself in the descending thoracic aorta, it is withdrawn into the abdomen and under fluoroscopic control, one attempts to catch the tip of the catheter in the mouth of a renal artery. If successful, the renal artery will hold the catheter tip whilst the curve of the catheter is withdrawn and the catheter will then flick straight (Fig. 14.4E). If a renal artery cannot be entered, then the catheter is withdrawn further and manipulated so that the sharp curve straddles the aortic bifurcation with the catheter tip passing into the contralateral common iliac artery (Fig. 14.4G). Further withdrawal of the catheter will then straighten out the kink of the catheter and then allow the straightened catheter to be passed upwards again into the aortic arch.

Whilst it is theoretically possible to form a knot in the catheter, the writer has not had this misfortune in more than a thousand left ventricular catheterizations performed in the manner described above.

Another difficulty may be encountered when the catheter tip enters inadvertently a coronary artery—usually the left one. This usually occurs after the catheter has curved back on itself on the aortic valve and it generally indicates that the preformed curve of the catheter is considerably less than half a circle. This complication will almost never occur if a pig-tail catheter is being used. The entry of the catheter into a coronary artery can usually be detected immediately at fluoroscopy as the catheter passes to the left instead of down into the left ventricle. It is important to keep a non-radio-opaque catheter full of contrast medium in order to detect this. The continuously observed E.C.G. may show an altered QRS or T wave; there may be a progressive bradycardia or an arrhythmia such as pulsus alternans or alternate extrasystoles. If a continuous pressure trace is being recorded, the pressure wave may become progressively diminished as the catheter passes down the narrowing coronary artery (Fig. 12.3): this is a very dangerous situation and the patient may complain of anginal precordial pain. The catheter must be *immediately*

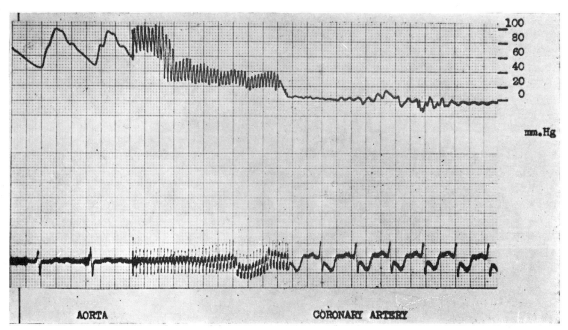

FIG. 12.3   *Coronary artery occlusion by catheter*. Grey Kifa catheter occluding left coronary artery of boy of 9 years. Upper trace —pressure manometry indicating cessation of flow through left coronary artery. Lower trace—E.C.G. (lead 2) demonstrating ST segment and T inversion during coronary occlusion. The catheter was withdrawn from the coronary artery immediately after the trace demonstrated here. After withdrawal of catheter there was initial bradycardia followed by return to normal E.C.G. and rate within 4 minutes.

N.B.—The recording paper speed was reduced to 1/10th normal rate near the centre of the trace. (Reproduced with permission of the Editor of The British Journal of Radiology.) R. G. Grainger (1965). Complications of cardiovascular radiological investigations. **38**, 201).

withdrawn from the coronary artery into the ascending aorta: after a few minutes rest, the catheterization can usually be continued without difficulty. The entry into the coronary artery can be confirmed fluoroscopically by injecting 2–4 ml of contrast medium but only if there is no fall in the continuously recorded pressure. The contrast medium used for this purpose should not be concentrated above 370 mg iodine per ml and should not contain a high percentage of sodium salt—in order to reduce to a minimum the risks of ventricular fibrillation. Conray 280, CardioConray and Urografin 60 or 76 are suitable media for this purpose and any risk incurred is extremely small.

Inside the left ventricle

When the catheter traverses the aortic valve, it enters the outflow tract of the left ventricle. This area is extremely sensitive to mechanical irritation and invariably ventricular extrasystoles occur immediately after catheter entry into the left ventricle (Fig. 13.3). The catheter is gently introduced further into the left ventricular cavity in an attempt to place the catheter tip in the centre of the ventricular cavity or towards the cardiac apex.

In the majority of patients, the extrasystoles cease as soon as the catheter tip has proceeded beyond the outflow tract and the operator can then adjust the catheter tip at relative leisure. The tip should be placed in the centre of the left ventricular chamber so that the injection of contrast medium will fill the chamber (both inflow and outflow) without inducing spurious mitral incompetence, which may be produced by injecting just anterior to the mitral orifice. A very stable position is that illustrated in Fig. 9 where the catheter curve is placed near the left ventricular apex and the catheter tip curves back to reach the mid-chamber.

In some patients, particularly those with rheumatic heart disease, the ventricular extrasystoles persist as the catheter is advanced further into the left ventricle. The patient will experience palpitation and may become apprehensive and even dyspnoeic as the cardiac output falls. The patient should then be reassured that the palpitation will soon cease and the catheter is left for a few seconds in the most suitable position that can be gained in the left ventricle. If, in the exceptional case, the catheter has entered the left ventricle with the guide wire protruding beyond the catheter tip, the guide wire is removed from the catheter as soon as the latter has entered the left ventricle. This is usually followed by cessation of the troublesome extrasystoles. If after about 20 s of catheter manipulation and trial of 'rest periods' within the left ventricle, the extrasystoles persist, the catheter *must* be withdrawn into the ascending aorta and left undisturbed for a few minutes. This invariably results in termination of the extrasystoles and the patient becomes relieved and regains confidence. A further attempt

at left ventricular catheterization is then made after the slow injection of 100 mg. of lignocaine through the catheter.

The author believes that in patients with rheumatic heart disease, the left ventricular outflow is more sensitive to mechanical irritation than is the outflow of the right ventricle. In a few patients this irritability is so great that no position can be found in the left ventricle at which the catheter tip may be placed without producing multiple extrasystoles. In these patients, it is advised that no injection of contrast medium be made, for there is an increased risk of producing ventricular fibrillation and also because the abnormal contractions of ventricular extrasystoles will not be an accurate guide to the usual cardiac action of the patient.

In placing the catheter in the optimum position within the left ventricle, it is essential to confirm that the catheter tip lies freely within the heart cavity and is not held rigidly by the papillary muscles against the endocardium. The more rigid catheters, particularly those of teflon, may actually penetrate the endocardium. This complication may sometimes be detected on the fluoroscopic screen by a sharp angular or rigid curve assumed by the catheter or because the catheter tip moves in unison with the adjacent heart wall rather than freely within the ventricular cavity. The free flow of blood through the catheter, the ease of saline injection and an undamped pressure trace are *no* criteria of the absence of this complication, for the side holes of the catheter may permit free access to the ventricular cavity even though the catheter tip may have penetrated the endocardium. A hand injected test dose of 5 to 10 ml contrast medium should always be made with the catheter in the position chosen for the major diagnostic injection of contrast medium. If the catheter tip has penetrated the endocardium, a small blob of contrast may persist in the ventricular wall at the end of the catheter and ventricular extrasystoles may be produced. Even a satisfactory hand test injection is *no absolute guide* to the absence of endocardial penetration. Fortunately, the soft pliable polythene catheters very rarely penetrate the endocardium and this is a major reason for the writer's preference for these catheters. In over five hundred left ventricular catheterizations using P.E. 240 soft polythene catheter, there has been only one instance of an intramural injection; using grey Kifa catheters, the incidence was about 1 to 2 per cent. Manufactured pig-tail catheters are very safe as the configuration and the flexibility of the terminal curve makes subintimal injection very unlikely.

An additional safety measure has been developed in this unit by the use of the cardiac catheter as an intracardiac electrode (Stentiford, 1968). For electric conductive purposes the catheter is filled with 5 per cent sodium bicarbonate and an E.C.G. trace is obtained using the catheter as an electrode. If the catheter tip has penetrated the endocardium, a bizarre QRST pattern with marked elevation of the ST segment is produced. The QRST complex becomes normal immediately the catheter tip disengages from the endocardium (Fig. 5.7).

This technique and the problem of the intramural injection is discussed further (Ch. 17).

A very high pressure injection (with rapid rise) may produce marked whipping of the catheter tip which increases the tendency to sub-intimal injection particularly in a small (infant) ventricle.

It is strongly recommended however that low-pressure injections should be made into the ventricles. A flow rate into the left ventricle of an adult should be no more than 8–12 ml/s and this is best achieved by an automated flow-controlled injector pump such as the Medrad, Contrac, Viamonte-Hobbs pump. The use of higher flow rates will probably cause ventricular extrasystoles which will distort the contraction pattern and may produce spurious mitral-valve incompetence.

References

BARON, M. G., WOLF, B. S., STEINFELD, L. & GORDON, A. J. (1963). Left ventricular angiocardiography in the study of ventricular septal defects. *Radiography* **81,** 223–235.

FIGLEY, M. M. (1964). Angiocardiography in valvular heart disease: morphologic and volumetric considerations. *Radiol. Clinics N. Am.* **2,** 409.

JACOBSSON, B. (1969). Platelet adhesion and aggregation following contact between blood and vascular catheters *in vitro. Scand. J. Haemat.* **6,** 216–220.

JACOBSSON, B., BERGENTZ, S. E. & LJUNGQVIST, U. (1969). Platelet adhesion and thrombus formation on vascular catheters in dogs. *Acta Radiol. Diagn.* **8,** 221–227.

JACOBSSON, B., PAULIN, S. & SCHLOSSMAN, D. (1969). Thromboembolism of leg following percutaneous catheterization of femoral artery for angiography. Symptoms and signs. *Acta Radiol. Diagn.* **8,** 97–107.

KJELLBERG, S. R., NORDENSTROM, B., RUDHE, U., BJORK, V. O. & MALMSTROM, G. (1961). Cardioangiographic studies of the mitral and aortic valves. *Acta Radiol.* Suppl. 204.

LIPCHIK, E. O., SHREINER, B. F., MURPHY, G. W. & DE WEESE, J. A. (1966). Angiocardiography evaluation of mitral valve stenosis. *Radiology* **86,** 839–842.

RAPHAEL, M. J. & ALLWORK, S. P. (1974). Angiographic anatomy of the left ventricle. *Clinical Radiology* **22,** 95–105.

13. Coronary Arteriography

Radiographic visualization of the coronary arteries has become a widely practised investigation as a result of surgical attempts to relieve angina pectoris. The operations performed have needed increasingly precise diagnoses as the surgeons have progressed from poudrage of the pericardium through endarterectomy to venous bypass grafts.

Radiology

The radiological equipment has to visualize small arteries against the background density of the thorax. The movement of the arteries due to the beating of the heart may reach 20 cm/s. Clear resolution of the coronary arteries therefore requires very short exposure times with high quality radiology. This is best achieved either by full size (e.g. 14 by 14 in) films on an A.O.T. changer or by pulsed cine equipment, although less sophisticated equipment can produce adequate results. Videotape monitoring of the cine is a useful accessory as this allows immediate assessment of the quality of the coronary angiogram but the 'stills' from the videotape are far inferior to 'stills' from cine films. In order to identify the main branches of the coronary arteries, exposures in at least two planes for each artery are needed. This involves at least four exposures, one for each coronary artery in each position. The movement of the patient into these positions is facilitated by the use of a rotating cradle in which the patient lies during the investigation, but its use entails increased radiation as the patient is lifted by the cradle to a greater distance from the X-ray tube than if the patient lies on the table top. High quality television screening is essential for positioning the catheter.

In order to identify the main branches of the coronary arteries, exposures in several projections are necessary. These are described in more detail later in this chapter. When using cine angiocardiography, frequent use is made of double image magnification which is helpful in elucidating lesions which appear doubtful on the single-image film. Particular difficulty may be experienced with lesions in the early part of the left coronary artery and its main branches. Oblique views taken 15° or so off-vertical with the camera moved headwards and the tube moved towards the feet may permit more certain diagnosis of lesions in this area (Eldh and Silverman, 1974; Aldridge et al., 1975). Multiple injections are therefore commonplace in making a satisfactory demonstration of abnormal coronary arteries and high-quality videotape is of the greatest value in deciding the scope of the investigation.

The movement of the patient into these positions may be achieved by a number of advances in technique which have recently become available. The simplest is the rotating cradle in which the patient can be rotated in a fixed axis under the camera. Alternatively the C arm is capable of rotating round the patient and also has the facility of permitting oblique views to be taken quickly. The main disadvantage of this apparatus is the necessity for changing the position of the camera if the view required necessitates swinging the C arm round the patient's head to the other side. A more recent development is the U arm. Here the tube and camera rotate on the same axis as the patient from a point some 3–4 ft rostral to the patient's head. The most recently developed machines also allow for oblique views in the sagittal plane as the tube and camera can be moved from the fixed vertical to oblique positions by a parallelogram arrangement of arms. These recent developments are described in Chapter 6.

Contrast media

The myocardium is very sensitive to disturbances in pH and electrolyte concentration. Marked changes in the electrocardiogram, and ventricular fibrillation may follow the injection even with the most suitable of the available contrast solutions (Fig. 13.1). Media containing a high sodium content should be avoided as their use leads to ventricular fibrillation in a significant number of cases. Not unexpectedly, contrast media entirely free of the sodium ion also cause an increase in complications, especially ventricular fibrillation. The optimal sodium ionic concentration is one about the same as that in plasma (140 mEq/1). The nearest approach to this is Triosil 370, but other useful media are Hypaque 65 and Urografin 76 (Verel et al., 1975).

Attention has been drawn to the risks of flushing the coronary arteries with physiological solutions of saline containing a high sodium concentration (Orvitt et al., 1972). We usually inject only contrast media into the coronary arteries. If flushing solutions are used they should contain a balanced mixture of ions, e.g. Hartmann's or Krebs' solutions, or alternatively, 5 per cent dextrose causes little disturbance if injected into human coronary arteries, although this is not the case in

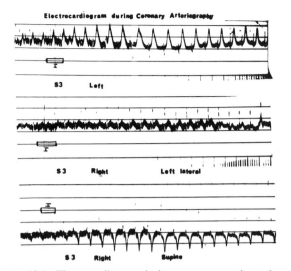

FIG. 13.1 Electrocardiogram during coronary arteriography. The three tracings show the typical T wave changes which may follow the injection of contrast medium into the coronary arteries. Upper trace—injection into the left coronary artery, patient supine. Middle trace—injection into the right coronary artery, patient in left lateral position. Lower trace —right coronary artery, patient in supine position. The marked difference in degree of the T wave inversion between the second and third injections is commonly observed.

experimental animals. Coronary arterial vasodilatation follows the injection of contrast media. A measurable increase in coronary blood flow was found to occur in 53 per cent of cases 5–10 s after injection. The flow returned to normal within one minute (Bassan *et al.*, 1975).

Catheters

Much early work of high quality was done by injecting contrast medium into the root of the aorta through a *loop catheter* of the type suggested by Bellman *et al.* (1960). The main disadvantages of this technique are the large volume of contrast medium injected and the manipulation of the catheter. The technique results in simultaneous filling of both coronary arteries, and does not give as good detail as selective coronary artery injection. Because of these disadvantages, aortic root injection has been largely replaced by selective injection of contrast medium into the individual coronary arteries by specially designed catheters.

Sones Catheters are plastic coated (woven) catheters made in 7F or 8F sizes. Both sizes taper towards the tip to 5F and have an end hole with two lateral holes placed about 2 mm from the tip. These side holes reduce the tendency of the catheter to obstruct the coronary artery. They are usually inserted by brachial arteriotomy but can also be introduced by Seldinger wire into the femoral artery. For satisfactory use the last few cm of the catheter

should be fixed in a suitable curve by a former when the catheter is autoclaved.

Judkins catheters are made from polyurethane tubing strengthened by fine spirally wound wires enclosed within the catheter wall. They are preformed into curves suitable for the right or left coronary artery (Fig. 13.2) and each catheter is available in three sizes. The size refers to the degree of terminal shaping of the tubing as all are of the same diameter. They end in a short narrow-angled tip with a single end hole. They are inserted by the Seldinger technique into the femoral artery using teflon coated guide wires. Standard steel guide wires will not easily negotiate the acute angle at the tip of these catheters and moreover the catheters tend to bind on the steel wires preventing easy manipulation.

A variety of *controllable tip* catheters is available for coronary arteriography, mostly based upon the Sones catheter. These catheters and their various control systems are very expensive and not very durable.

The *choice of catheter* for coronary arteriography appears to be very much one of individual taste and use. We have used Judkins catheters almost exclusively and have found them easier to control than the Sones catheter. Others have had the contrary experience, preferring the Sones which is easier to introduce into the right coronary artery. We have not used the controllable catheter sufficiently often for coronary work to feel confident with it. The need to withdraw the controlling

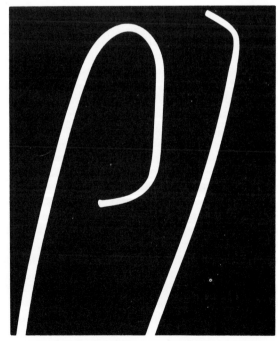

FIG. 13.2 Terminal curves of Judkins catheters. Left coronary catheter to left, right coronary catheter on the right.

guide wire before making a test injection has seemed to us to more than counter its advantage of having a controllable tip.

Precautions during coronary arteriography are important and should be taken in advance. In our experience ventricular fibrillation is a common-place event in this investigation (at least compared to its frequency in other catheter procedures). A D.C. defibrillator must be ready for instant use throughout the investigation, and all members of the catheter team including all the nursing staff present should be familiar with its use. A firm stool about 10 inches high should be kept near the X-ray table to give a higher stance for performing external cardiac massage since it is difficult for anyone of average height to give effective massage from floor level to someone on an X-ray table. If the patient is not investigated under general anaesthesia, an anaesthetist should be warned for emergency call. At all times the E.C.G. must be observed by an experienced technician who will give instant warning of any cardiac irregularity. In addition a doctor observes the E.C.G. throughout the course of any injection into a coronary artery. Ventricular fibrillation is more frequent following and during *right* coronary artery injection.

We have found the intravascular injection of Lignocaine 100 mg reduces the incidence of ectopic beats and of ventricular fibrillation. The effect lasts for 30 to 45 minutes and the drug is conveniently given through the same catheter into the descending part of the thoracic aorta at intervals during the investigation.

Throughout the catheterization, the catheter pressure is monitored. The catheter is connected to a three-way tap. One junction of this tap is used for the injection of contrast medium, the other is connected to a pressure transducer by plastic tubing. This should be at least 1 metre long to permit pressure monitoring during movement of the patient on the X-ray table. The pressure should be observed at all times during catheter manipulations. This is essential for both coronary arteries but the right coronary is more easily occluded by the catheter. The pressure monitoring should only be omitted during the actual injection of contrast medium and must be switched on *immediately* afterwards.

General anaesthesia for coronary arteriography is not usually needed since the procedure is painless. However, if external cardiac massage is performed in a conscious patient to maintain the circulation during rapid ventricular tachycardia or fibrillation, few investigators would continue the catheterization. When investigating patients who have long-standing angina with severe symptoms, we have preferred a general anaesthetic as ventricular fibrillation has frequently occurred. It has been possible to restore normal rhythm and complete the investigation despite several episodes of fibrillation.

Many investigators routinely inject Heparin (5000 U.) into the circulation through the coronary catheter when it is in the descending aorta as prophylaxis against thrombosis during investigations.

Catheterization

With the Judkins catheter, the left coronary artery is much more easily entered than the right. Either may be attempted first. The general tactic is to first identify the level of the aortic root on the screen by advancing the catheter until the valve is reached. The catheter tip is then introduced into the appropriate sinus of Valsalva and moved up or down until it passes into the desired coronary artery.

The sizes of catheter are intended to suit different diameters of aorta. Unless the aorta is obviously dilated, it is usually best to try the middle size first. The *left coronary catheter* is made with an almost complete loop at the patient end (Fig. 13.2) so it is necessary to pass it up on the guide wire. The guide wire is introduced by the Seldinger needle and the femoral puncture dilated with a plastic catheter dilator since the Judkins catheters do not end with a fine introducing edge. The left coronary catheter is then introduced and passed up with a few cm of the guide wire projecting through its advancing end. The patient is screened supine or rotated slightly. When the guide wire reaches the aortic arch the soft tip of the wire will usually find its way round into the ascending aorta. If, however, it enters one of the branches of the aortic arch and can be seen to pass into the neck or towards one of the shoulders, the catheter should be drawn back and the guide wire drawn back into the catheter. The natural curl on the catheter can then be used to direct it over the arch into the ascending aorta. It is important to withdraw the guide wire only one or two cm into the catheter. If drawn back too far, the catheter will be likely to form into its loop as it is advanced.

Once in the ascending aorta the guide wire is withdrawn and the catheter is advanced with its concavity coinciding with that of the arch. The catheter pressure is monitored continuously. In about half the cases the catheter will enter the left coronary artery first time and the investigator must be aware of this possibility. A fall in the pressure recorded may indicate that the coronary artery is blocked by the catheter (Fig. 12.2). Should this happen the catheter must be gently drawn back until a normal aortic pressure is recorded, *before* injecting a test dose of contrast medium. Injecting contrast medium into a blocked coronary artery is making bad worse and makes ventricular fibrillation almost a certainty.

More commonly the catheter tip enters the left coronary without obstructing it and its likely position is judged by experience (Fig. 13.3). One or two ml of contrast medium are gently injected by hand through the catheter. If the catheter is in the artery the outline of the

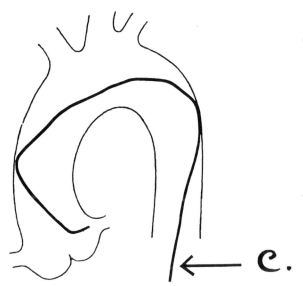

FIG. 13.3 Left coronary catheter (C) in position in the left coronary artery.

artery is seen on the fluoroscopic T.V. screen. If it is not, the contrast medium will be swept up the aorta.

Occasionally the left coronary artery is difficult to catheterize. This is usually because the first few cm of the aortic wall run almost horizontally so that the coronary artery takes an almost vertical course at its origin. The larger or smaller curve catheter may enter it, but sometimes even this is not possible. The catheter may be given an additional bend about 2 cm. from its tip to increase its curvature. If this fails the catheter tip should be placed as close to the origin of the artery as possible whence a large hand injection of about 10 ml contrast medium will usually give adequate pictures. After securing adequate left coronary angiograms (and checking them on videotape), the catheter is then withdrawn over the Seldinger wire.

The *right coronary artery* catheter is then inserted over the same wire. This catheter is easily manipulated into the ascending aorta by drawing the guide wire back from the tip and advancing the catheter with the angled tip pointed to the inner aspect of the curve of the aortic arch. Once in the root of the aorta the catheter is rotated through 180° so that the tip projects forwards and laterally to the right. It is usual to rotate the patient to L.A.O. for this. It is usually possible to recognize its entry into the right coronary artery by a sudden· lateral and downwards movement as it is gently moved up and down the aortic wall (Fig. 13.4). Again the coronary arterial pressure is carefully monitored throughout the movements of the catheter. Small injections of contrast will enable the artery to be localized, but the insertion of the catheter is more difficult than in the case of the left coronary artery.

Two factors largely contribute to this difficulty. One is the tendency of the catheter to enter the posterior sinus of Valsalva. It is very difficult to be sure of this when screening in the antero-posterior plane and it is surprising how often rotation of the patient into the lateral position will show that the catheter tip is pointing backwards and to the right instead of forwards and to the right despite the operator's conviction to the contrary. Screening in the L.A.O. position reduces the difficulty once the operator is orientated to the changed relations with the heart.

The second factor which makes the investigation difficult is the occasional tendency of the catheter tip to jump from the sinus of Valsalva to a point some 5 to 6 cm up the aorta each time it is slowly drawn back from the region of the aortic valve. In such circumstances it may be possible to enter the artery by pushing the catheter down the arch and drawing it back again gently rotating it between each sweep. If this does not work, it is not infrequently possible to get into the artery by passing the catheter on into the left ventricle, rotating the tip to what is hoped is the right position and then very slowly easing it out of the ventricle. If successful, the catheter tip jumps straight into the origin of the artery. Careful pressure monitoring is needed with the technician fully aware of the nature of the manoeuvre since the sudden transition from the ventricular trace to a low arterial pressure may indicate the catheter has blocked the coronary artery. Failure to enter the right coronary artery is more commonly due to incorrect positioning of the catheter than to using the wrong catheter. It is desirable to go on trying

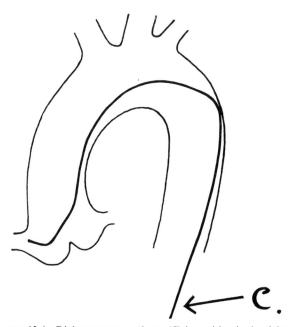

FIG. 13.4 Right coronary catheter (C) in position in the right coronary artery.

for much longer before deciding to change to a different curve.

The Sones catheter is generally accepted to cause fewer complications in the performance of coronary arteriography than does the Judkins catheter. This may well be the result of the lateral slots near the tip of the Sones catheter which allow blood to reach a narrow coronary artery that would be occluded by a Judkins catheter. However, this advantage must be weighed against the need to cut down on the brachial artery for the Sones technique and the time needed for repair of the artery after the investigation. Brachial arterial occlusion may occur following the investigation and while the rich anastomosis around the elbow-joint protects the forearm from major disaster, it limits the capacity for sustained work with the affected forearm (usually the right).

The insertion is usually performed from the right forearm. The brachial artery is identified at the antecubital fossa by palpation and dissected out through an incision which the author (D.V.) prefers to make in the line of the artery. It is usually possible to plan the site of the incision to avoid major veins. The artery is secured by snares in a length where no posterior branch enters between the snares and it is then opened as described (p. 78). Because of the arterial anastomosis at the elbow any branch entering between the snares will bleed profusely, and retrograde bleeding from the distal limb will also occur if it is not secured by a snare. Some make a practice of injecting heparin into the distal part of the brachial artery to lessen the risk of thrombosis but the author has not done this and has not observed thrombosis at the site of the arteriotomy. Any heparin, or other fluid will be dispersed rapidly by the anastomotic blood flow as can be easily demonstrated by releasing the lower snare following such an injection. Blood, not heparin, is seen to flow from the vessel.

Bleeding from the proximal end of the artery is controlled by a snare. If a pig-tail catheter is to be used for left ventricular angiocardiography, the tip of the catheter may be straightened by inserting a guide wire into the catheter as far as the tip. If this is not done there may be some bleeding while the curled tip is persuaded to enter the artery. The snare is loosened as the catheter is passed up and is adjusted so that the catheter moves easily without haemorrhage occurring. Any spasm induced by the snare or passage of the catheter will usually respond to the injection of some contrast medium into the arterial lumen just above the arteriotomy, and more contrast should be applied to the outside of the artery at the site of the spasm. After left ventricular angiocardiography the catheter is changed for the Sones which, inserted from the right arm, will usually reach the ascending aorta without difficulty.

Once in the aorta the level of the valves is identified by passing the catheter down until it either bends at the tip indicating that it has impinged on a valve cusp, or the pressure trace from the catheter indicates that it has entered the ventricle. The right coronary artery is usually the easier to enter with the Sones catheter. With a patient in the L.A.O. position the catheter is curved to point laterally to the right and, usually, slightly inferiorly. It will usually enter the coronary artery with little difficulty. Occasionally a curve may need to be set in the end of the catheter by alternate immersion in hot and cold water.

The left coronary artery is often more difficult to enter with the Sones catheter, particularly when its initial course is almost vertical. Here it may be necessary to produce a tight U-shaped curve on the catheter, either by flexing it in the root of the aorta against the valve cusps or with hot and cold water as described earlier (p. 78).

Injection of contrast medium for visualization of the arteries ideally requires preliminary checking of several important points. Both coronary arteries may divide immediately after their origin. In addition there may be narrowing at the very origin. The catheter must not be inserted so far that the first branch of the coronary artery is not visualized, and ideally some of the injected contrast should reflux into the aorta, so visualizing the origin of the artery. One or two test injections are made in the P.A. position to see if an optimal position is possible.

The screen should be positioned so that the origin of the artery is in the upper part of the field. In positioning for the right coronary artery, the catheter tip must be in the left upper quadrant. Both the branch to the pulmonary conus and the coronary sinus branch usually come off this artery and pass upwards above the level of the coronary origin. In the left coronary artery there are rarely any branches passing upwards so the catheter tip may be placed nearer to the top of the screen. The screen should include the whole of the heart to reveal any unexpected anastomoses which may have formed. In a large heart or if a five-inch image intensifier field is used, 'panning' of the screen along the course of the coronary artery is necessary during cine recording.

If the catheter has been inserted without reducing the pressure below aortic level, it is advisable to proceed at leisure. A test injection is made to make sure that the contrast is rapidly cleared from the coronary tree and that the screen position is suitable. We usually run a P.A. exposure of the artery on cine and videotape in deep inspiration and check the run on the videotape. A gentle injection of 6 to 10 ml by hand is given over 2 to 3 seconds. The patient is then rotated to the left anterior oblique position, while the pressure is carefully watched lest the movement forces the catheter further into the coronary artery with a fall in pressure. The screen position is readjusted and the run repeated. A lateral run is then made with the same precautions. All exposures for recording are made in deep inspiration to clear the liver shadow as far as possible from the field. If any doubtful area is seen on the videotape replay, a further run is made on double image centered on the area in question. If the apparatus permits, oblique double-image views are taken routinely of the early course of the left coronary artery. After obtaining adequate angiograms, the catheter is withdrawn.

When the introduction of the catheter causes a fall in coronary artery pressure to half the aortic pressure, the investigation is much less easy and much more dangerous. The catheter must remain in the artery for the briefest possible time. The left coronary artery can usually be visualized by the following method. The patient is positioned for the cine run with the catheter just above the orifice of the coronary artery. When the position is satisfactory the catheter is advanced into the artery, 6 to 10 ml of contrast injected over 2 to 3 seconds, and the catheter immediately withdrawn. This technique is occasionally possible with the right coronary artery, but usually the position is not sufficiently certain for this to be done. It may be possible to catheterize the artery with the patient in the left anterior oblique position or the lateral position and so allow a brief cannulation for the injection. In both cases, shortening the tip of the Judkins catheter by cutting off 1–2 mm. with a scalpel may allow entry to the coronary artery without a significant fall in pressure. If this is impossible, the artery may be filled by an injection of 10 to 20 ml of contrast given rapidly into the right coronary sinus of Valsalva. In this technique the successful recording of coronary arteriograms depends greatly on the skill of the radiographer and the equipment at his disposal.

Throughout these injections the *electrocardiogram must be closely observed*, preferably by a medically qualified member of the team. The member of the team making the injection observes the passage of the contrast medium through the coronary arteries. At the end of the injection, the contrast medium should clear from beyond the tip of the catheter. If it does not, it is likely that the catheter is obstructing the artery and should be immediately withdrawn. Often injection into the left coronary artery is followed by visible filling of the coronary sinus which may be recorded if desired. 'Panning' along the course of the coronary artery will be essential if the five- or six-inch intensifier field is used and this requires practice by a member of the team familiar with the anatomy and the equipment.

A left ventricle angiocardiogram is recorded in the right anterior oblique position to assess left ventricular function. If this is grossly impaired, further investigation may be unnecessary.

The main complications of this technique have been mentioned. Ventricular fibrillation is comparatively common (especially from right coronary catheterization), asystolic arrest less so. Runs of extrasystoles or ventricular tachycardia may occur and are alarming signs

and symptoms. Their frequency, as mentioned, may be reduced by injections of lignocaine. All these may be aborted by asking the conscious patient to cough. Failure of ventricular output requires immediate cardiac massage but the effect of forced coughing, if successful, may render this unnecessary. After every coronary artery injection, the patient may be made to cough vigorously for a few seconds. This increases coronary blood flow and increases cardiac output. However, it is essential that the confidence of the patient is maintained. With some patients it is better to avoid repeated requests to cough and proceed with a casual conversation designed to suggest that little of moment is likely to occur. Should a gross irregularity causing functional standstill be seen on the monitor, there is about 15 seconds during which the patient may be asked to cough. In every case the injection of contrast should be seen to be followed by its rapid clearing from the coronary artery. If this does not occur, the catheter should be *instantly withdrawn*.

Other hazards include damage to the intima of the coronary artery by the tip of the catheter, a build up of thrombus within the catheter which may cause embolism, and rarely intramuscular injection of contrast medium. It must be stressed that all catheter manipulations and contrast injections must be made gently. These catheters seem more liable to induce clotting than simple polythene or Kifa catheters and they must be perfused with physiological fluid or contrast medium every few seconds. Our experience in this respect differs from that of Nejad et al. (1968) who investigated the formation of surface cotting on various catheters in dogs.

Assessment of the results of angiography depends upon a thorough knowledge of the anatomy of the coronary arterial tree and its variations. Double origins are more common for the branches of the right coronary artery, the conus branch originating separately in 10 per cent or more of cases. The work of Paulin (1966), using aortic injections with a loop catheter, should be consulted by all embarking on coronary angiography. His monograph, besides providing a clear analysis of the anatomical variations, is illustrated by a series of angiocardiograms which investigators using more sophisticated and recent techniques of injection and radiography will be pleased to equal. Identification of particular branches depends upon comparing the cine runs obtained in two or three planes.

The selective coronary angiographic method and interpretation as discussed in Judkins' theses have become widely accepted.

Coronary artery anatomy

The coronary arteries derive their name from their resemblance to a royal crown (*corona*, L., a crown). This well describes the basic pattern of the arterial supply to the heart. An arterial ring encircles the heart in the atrio-ventricular groove, and branches pass from this at intervals over the exterior of the ventricles towards the apex of the heart. The classical anatomy textbook names only two of these arteries which supply the ventricle largely because the distribution of the arterial supply varies greatly in detail. The recently developed techniques of coronary artery surgery, however, have necessitated precise localization and characterization of coronary arterial lesions, and several differing systems of nomenclature for the branches of the coronary arteries have come into use in the past ten years. Kaltenbach and Spahn (1975) compare nine different systems.

The anatomy and function of the heart primarily determine the distribution of the coronary arteries. Blood has to be supplied to the ventricles, more being needed by the thicker-walled left ventricle than is required to maintain the right, and an adequate supply has to reach such structures as the sino-atrial node, the A.V. node and the ventricular septum. In considering the detailed anatomy in an individual case, the general pattern is based on the original concept of the anatomist, that is, that the right and left coronary arteries pass round in the atrio-ventricular groove to meet at the back of the heart where the interventricular septum intersects the atrio-ventricular groove. This point is anatomically described as the posterior crux, and is commonly alluded to as simply the 'crux' since the anterior crux usually has no particular significance lying as it does in the area between the origins of the two coronary arteries from the aorta.

The nomenclature used for the coronary arteries and their branches which is now in common use is a mixture of terms derived from classical anatomical studies, surgical anatomy, and the radiological appearance. In this brief account the synonyms for the arteries are not given: a comprehensive account may be found in the paper by Kaltenbach and Spahn (1975) already mentioned. Some terms in general use require explanation if the system is to be comprehensible.

1. Arteries supplying the ventricle are said to 'descend' towards the apex of the heart.

2. The superior (left) border of the heart is named the 'obtuse margin'.

3. The inferior (right) border is termed the 'acute margin'.

These terms derive from the appearances seen at operation or on radiographic visualization of the heart.

LEFT CORONARY ARTERY

The left coronary artery arises from the left sinus of Valsalva and runs forwards between the main pulmonary artery and the left atrial appendage. The first major branch is usually the anterior interventricular artery which descends to the apex along the interventricular septum giving off branches to the left and right ventricles and to the septum. This is usually called the *anterior descending* branch and branches to the left ventricular surface are usually large and are termed *diagonal* branches. Not infrequently, the anterior descending artery divides into two branches, one lying in the interventricular groove, and the other the diagonal, coursing towards the apex over the left ventricle. The left coronary artery continues backwards in the atrioventricular groove where it is usually called the *circumflex* branch of the left coronary artery. There is usually a large branch from this part of the artery which courses along the upper border of the left ventricle and is termed the *obtuse marginal* branch. The left coronary artery is often larger than the right but the circumflex artery reaches the (posterior) crux and turns down towards the apex of the heart as the posterior interventricular artery or *posterior interventricular* branch in only 20–30 per cent of cases. When this occurs the left coronary artery is said to be 'dominant'. The left coronary artery gives branches to the left atrium and occasionally to the pulmonary conus. The atrial branch of a dominant left coronary artery may supply the blood to the sino-atrial node—the *sinus branch*. This occurs in about 40 per cent of cases.

RIGHT CORONARY ARTERY

The right coronary artery originates in the anterior sinus of Valsalva. It passes forwards and to the right between the root of the pulmonary artery and the right atrial appendix to descend in the atrio-ventricular groove in the front of the heart. It usually has one major branch which runs along the antero-inferior margin of the heart towards the apex. This is usually called the marginal or *acute marginal* branch. The right coronary artery commonly terminates in the atrio-ventricular groove when the left coronary artery is dominant. More often, however, the right coronary artery is dominant, and in this circumstance it reaches the crux and forms the *posterior interventricular* artery. The right coronary artery gives rise near its origin to the right atrial branch which usually (60 per cent) supplies the sino-atrial node, and is also the usual source of the *conus artery* to the pulmonary conus.

All branches of both arteries coursing over the ventricles give rise to arteries entering the ventricular wall and, where it is adjacent to the overlying artery, to the branches supplying the septum.

Identification of lesions in coronary arteries

Atheromatous lesions in the coronary arteries may appear as localized constrictions reducing the vessel lumen in all projections, or, if largely confined to one side of the artery, may be apparent only on one projection, and in another be missed despite careful scrutiny. Furthermore, vessel movement may make a short lesion difficult to see. It not infrequently happens that such a lesion may be seen on a few frames only of the cine taken in one projection as it moves into and out of the shadow cast by another artery. This is particularly likely to happen with lesions in the early part of the obtuse marginal artery which may be overlaid in the P.A. view by the anterior descending artery or by diagonal branches. Such a lesion, if short, may be invisible in the oblique projections since the X-ray beam may not fall at right angles to the lesion but be so much in the line of the artery that the vessel appears to be intact. Cranio-caudal tilt views are most valuable. Slower filling of the segment beyond the narrowing may be a clue to its presence if the cine is viewed by single frames, but slow filling is a very unreliable guide. Identifying stenotic areas in coronary arteries can be an uncertain business. While some lesions are so clearly demonstrated by the technique that they are obvious on a test injection, others defy identification. Increasing experience in this field leads to caution, coupled with a conviction that the method only shows up the more gross lesions.

Coronary occlusions may be evident in the sudden termination of a major artery in a leash of collaterals, by the absence of an expected vessel, or by retrograde filling of a blocked artery from another branch. The last requires a cautionary note. It frequently happens that such a vessel when filled retrogradely appears to have a very narrow lumen. For example, the anterior descending artery not infrequently blocks just at its origin and fills retrogradely from the acute marginal branch of the right coronary artery, appearing threadlike. When explored surgically it usually turns out to have normal lumen beyond the block but the flow in the collateral supply was not enough to distend the system adequately. It is important to appreciate that the assessment of vessel-size beyond blocks and major narrowings is unreliable. Low flow may give a misleading appearance suggesting that the damage to the vessel is much greater than it really is.

Radiological identification of the branches of the coronary arteries

The variability of the coronary arterial tree makes identification of a particular branch affected by disease a difficult matter. This difficulty is increased by the nature of the image obtained by radiography since the shadows of the coronary arteries are superimposed. The problem is greatest with the left coronary artery. A further problem is that significant atheromatous narrowings in the arteries may be very short and may only show clearly in a single projection. The use of double image may clarify difficult areas, and the use of four projections, L.A.O., P.A., R.A.O. and left lateral, in difficult cases will usually resolve uncertainties in the localization of lesions. While four projections may be needed for the left coronary artery, two (R.A.O. and P.A.) usually suffice for the right (see Figs. 13.5–13.10). Additional cranio-caudal tilt views are very valuable for the left main coronary artery and the origin of its branches.

Sequence of investigation

In performing coronary arteriography it is usual to in-clude a left ventricular angiocardiogram. This permits an assessment of left ventricular function together with the identification of areas of poor contraction (dyskinesia), absent contraction (akinesia) or paradoxical expansion (aneurysm). This assessment by visualization is supplemented by an estimate of ventricular shortening obtained by echocardiography.

Since the left ventricular angiocardiogram may reveal dilatation with poor contraction and an end-systolic volume so great as to preclude surgery, this investigation is logically performed first, a gross degree of disease rendering further investigation unnecessary.

The left ventricular angiocardiogram is performed in the R.A.O. position and a convenient sequence (on the table on which the patient has to be rotated) is to change to a left coronary-artery catheter without moving the patient, visualize the artery on normal image, and if the videotape record suggests it, obtain an enlarged view of any doubtful area on double image. The P.A. view is then obtained followed by left lateral and L.A.O. again using single image followed by double image if indicated. Double image, with panning, should be used whenever possible.

The right coronary catheter is then inserted and the artery catheterized as it is most easily entered in the L.A.O. position. After views in the L.A.O. position, the P.A. projection is obtained. Should the appearances be in doubt, further positions may be visualized but usually this is unnecessary.

Identification of Branches of left coronary artery

The circumflex branch can be identified with confidence in the P.A. view if the cine is run until the coronary sinus is seen to fill. Since this structure also lies in the left atrio-ventricular groove it gives the line of the circumflex artery. In oblique and lateral views it forms the most posterior branch of the L.C.A. (see Figs. 13.5–13.10). Sometimes this circumflex branch is very narrow and does not reach the crux.

The anterior descending branch of the left coronary artery is often difficult to distinguish in the P.A. view from the *obtuse marginal branch* as their origins are

FIGS. 13.5 to 13.10   Diagrams of the coronary arteries as they commonly appear in the most frequently used projections. FIG. 13.5, Left coronary artery, postero-anterior projection; FIG. 13.6, left coronary artery, lateral projection; FIG. 13.7, left coronary artery, left anterior oblique projection; FIG. 13.8, left coronary artery, right anterior oblique projection; FIG. 13.9, right coronary artery, left anterior oblique projection; FIG. 13.10, right coronary artery, right anterior oblique projection. Abbreviations: AM, Acute marginal; AV, A-V nodal branch; CO, conal branch; CX, circumflex artery; D, diagonal artery; LAC, left atrial artery; LAD, left anterior descending; OM, obtuse marginal; PD, posterior descending; PL, postero lateral; S, septal; SA, sino-atrial branch.

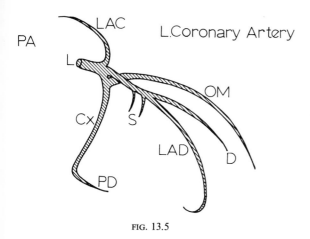

PA

L.Coronary Artery

FIG. 13.5

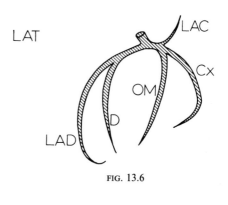

LAT

FIG. 13.6

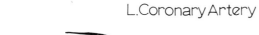

L.Coronary Artery

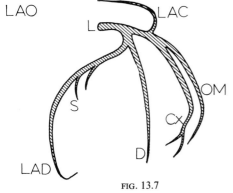

LAO

FIG. 13.7

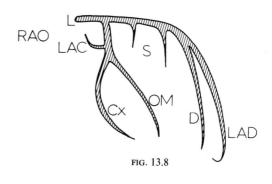

RAO

FIG. 13.8

R.Coronary Artery

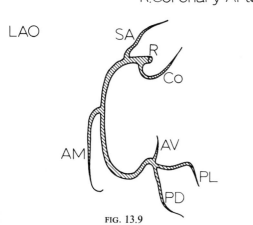

LAO

FIG. 13.9

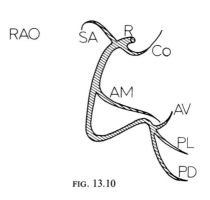

RAO

FIG. 13.10

usually close together and both run to the apex of the heart. As a rule, the obtuse marginal branch will have the more superior course, but this is not always so, the anterior descending not infrequently having a branch which appears in this projection to lie above the acute marginal whose oblique branches descend posteriorly over the surface of the left ventricle and so often appear to interlace with those of the anterior descending, and occasionally with the circumflex. The position is usually clarified in the lateral and oblique views where the anterior descending artery can be seen to lie in front with the obtuse marginal behind and above it. Not infrequently the anterior descending artery divides soon after its origin into two approximately equal branches, one running in the interventricular groove and the other on

the left ventricle. This can cause some discussion when the angiocardiograms are viewed as the interpretation can be difficult.

Identification of branches of the right coronary artery

The right coronary artery runs in the right atrioventricular groove towards the crux, giving off a major branch to the right ventricle (the *acute marginal*) and ending either by forming an anastomosis with the left coronary artery in the atrioventricular groove which is usually not visible on angiocardiography or, if it is the dominant artery, by turning down in the postero-inferior interventricular groove as the posterior interventricular artery. It is usually easy to distinguish them by oblique and P.A. views: rarely a lateral view is needed.

References

ALDRIDGE, H. E., McLOUGHLIN, M. J. & TAYLOR, K. W. (1975). Improved diagnosis in coronary cinearteriography with routine use of 110° oblique views and cranial and caudal angulations. *Am. J. Cardiol.* **36,** 468.

BASSAN, M., GANZ, W., MARCO, H. S. & SWAN, H. J. C. (1975). Effect of intracoronary injection of contrast medium on coronary blood flow. *Circulation,* **51,** 442.

BELLMAN, S., FRANK, H. A., LAMBERT, P. B., LITTMAN, D. & WILLIAMS, J. A. (1960). Coronary arteriography. I. Differential opacification of the aortic stream by catheters of a special design. *New Engl. J. Med.* **262,** 325.

ELDH, P. & SILVERMAN, J. F. (1974). Methods of studying the proximal left anterior descending coronary artery. *Radiology,* **113,** 738.

HYNES, D. M., VEREL, D., MOORE, R. D. & BATES, P. F. (1969). The use of the 70 mm camera for coronary arteriography. *Br. J. Radiol.* **42,** 736.

JUDKINS, M. P. (1967). Selective coronary arteriography. A percutaneous transfemoral technic. *Radiology* **89,** 815.

JUDKINS, M. P. (1968). Percutaneous transfemoral selective coronary arteriography. *Radiol. Clin. N. Am.* **6,** 467.

KALTENBACH, M. & SPAHN, F. (1975). Koronarographische Nomenklatur und Typologie der Koronararterien des Menschen. *Zeitschr. für Kardiologie,* **64,** 194.

NEJAD, M. S., KLAPER, M. A., STEGGERDA, F. R. & GIANTURCO, C. (1968). Clotting on the outer surfaces of vascular catheters. *Radiology,* **91,** 248.

PAULIN, S. (1964). Coronary angiography. A technical, anatomic and clinical study. *Acta Radiologica,* Suppl. 233, Stockholm.

SONES, M. F. & SHIREY, E. K. (1962). Cine coronary arteriography. *Med. Concepts Cardiovasc. Dis.* **31,** 735.

VEREL, D., WARD, C. & AMAN, M. (1975). Comparison of Triosil 370 with Urografin 76 and Hypaque 65 for coronary arteriography. *Br. Heart J.* **37,** 1049.

Also see References in Chapter 6 (Contrast Media) and Chapter 17 (Complications).

14. The Standard Angiocardiographic Injections

One of the fascinations of cardiac catheterization, both of the venous and of the arterial pathways, is the unpredictability of the various situations that may arise during the catheterization. The operator must be prepared to modify the examination and to exploit to the full any unexpected course which the catheter may take. Whilst encouraging this individual approach to any diagnostic problem, the operator must have a basic routine procedure on which to base his catheterization technique.

Left heart injections

During selective left heart angiocardiography, there are three fundamental sites at which the diagnostic injections are made.
1. Left ventricle.
2. Ascending aorta.
3. At the junction of the aortic arch and the descending aorta.

Not all of these injections may be needed in any particular patient.

The order in which these injections are made can be varied, but the writer prefers to catheterize the left ventricle and make the diagnostic intraventricular injection at the very onset of the procedure when the patient is fresh and at his best.

1. THE LEFT VENTRICULAR INJECTION

The tip of the catheter is placed towards the centre of the ventricular cavity near the apex as previously described (p. 105). Particularly in rheumatic heart disease, the irritability of the left ventricle may be such that the only position in which the catheter tip may be tolerated is at a situation which is not ideal, such as just below the aortic valve or directed towards the lateral wall of the ventricle. In these cases, the diagnostic injection of contrast medium should be made at these sites after confirming that the catheter tip lies freely in the ventricular cavity (p. 105).

The volume of contrast medium used depends on the size of the patient and of the left ventricular cavity, and of the cardiac output. In children, 1 ml/kg body weight is an average volume, with 4 ml as a minimum. In adolescents 30 ml is the usual volume, whilst in adults 40 to 50 ml or even 60 ml may be injected into the ventricle.

The proprietary make of contrast medium will depend on individual preference: through large bore catheters Hypaque 85, Urografin 76 or CardioConray are very suitable media. When catheterizing a small infant with a very small bore catheter (e.g. size 5 or 6), an increased flow rate of iodine can be achieved using the less viscous Conray 420 (or even Hypaque 45), with a corresponding improvement in radiographic contrast. Further details of contrast medium are discussed on page 60 *et seq.*

The pressure selected for the injection will also depend on the catheter used as the thinner-walled polythene catheters are considerably weaker than the Kifa-Odman catheters which are in turn, more easily burst than woven nylon, polyurethane or teflon catheters. If the injection pressure into the ventricle be too high, more extrasystoles will be produced probably by catheter whip, and higher pressures should therefore be avoided. In order to obtain an adequate flow rate with a low injection pressure, it is important to use the *largest internal diameter catheter which is practical.*

The objective is to inject 30 to 50 ml of contrast medium in 3 to 5 seconds into a normal-sized adult left ventricle providing a flow rate of about 8–12 ml/s. It is important not to inject at a greater rate than this for ventricular extrasystoles will probably be produced and this may result in spurious mitral-valve incompetence.

Recently introduced sophisticated pumps e.g. Contrac, Cordis, Medrad, Viamonte-Hobbs, enable one *to dial the required flow rate* as the pump computer or feed back mechanism takes into account the many variable factors such as catheter bore, length, viscosity, etc. Some of these pumps have an adjustment to reduce the acceleration at the beginning of the injection: this slow rise should be used for intraventricular injections as it reduces catheter whip. The bursting pressure of catheters constructed of the various possible materials should be determined for the particular pump which is being utilized. These flow-rate controlled pumps are a major advance, particularly for intraventricular injections as they permit one to avoid or to minimize the occurrence of disturbing extrasystoles.

The full-sized angiogram films are commenced automatically and synchronously with the onset of the injection by an electrical linkage. When cine-angiocardiography is being employed there is a short 'warm up' period of 2 to 3 seconds after pressing the contact switch before the cine-radiographs and the television monitor have gained peak performance. It is therefore strongly recommended that the contact switch for the cine-recording should be closed first and the angio-cardiographic injection should be delayed, perhaps 2 to 4 seconds, until the television monitor has gained a satisfactory image

The duration of the radiography is usually about 4 to 6 seconds. With full-sized radiographs, a rate of 3 to 5 films/s is usually adequate for diagnostic purposes and accordingly 12 to 20 films are loaded into each cassette. With cine-recording, 32 frames/s can be used in adults but for infants and children a faster speed (up to 50 frames/s or more) is used to allow for the more rapid heart action. When the cine-recording is being monitored on a television screen, the cut-off point, and therefore the duration of the cine-recording is easily decided—but one should allow 1 to 4 s recording after the heart and aortic arch are cleared of the diagnostic bolus of contrast medium. This enables one to confirm valve or heart wall calcification.

The position of the patient and the radiographic projection employed will depend on the clinical problem being investigated and will be discussed further under the relevant sections. For 'routine' technique, the author prefers a true A.P. and lateral exposure on the bi-plane full-sized film changer; and the right anterior oblique projection for the first cine-angiographic injection. Other radiographic projections are taken as and when required as indicated in subsequent sections.

When employing cine-angiocardiography, the diagnostic interpretation of the left ventricular injection can almost always be made by direct observation of the television monitor. If there is a video-tape linkage, an immediate play-back will be available for confirmation (or otherwise) of the initial impression. A decision can be made immediately, as to whether a further left ventricular injection, probably in another radiographic projection will be needed in order to establish the diagnosis.

If full-sized angiographic films are being used, no direct television monitoring will be available, and the diagnostic value of the injection will only be assessed when the films are processed. For this reason, either speedy hand-processing or, preferably, automatic processors using a 90 s cycle should be used. In the writer's unit, 90 s automatic roller processing has very successfully replaced our previous manual processing. During this period, the catheter tip is left in the left ventricle provided that the patient is comfortable and that extra-systoles are not being produced. If the first left ven-tricular angiocardiographic injection is found to be in-conclusive or provides incomplete information, a further angiographic series may be taken of a (modified) second left ventricular injection, provided that the first injection has not seriously disturbed the patient.

Unfortunately, a satisfactory angiocardiographic in-jection into the left ventricular cavity may produce one or more ventricular extrasystoles (Fig. 14.1). This is due to the *mechanical* effect of jets of fluid and of the movement of the catheter tip caused by the injection, for a rapid hand injection of 10 ml saline produces the same ven-tricular response as an equal volume of contrast medium (Fig. 14.2). Pump pressures should therefore not be too high and the 'slow rise' should be used on pumps with this facility. These extrasystoles distort the angiocardio-graphic appearances and are best avoided by using a flow rate of no greater than 8–12 ml/sec. This is best achieved by utilizing a flow-controlled pump. The cine-recording provides visual evidence of any abnormal heart action produced by the injection and this is confirmed by the E.C.G. recording. Cine-recording is a much more accurate method than full-size films in detecting mitral incompetence produced by extra-systoles.

After the left ventricular angiocardiographic injection and when the cardiac action has settled, a pressure trace recording is taken with the catheter tip in the left ventricle. Having checked this record and the diagnostic adequacy of the angiocardiographic films or videotape recording, the catheter is slowly withdrawn during continuous pressure recording. As the catheter tip reaches the left ventricular outflow, extrasystoles are almost always produced but they cease as soon as the aortic valve is traversed. The pressure recording is continued into the ascending aorta so that any gradient within the left ventricle or at the aortic valve will be recorded (Fig. 14.3).

If oximetry readings are indicated, a blood sample is taken from the left ventricle before catheter withdrawal.

A satisfactory left ventricular angiogram will cause complete radiographic opacification of the entire cham-ber during at least one normal ventricular contraction. The presence of mitral incompetence (Fig. 110), ven-tricular septal defect (with left to right shunt, Fig. 47), a left ventricular—right atrial shunt (Fig. 46), intraven-tricular filling defects and obstructions (Fig. 111), will be demonstrated should they be present. The end-diastolic and end-systolic volumes of the left ventricular cavity and the thickness of the left ventricular wall can be assessed from a satisfactory left ventriculogram. This assessment is more realistic and more valid from cine-recordings than from full-sized films which may not record the extremes of systole and diastole.

The aortic valve is visualized both in A.P. and lateral projections and the presence of aortic valve stenosis may be demonstrated. The ascending aorta, aortic arch and descending aorta with their branches are well seen after left ventricular angiographic injection.

2. ASCENDING AORTIC INJECTION

After the production of a satisfactory left ventriculo-gram (as checked by television monitoring, video-tape or processed full-size radiographs), the catheter is withdrawn into the ascending aorta. In many of the clinical con-

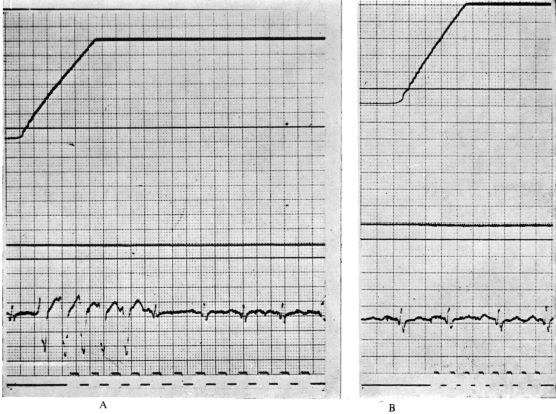

A   B

FIG. 14.1 *Left ventricular and Ascending Aortic Angiographic Injections.* 7 kg/cm^2 Gidlund pump. Grey Kifa catheter.
A. *Left Ventricular Injection* (35 ml Angio Conray).
The upper trace indicates the rate of emptying of the Gidlund syringe. (5 large squares = 1 s). The injection took 1·1 s.
The middle trace is the E.C.G. record. Note five ventricular extrasystoles occur, commencing with the onset of the
injection. Normal contractions follow. The lower trace indicates the radiographic exposures, taken at 3 per s.
B. *Ascending Aortic Injection* (30 ml Angio Conray).
The injection takes 0·8 s. Note absence of extrasystoles or of E.C.G. change throughout the injection. Radiographic
exposures at 5 per s.
(Reproduced with permission of the Editor of *The British Journal of Radiology.* Grainger, R. G. (1965) Complications
of cardiovascular radiological investigations. **38,** 201).

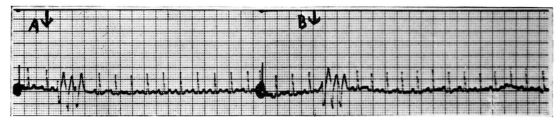

FIG. 14.2 *Left Ventricular Injections of Saline and Contrast Medium.* Identical extrasystole pattern following hand injections of 10 ml saline and 10 ml Conray 280 into left ventricle (same patient). A. 10 ml saline injected by hand through
the catheter into left ventricle. B. 10 ml Conray 280 injected by hand through catheter into left ventricle. (Reproduced
with permission of the Editor of *The British Journal of Radiology.* Grainger, R. G. (1965) Complications of cardiovascular radiological investigations. **38,** 201.)

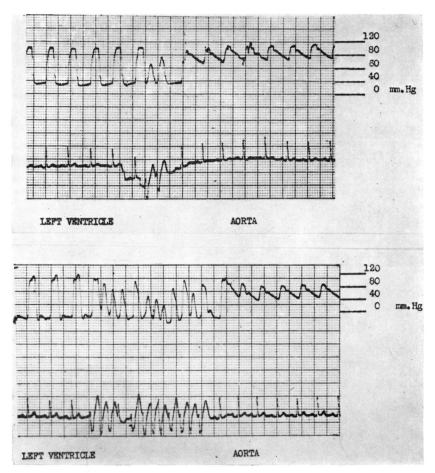

FIG. 14.3 *Withdrawal of Catheter from Left Ventricle through Aortic Valve into Ascending Aorta.* Two withdrawals in the same patient, indicating variable irritability of the outflow tract of the left ventricle. During the upper tracing, there were two ventricular extrasystoles. During the lower tracing, there were eleven ventricular extrasystoles. (Reproduced with permission of the Editor of *The British Journal of Radiology.* Grainger, R. G. (1965) Complications of cardiovascular radiological investigations. **38,** 201.)

ditions being investigated, it is desirable to make an injection of contrast medium at this site.

For the investigation of aortic valve incompetence, the site of election for the catheter tip is about 4 cm above the aortic valve. This position is gained under fluoroscopy: if using non-radio-opaque catheters, they are filled with contrast medium in order to render them visible under fluoroscopy. It is most important to avoid making the angiographic injection into the mouth of a coronary artery: a test hand injection of contrast medium should always be made. The catheter tip should be directed downwards, towards the aortic valve. If the catheter tip has become sharply curved (as occasionally happens after withdrawing from the left ventricle), the tip may be directed upwards and away from the valve (Fig. 14.4A) so that an injection of contrast medium will not ade-

quately demonstrate the aortic face of the aortic valve. A small hand injection of contrast medium will reveal the situation and demonstrate the direction of the injected stream. If the situation be adverse and the catheter tip be curved away from the aortic valve, attempts are made to improve the catheter position. The technique is to withdraw the catheter into the aortic arch where it may straighten, or to hook the catheter into the origin of one of the major aortic arch branches (Fig. 14.4) and so uncoil the terminal loop. The catheter is then advanced again into the ascending aorta, this time with the tip directed, as required, at the aortic valve. If this manoeuvre is unsuccessful, the catheter is withdrawn into the abdominal aorta and an attempt is made to enter the catheter tip into a major aortic branch (such as the renal artery). If this is still unsuccessful, the catheter may be

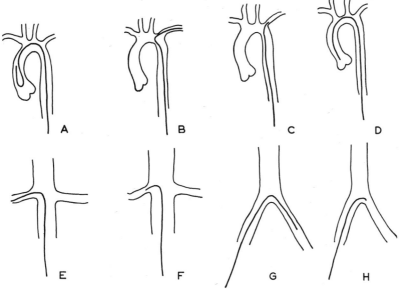

FIG. 14.4 *Uncoiling a Catheter Loop.* A. The catheter tip is turned back on itself and does not point towards the aortic valve. Different techniques to uncoil the catheter tip are presented in the other diagrams. B. The catheter is withdrawn and an attempt is made to catch the distal limb in one of the aortic arch branches (e.g. left subclavian). C. The catheter is withdrawn from position B until the end is uncoiled. D. When it is uncoiled, the catheter is then advanced again until it lies (uncoiled) just above the aortic valve, as required for an ascending aortic injection. E. & F. If the catheter cannot be 'caught' in a head artery, the catheter is further withdrawn and an attempt is made to catch the distal loop in a renal artery. (E). Further withdrawal uncoils the loop. (F). The catheter can then be advanced again to reach the position D. G. & H. If the renal arteries cannot be utilized, the loop is withdrawn further and an attempt is made to straddle the aortic bifurcation. (G). Further withdrawal of the catheter will straighten the catheter (H), which can then be advanced to gain position D.

withdrawn further so that the catheter curve straddles the aortic bifurcation. Once the catheter tip has 'caught' in the mouth of a branch artery, or has straddled the aortic bifurcation, further careful withdrawal of the catheter will straighten out the curve and the catheter tip will again point towards the heart (Fig. 14.4). It may then be advanced again round the aortic arch to reach the position of choice for an injection into the ascending aorta.

Re-insertion of the guide wire may help to straighten an undesirable catheter curve, but even a flexible plastic-coated guide wire may not pass through a catheter which has curved sharply back on itself within the aortic lumen. A pig-tail polyurethane catheter will retain its terminal curve and is unlikely to double back on itself. This type of catheter, although more costly, is very suitable for left ventriculography and ascending aortography.

Having gained a catheter position 4 to 6 cm above the aortic valve, with the exit holes directed at the aortic valve, a hand test injection of 5 to 10 ml of contrast medium is made to ensure that the catheter tip lies freely within the aortic lumen and not in the mouth of a coronary artery.

The usual volume of contrast medium injected in the ascending aorta is 30 ml, occasionally 40 to 50 ml. The same medium is used as for the left ventricular injection, e.g. CardioConray, Urografin 76, Hypaque 85. The pump pressure is adjusted to provide a flow rate of about 30 ml/s. The pressure of injection on the Gidlund pump dial is 4 to 8 kg/cm^2 depending on the type of catheter. High pressure aortic injections will not cause extrasystoles. Radiography should commence with the onset of the angiographic injection and continue for 3 to 5 seconds (but see p. 118 for cine).

This contrast medium injection rarely causes an alteration in the cardiac rhythm (Fig. 14.1) but quite frequently there is a change in the T wave or ST segment due to flooding of the coronary arteries (and consequently the myocardium) with contrast medium. High concentrations of sodium contrast media (e.g. Conray 480, Conray 420, Triosil 75) are not preferred for this injection as they are more likely to cause ventricular fibrillation than media with a lesser sodium ion concentration (e.g. CardioConray, Urografin 76, Hypaque 65 or 85). See page 60.

The change in the E.C.G. usually lasts less than 2 minutes.

A satisfactory ascending aortic injection will cause complete opacification of the ascending aorta, arch and upper descending aorta. The contrast medium will pass retrogradely during diastole to reach the aortic valve, the aortic surface of which must be clearly demonstrated. If the monitor, videotape or processed full-size films do not demonstrate these features, then a further injection should be made after adjusting the unsatisfactory factor. This is usually the position of the catheter tip, as from too high a position the contrast medium may not reach the aortic valve and may not therefore demonstrate aortic incompetence: too low a position of the catheter may interfere with aortic valve closure and may induce apparent aortic valve incompetence when none is present.

The usual radiographic projection advised is the left lateral or left anterior oblique if only one plane radiography (e.g. cine radiography) is being used. For bi-plane studies, A.P. and lateral projections may be used, but the aortic arch is often rather a 'tight' curve and the ascending aorta and aortic valve may partly overlap the descending aorta in the true A.P. plane (Fig. 31). To avoid this, the patient should be turned 10 to 20° to the right, left side up to produce a slight LAO position for the A.P. projection (p. 132).

A satisfactory ascending aortogram will demonstrate the competence or incompetence of the aortic valve, aorto-pulmonary shunts, supravalvar aortic stenosis, coarctation or other abnormality of the aorta and its branches.

Cine-recording is much to be preferred for the detection of aortic incompetence or aorto-pulmonary shunts. Full-size films may be preferred for most other aortic abnormalities.

DESCENDING AND AORTIC ARCH INJECTION

This injection is usually designed to demonstrate a left to right shunt through a patent ductus arteriosus. The shunt may be adequately shown by the preceding injection but frequently better visualization is obtained by placing the catheter tip just below the origin of the left subclavian artery.

It is essential that the catheter tip does not lie within the origin of the left vertebral artery for then the injection of the diagnostic bolus of contrast medium may produce severe and perhaps fatal dysfunction of the vital centres in the medulla. Fluoroscopy of the catheter position is no certain guide in avoiding this hazard, which can only be prevented by *always* making a small hand injection of contrast medium whenever the catheter tip is placed near the origin of the subclavian artery.

The pressure of injection, the volume and type of contrast medium and the duration of radiography are as for the ascending aortic injection. The best projection for seeing the ductus itself is the left anterior oblique but, if the ductus is small or the shunt transmitted is small, this projection may be unsuccessful. The optimal projection for demonstrating the presence of a small left to right shunt is the A.P. (or P.A.). In this projection, the main pulmonary arteries are well seen and any minor opacification of them can be detected, particularly on cine-recording. It is therefore essential to include an A.P. (or '20° off A.P.' patient rotated to right) projection before the absence of a shunt through a patent ductus can be assumed.

This injection causes no E.C.G. disturbance.

A satisfactory injection will demonstrate the entire aortic arch and the origin of its major branches. The normal bronchial arteries are often not visualized without selective catheterization. The descending aorta and its branches are visualized on the later films.

Aortic arch injections are also frequently made in patients with symptoms of cerebral ischaemia in order to visualize the thoracic and cervical portions of the carotid and vertebral arteries. The catheter tip should be placed at the beginning of the aortic arch; the innominate artery will always fill if an adequate bolus of contrast medium is delivered at this site. The optimum projection is with the thorax at 45° left anterior oblique, with the head rather more lateral, patient looking well to the right with the chin up and head extended. Full-size films should be taken in this projection; bi-plane films are unnecessary. The centre of the film should be much higher than usual, for the field should include only the upper half of the aortic arch but as much as possible of the neck. The radiographic exposure is critical as the beam must be sufficiently penetrated to show the aortic arch and sufficiently 'soft' to demonstrate the vessels of the neck. Because of this, and because of the many confusing bone opacities in the upper thorax, the *subtraction* technique (Fig. 113) is most helpful in this investigation. A plain film for subtraction purposes is best obtained at the beginning of the aortogram series, immediately before the injection of contrast medium.

Right heart injections

During right heart catheterization, angiocardiographic injections are made most frequently (in descending order of frequency) into the following sites:

1. The right ventricle.
2. The pulmonary artery.
3. Any left heart chamber which is entered by the catheter.
4. The right atrium (occasionally).
5. The venae cavae.
6. The pulmonary veins.

1. THE RIGHT VENTRICULAR INJECTION

The tip of the catheter is usually placed towards the apex of the right ventricle, that is, in the middle of its cavity. This injection site generally ensures that the whole of the right ventricle is opacified, including its inflow tract and the ventricular aspect of the tricuspid valve. The outflow tract is opacified when the ventricle contracts and ejects the contrast medium through the pulmonary valve into the pulmonary artery.

If the abnormality is thought to be at or near the pulmonary valve or if the right ventricular injection is being made in order to visualize the *left* heart, then it is generally advisable to place the catheter tip in the right ventricular outflow and to inject the contrast medium two or three cm below the pulmonary valve. This will provide improved detail of the right ventricular outflow, pulmonary vessels and the left heart, because less dilution of the contrast medium is likely. The presence of the catheter tip in the right ventricular outflow may however cause a local contraction of the outflow muscle producing a false appearance suggesting infundibular obstruction.

The type and volume of contrast medium and the pressure of its injection is the same as for left ventricular injections (p. 118).

The duration of radiography depends on the cardiac problem being investigated. For demonstration of the *right* ventricle, pulmonary valve and pulmonary artery, a period of 3 to 5 seconds radiography is quite adequate but if opacification of the *left* heart is required, usually to detect a left to right shunt, then the radiography should be continued for at least 12 seconds.

The frequency of radiographic exposure (on full-sized films) also depends on the particular investigation. For demonstration of the right ventricular outflow, pulmonary valve or the main pulmonary arteries, exposures at 3 to 5 per s for 2 or 3 seconds are usually satisfactory. The frequency of exposure can then be reduced for the later films as rapid exposures are not necessary to visualize the pulmonary veins and the left heart. After the initial 2 or 3 seconds, the frequency can then be reduced to 1 or 1·5 per s for the next 8 to 10 seconds. Usually 18 to 24 exposures in each plane is quite adequate.

If the objective of the injection is to detect a left to right shunt, then a film frequency of 1·5 or 2 films a second for 12 seconds will be adequate.

The majority of right ventricular angiocardiograms are performed for the investigation of congenital heart disease, often in infants or children. As the requirement is for detailed anatomical demonstration, full-sized radiographs may be considered advisable, preferably bi-plane. Cine-recording is, however, a much more sensitive method of demonstrating a small shunt.

The optimal projections for bi-plane right ventricular angiography are true A.P. and lateral. The lateral projection is of much greater value for the right ventricle, as it is not obscured by the dorsal spine, and the pulmonary valve is particularly well seen, unobscured by other soft tissue or bony shadows (Figs. 57 and 58). The appendage of the right atrium is large and projects forwards to appear superimposed exactly on the pulmonary valve on the lateral radiograph. If the right atrial appendage contains contrast medium, the detail of the pulmonary valve and right ventricular outflow will be completely obscured. It is therefore most important *not* to inject the contrast medium into the right atrium if it is intended to visualize the right ventricular outflow. If it is not possible to enter the right ventricle with the catheter, and if the injection *has* to be made into the right atrium, then the right anterior oblique projection will demonstrate the right ventricular outflow to the best advantage.

The forceful injection of contrast medium into the right ventricle usually causes a few ventricular extrasystoles as described for left ventricular injections. During this period, irregular contractions of the ventricle may cause unusual ventricular angiographic appearances which should be discounted.

2. THE PULMONARY ARTERY INJECTION

The catheter tip is passed through the right atrium, the right ventricle and across the pulmonary valve into the main pulmonary artery. This position is confirmed by screening and by pressure recording (Ch. 10). The angiocardiographic injection is made with the catheter tip in the main pulmonary artery, midway between the pulmonary valve and the bifurcation of the main pulmonary artery. The volume of contrast medium to be injected, the programme of the radiographic exposures and the radiographic projections utilized are dependent on the objective of the catheterization procedure.

If the angiocardiogram is being performed to investigate the anatomy of the pulmonary arteries, such as in pulmonary thrombo-embolic disease, or in stenosis of these arteries, then a relatively small volume of contrast medium (20 to 40 ml) is usually adequate for an average-sized adult with a normal (or reduced) pulmonary blood flow. Improved detail will be achieved by injecting 15–25 ml separately into the right and left main pulmonary arteries. As anatomical detail is the principal requirement, full-sized films are taken at 4 or 5 per s for 2 or 3 seconds followed by a slower rate for a further 2 or 3 seconds. Antero-posterior radiographs will generally be adequate, for in the lateral projection, the circulations of the two lungs are partly super-imposed. If the angiocardiogram is being performed to demonstrate the *left* heart, then a larger volume of contrast medium should be injected into the pulmonary artery—say 40 to 60 ml for an average-sized adult. If anatomical detail of a left-sided lesion such as aortic coarctation is required, then full-sized radiographs should be taken. The optimal projections are usually antero-posterior and lateral. The radiographic programme must be sufficiently prolonged to visualize the *left* heart—usually 10 seconds is adequate but up to 20 seconds may be necessary. A sequence of 3 films per s for 1 second (to visualize the pulmonary arteries) followed by 1 to 2 films per sec for 10 to 15 seconds will generally be found satisfactory, depending on circulation time.

If the patient is being investigated for an anticipated left to right shunt, a larger volume of contrast medium, up to 60 ml (or even 70 ml) may be necessary as the pulmonary blood flow may be much increased, causing considerable dilution of the medium. In the author's experience, bi-plane angiocardiogram films in A.P. and lateral projection provide a very reliable method of investigating a possible left to right shunt during right heart angiography (e.g. Figs. 41, 42, 45). Cine-angiography will often detect a very small shunt which may be equivocal on the large films.

3. LEFT HEART CHAMBERS

These may be entered by the catheter during right heart catheterization as the catheter may pass through a foramen ovale, an atrial or ventricular septal defect (Figs. 29, 44). A patent ductus arteriosus may also be traversed with the catheter passing from pulmonary artery to aorta (Fig. 11). Aortic entry should be confirmed by pressure measurement or by passing the catheter below the diaphragm. Advantage should be taken of the catheter entry into left heart chambers, by obtaining pressure measurements and oximetry readings of every chamber entered. Angiocardiographic injections may also be made into the left heart chambers (during right heart catheterization) in order to visualize the anatomy of the left heart or to investigate the presence of a left to right shunt (e.g. Figs. 28, 29, 31, 34, 44, 46).

The details of left-sided angiocardiographic injections are discussed on page 118 *et seq.*

4. RIGHT ATRIUM

Right atrial injection of contrast medium may be required in order to investigate the possibility of a right to left atrial shunt or to assess the tricuspid valve and its drainage (Fig. 75). The latter assessment may be required in transposition of the great vessels as it will differentiate the physiological circulation in corrected transposition (right atrium supplying left ventricle) from uncorrected transposition, in which right atrial blood passes into the anterior (right) ventricle and thence into the transposed aorta (Figs. 70–74).

In Ebstein's anomaly and tricuspid atresia, right atrial angiocardiography will demonstrate the disordered anatomy of the right atrium and the tricuspid valve and the route of blood through the heart chambers (Figs. 76–78).

The antero-posterior and lateral projections are preferred with full-sized angiocardiographic films. The right anterior oblique projection will usually project the tricuspid valve in profile but the valve is often well seen in the A.P. and especially in lateral films (Fig. 26A).

5. VENAE CAVAE

Vena caval injection of contrast medium may be indicated if aberrant systemic venous drainage is suspected. Occasionally the inferior vena cava is absent and the venous return from the lower half of the body is conveyed by an enlarged azygos vein which runs along the posterior thoracic wall before arching over the right hilum to enter the superior vena cava. This anomaly makes cardiac catheterization from the leg veins very difficult or even impossible. The anatomy is well demonstrated by an angiographic injection into the azygos vein (Fig. 37A and B). Antero-posterior and lateral angiocardiograms are preferred. Left-to-right intracardiac shunts frequently accompany this anomalous venous drainage.

6. THE PULMONARY VEINS

These are often entered by the catheter during right heart catheterization. There are two possibilities, either (a) the pulmonary vein drains directly into the right atrium (aberrant pulmonary venous drainage) or (b) the catheter passes from the right atrium through a foramen ovale or ASD into the left atrium and thence into a normally draining pulmonary vein.

The differentiation between these two possibilities *cannot* be made by study of the catheter position and its course (Fig. 3). The only radiological method which permits differentiation is to inject contrast medium into the pulmonary *vein* and to note the chamber into which it drains. Antero-posterior angiocardiographic films or cine-recording are preferable for a period of 2 to 3 seconds. Whilst a small hand injection of contrast medium may be sufficient, it is often advisable to inject 20 to 30 ml by pump at low pressure into the pulmonary vein which has been entered by the catheter (Figs. 38, 39, 40). Unless this radiological information is obtained at this stage, it is likely that confusion will arise in the differentiation of aberrant pulmonary venous drainage from a normal pulmonary vein entered by catheter via an atrial septal defect. Pulmonary veins which drain anomalously into the right atrium are often impossible to diagnose during the laevo-phase following right-heart injections. In infants with pulmonary artery atresia, a forceful injection into the pulmonary vein will often cause retrograde opacification of the pulmonary *artery*, indicating the degree of atresia.

15. Clinical Angiocardiographic Investigations

Every patient poses his own specific diagnostic problems and unless an individualistic approach is adopted by the investigator, serious deficiencies in the information obtained will be inevitable. Nevertheless, this personal and individualistic approach must be firmly based on a well tried and proven technical routine. Many patients present with similar diagnostic problems and some of these are discussed here. It is again emphasized, however, that every patient and his individual clinical problems must be fully appreciated by the investigator *before* the catheterization is commenced.

The actual radiographic technique utilized for the angiocardiographic procedure will depend on the clinical problem and on the radiographic facilities available. As discussed previously, it is best to have both cine-recording and full-sized bi-plane or miniature photo-fluorogram (70 or 100 mm) facilities available on the same catheterization table. Frequently this ideal is deliberately not pursued because it may be preferable in an investigation unit to have two separate catheterization installations—one for cine-recording with photofluorography, and the other for full-sized bi-plane angiocardiography. This arrangement permits the investigation of more patients when finances are limited. It should usually be possible to transfer the patient from one table to the other should both facilities be required. A video-tape recorder will be particularly valuable in this kind of installation as it permits video-cine recording in each room.

The decision as to which radiographic facilities are likely to be needed should be made before the catheterization is commenced. Cine-angiocardiography is preferred for the investigation of rheumatic valve disease, left-to-right shunts, myocardial function and contractility. Full-sized angiocardiographic facilities provide a very valuable gain in anatomical detail in the investigation of cyanotic congenital heart disease. For coronary arteriography, good quality, single-plane cine using a 5- or 6-in intensifier field is much preferred, but added information may be gained by miniature (70 or 100 mm) or full-sized radiographs.

In the following sections, the preferred technique will be indicated but frequently either method will be satisfactory.

SELECTIVE LEFT ANGIOCARDIOGRAPHY

RHEUMATIC HEART VALVE DISEASE

Patients with rheumatic valve disease are referred for catheterization and angiography of the left heart in order to assess the efficiency of the mitral and aortic valves. It may also be necessary to visualize the coronary arteries in an attempt to assess the significance of coronary atheroma for example in patients with angina and aortic valve disease.

In our unit, surgeons now request coronary arteriography prior to surgery of the aortic valve.

Mitral regurgitation (but not stenosis), aortic incompetence and stenosis may be evaluated by retrograde left ventricular and aortic angiocardiography.

Cine angiography permits a considerably quicker examination (because an immediate diagnosis can be made on the television monitor), and it allows better appreciation of the significance of extrasystoles in the assessment of mitral incompetence. Television monitoring and cine-recording during the angiocardiographic injection is therefore the technique preferred by the author.

The first angiocardiographic injection is best made into the left ventricle as previously described. For the detection of mitral incompetence, the right anterior oblique projection is preferred. This projection provides better visualization of the leaflets of the mitral valve so that its detail may be better assessed, but in this position the left atrium lies superimposed obliquely on the dorsal spine and minor opacification (because of slight mitral incompetence) may not be clearly demonstrated on big films. The true left lateral position does not project the mitral valve tangentially and the valve is therefore not well visualized, but minor opacification of the left atrium can be more easily recognized if large films are being used. The author may therefore prefer the left lateral projection if large films are being employed: R.A.O. projection is much preferred for cine-angiocardiography since it displays the left ventricle lengthwise with minimal fore-shortening. It has been claimed (Demany, Kay and Zimmermann, 1966) that angiocardiography in the right anterior oblique projection may distinguish the mobile stenotic mitral valve from the rigid stenotic valve. This is very useful information for the surgeon. The R.A.O. projection is generally regarded as the first choice for left ventricular angiocardiography for assessment of the mitral valve. The L.P.O. projection provides an equivalent view and Lipchik et al. (1966) suggest an additional tilt of the tube towards the head of the patient as providing the optimal view of the mitral valve.

If the angiocardiographic ventricular injection causes multiple extrasystoles, the arrhythmia will be recognized on the television monitor and/or on the E.C.G. tracing. A few extrasystoles are usual but they rarely cause 'spurious' significant mitral incompetence (Nagle, Walker and Grainger, 1968). A small puff of contrast medium may pass retrogradely through the normal mitral valve, particularly during or immediately after a burst of extrasystoles but there is rarely any doubt that this is not significant. If there is any question of diagnostic errors being made because of extrasystoles, a second lower pressure ventricular injection delivering say 10 ml/s, should be considered if the first one has not disturbed the patient. The television monitor (and subsequently the cine-recording or videotape), provides a much more informative picture of extrasystoles and their influence than do full-sized films. Cine-radiology is therefore greatly preferred to full-sized film angiocardiography in the investigation of rheumatic valve disease.

Films should be taken for 4 or 5 seconds during which time the left ventricle will have cleared of contrast medium. The details of the ventricular injection and film programming are discussed on page 117.

Having achieved a satisfactory left ventricular injection and having established the diagnosis of mitral competence (or incompetence) by television monitoring, video-tape, or checking of the radiographs, the catheter is then withdrawn from the left ventricle.

A pressure recording is taken with the catheter in the left ventricular cavity and during catheter withdrawal. As the catheter tip passes through the left ventricular outflow, a few extrasystoles are usually produced: this will cause a spurious pressure tracing. As soon as the aortic valve is traversed, the extrasystoles cease (Fig. 14.3). The aortic systolic pressure is then compared with the left ventricular systolic pressure (measured during normal ventricular activity). A difference of more than 5 mmHg in the two systolic pressures indicates a degree of stenosis at the aortic valve.

The catheter tip is then placed 4 to 6 cm above the aortic valve and an aortic injection of contrast medium is made as previously described (p. 120). Films are only required for 3 or 4 seconds. The preferred projection for the detection of aortic incompetence is the left lateral position for the aortic valve and the left outflow tract both lie in front of the dorsal spine and are not well seen on A.P. films. The contrast medium may not reach the aortic valve cusps, e.g. the injection may be delivered too high in the aorta, the injection pressure may be too low or the catheter tip may be curved back on itself (p. 121). If the contrast medium does not reach the valve, the defective technique is amended and a further injection made.

Alternatively, the catheter, particularly some pig-tail varieties, may jerk downwards 4–6 cm at the beginning of the injection and come to lie on the aortic valve or may even prolapse through it, producing spurious aortic incompetence. The diagnostic adequacy of the injection is checked on the television monitor or radiographs, particular attention being paid to the contrast medium reaching and fully delineating the aortic surface of the aortic valve (Figs. 85–87), without the catheter deforming the valve. If the angiographic technique is seen to be satisfactory, the catheter is withdrawn from the peripheral (usually femoral) artery and the catheterization is terminated. Extrasystoles do not occur during aortic injections and will not confuse the radiographic recording.

Cine-recording is preferable and is much more sensitive for the assessment of aortic incompetence. It is very important to position the image intensifier so that the aortic valve is situated near the top of the field so that the whole of the left ventricle can be visualized. A common mistake is to centre the intensifier over the aortic valve so that the left ventricle is not well shown.

LEFT TO RIGHT SHUNTS

A frequent reason for performing left heart angiography is in the investigation of left to right shunts. This may be the first investigation undertaken if, for example, a patent ductus arteriosus or a ventricular septal defect is clinically suspected and confirmation is required prior to surgery.

In some patients, a previous right heart catheterization may have demonstrated a left to right shunt (either by oximetry or angiography) but the site of the shunt may have been uncertain. A subsequent left angiocardiogram will define the site of the heart defect and shunt.

In patients who are to be submitted to open heart surgery, it is essential to exclude a patent ductus for, during the retrograde aortic perfusion, the patent ductus will leak blood into the pulmonary artery and will prevent successful perfusion. If a patent ductus be present, it must be ligatured before the perfusion is set up. If there is any reason to suspect that the ductus is patent in addition to other cardiac defects (for which the open heart surgery is being undertaken), then a retrograde aortogram should be undertaken to decide the state of the ductus. If the ductus proves to be patent, then the surgeon will ligature the ductus before setting up the perfusion.

The angiocardiographic technique to be employed will depend on the clinical situation to be investigated.

Cine-angiography is preferred to full-size film angiography for the demonstration of left to right shunts. The contrast medium and pressure of injection are the same as for the investigation of rheumatic valve disease and are discussed on pages 117–124. The volume of contrast medium may have to be increased to 40 to 50 ml if there is a large left to right shunt in order to achieve adequate visualization of the left heart chambers.

Patent ductus arteriosus

This is the simplest investigation being discussed here. The catheter tip is placed in the descending limb of the aortic arch at about the level of the origin of the left subclavian artery. The angiographic injection (30 ml in the adult) is made at this position. As previously stressed, it is essential to ensure that the catheter tip has not entered the left subclavian and left vertebral artery origin—delivery of the diagnostic angiographic injection into the vertebral artery could be fatal. The only way to eliminate this hazard is to inject a small test dose of contrast medium by hand during fluoroscopy immediately before making the diagnostic injection.

The best projection for the demonstration of a shunt through the ductus is the antero-posterior (or P.A.) for any contrast medium entering the pulmonary artery can be readily recognized as it pulses towards and through the lungs. In this (A.P. or P.A.) position, the actual ductus will not be seen but its presence can be inferred when the shunt is recognized (Fig. 51). For actual visualization of the ductus, a lateral or left anterior oblique radiographic projection is preferred (Figs. 50, 96). Radiographs are required for only 3 to 4 seconds during and after the angiographic injection.

The ductus arteriosus is almost always on the same side as the aortic arch and therefore will be detected if the contrast medium injection is delivered into the descending limb of the aortic arch. In a few rare cases, the ductus may arise from the subclavian artery on the side opposite to the aortic arch and a systemic-pulmonary artery communication at this site would remain undetected by the injection technique just described. These rare instances usually occur in patients with pulmonary stenosis and a right to left ventricular shunt (often of Fallot type) and the aortic anatomy may well have been demonstrated by a previous right angiocardiogram. If this anomaly is being sought by retrograde aortography, the diagnostic injection of contrast medium should be made in the *ascending* and not the descending limb of the aortic arch.

If the ductus is patent, it is often possible to pass the tip of the catheter from the aorta into the duct. This manipulation is much easier if the catheter end has previously been formed into a $\frac{3}{8}$ of a circle curve as described previously. The catheter is rotated (each way) and man-ipulated repeatedly up and down a few centimetres in the descending limb of the aortic arch just below the origin of the left subclavian artery. If the catheter tip 'catches' and moves to the right or left or anterior to the aortic line, then it has probably entered the ductus. This can be confirmed by taking a pressure measurement, or (less readily) by withdrawing a sample of blood for oximetry. If the ductus has been entered, the catheter can usually be advanced into the main pulmonary artery (Fig. 48) and, if required, a pulmonary angiogram can be performed. In some patients the catheter may be passed retrogradely through the pulmonary valve into the right ventricle (Fig. 48). The pressure in the pulmonary artery should always be measured so that the aorto-pulmonary gradient can be determined and the peripheral pulmonary arteriolar resistance can be assessed.

In some patients the peripheral pulmonary vascular resistance is equal to systemic vascular resistance and the pulmonary artery blood pressure equals aortic pressure. This state of balanced pressures with bi-directional shunt through the ductus is called the 'hypertensive' or Eisenmenger ductus and the shunt may be equally well demonstrated by aortic or pulmonary artery injection of contrast medium.

If there is a suspicion of arterial desaturation due to a right to left shunt, a sample of blood from the descending aorta should be also taken for oximetry.

The bronchial arteries take origin from the upper part of the descending aorta near to the ductus origin. A hand injection of 2 or 3 ml contrast medium during careful fluoroscopy will distinguish whether the catheter has entered the ductus or a bronchial artery.

Other aorto-pulmonary shunts

The patent ductus is by far the most frequent aorto-pulmonary shunt but other sites of communication are occasionally encountered.

1. *Aorto-pulmonary window*. An aorto-pulmonary artery window is a rare anomaly which can only be diagnosed convincingly by catheterization and selective angiography. An injection at the level of the ductus will not demonstrate this left to right shunt (Fig. 52A). If an A-P window is suspected, then the catheter is passed round the aortic arch into the first part of the ascending aorta where a second angiographic injection is made. The shunt is usually large and will be detected in both A.P. and lateral projections. As the condition is one of considerable rarity, full-sized bi-plane film angiography will be advisable for full anatomical detail and pictorial purposes (Fig. 52), but cine-angiography will also demonstrate the lesion well.

2. *Truncus arteriosus*. In the aorto-pulmonary window, the ascending aorta and the pulmonary artery are distinct vessels with their own semi-lunar valves. In a truncus arteriosus, the ascending aorta and the main pulmonary

artery are combined into a single large artery (the truncus) from which the pulmonary arteries arise (Fig. 82). Very rarely, the pulmonary artery to only one lung so arises (Figs. 83, 84) and this anomaly may be termed 'hemi-truncus'.

Retrograde aortography may be indicated in the investigation or confirmation of a truncus. Full-sized films are suggested in order that full anatomical detail be obtained. The angiographic injection is made into the ascending aorta and 40 to 50 ml of contrast medium may be required in the adult, but the patient is usually a child (1 ml/kg body wt.). Selective angiographic injections may usefully be made into the 'bronchial' arteries of truncus type IV or pseudo-truncus.

The majority of patients with persistent truncus present in childhood and a right heart catheterization and angiography will usually establish the diagnosis without need of retrograde left-heart catheterization.

In some patients with a truncus or A-P window, there may be such streaming of the blood flows, that a right ventricular injection may not fully demonstrate the aortic element as most of the contrast medium may be ejected into the pulmonary artery component. An angiographic injection into the base of the ascending aorta will demonstrate the correct anatomy but care must be taken that the injection is delivered immediately above the semilunar valves, proximal to the origin of the abnormal pulmonary arteries (Fig. 82).

3. *Coronary artery fistula*. A coronary artery, arising normally from the ascending aorta, may run an abnormal course and terminate in a right heart chamber or the pulmonary artery. These coronary arteries are often dilated, tortuous, varicose and sometimes aneurysmal, but even without these complications they may transmit a considerable left to right shunt accompanied by an unusual (continuous) murmur. A coronary artery fistula is readily diagnosed by an angiographic injection into the ascending aorta. Full-sized angiocardiographic films are advised in both A.P. and lateral projections. Selective catheterization of the abnormal coronary artery by the original or by a coronary catheter will permit selective coronary angiography which will provide much improved detail (Fig. 104). The volume injected will depend on the size of the coronary artery, 8 ml for a normal artery. Because of the possible danger of high concentrations of sodium ion causing ventricular fibrillation, it is advisable to use a low sodium contrast medium e.g. Cardio-Conray, Hypaque 65, Urografin 76 or Triosil coronaire.

4. *Operative aorto-pulmonary shunts*. A previous Taussig-Blalock anastomosis (subclavian artery to pulmonary artery branch), or a Pott's operation (descending aorta to pulmonary artery branch), or a Waterston-Cooley operation (ascending aorta to right pulmonary artery) provide a therapeutic left to right shunt in order to increase the blood flow to ischaemic lungs.

Retrograde aortography will demonstrate the operative technique which has been employed and the degree of patency of the anastomosis. The angiographic injection is made as for investigation of patent ductus or truncus depending on the site of the operative shunt, using a large volume e.g. 40 ml of contrast medium in the adult. Full-sized angiographic films are desirable for demonstration of the anatomical detail; A.P. and lateral projections are advised.

The natural tendency is for the Blalock anastomosis to become smaller relative to the growing heart size. The Pott's operation, on the other hand, not uncommonly develops into an embarrassingly large left to right shunt and occasionally into an aneurysmal dilatation of the pulmonary artery. Eisenmenger Reaction is a frequent complication.

During the passage of the catheter up the aorta, it is often possible to enter the curved tip of the catheter through a Pott's anastomosis into the pulmonary artery. If this manoeuvre is successful, pressure measurements should be taken in the pulmonary artery, and oximetry analysis of blood from the pulmonary and descending aorta should be made. An angiographic injection into the pulmonary artery will demonstrate the pulmonary vasculature. The A.P. or P.A. (patient supine) is the most valuable projection, and the full-sized radiographs will provide a useful improvement in detail compared with the cine-recording.

Following the Waterston-Cooley operation, there is usually considerable deformity and some stenosis of the pulmonary artery at the site of the anastomosis. The shunt is usually mainly into the right pulmonary artery and this shunt is best demonstrated by left ventriculography or aortography. The left pulmonary artery is however best shown by right-heart angiocardiography.

Ventricular septal defect

Ventricular septal defect will transmit a left to right shunt unless there is an obstruction at the outflow of the right ventricle or pulmonary artery. The left to right shunt through the ventricular septal defect can be well demonstrated by left ventriculography.

The angiographic injection is made with the catheter tip in the mid left ventricle as previously described. The optimal projection is the left anterior oblique as, in this position, the ventricular septum is usually in the plane of the incident X-ray and will be best demonstrated. The jet of contrast medium will be seen in this projection to traverse the defect and pass forwards into the right ventricle. An additional cranio-caudal tilt of the tube may provide an even better view of the interventricular septum (Raphael & Allwork, 1974; Lipchik *et al.*, 1966).

If the left lateral projection be used, the interventricular septum will often lie very obliquely to the X-ray beam and it may be completely invisible even on excellent quality angiograms. If there be a large (left to right) ventricular shunt, it may therefore be impossible in the lateral projection to decide whether there are two ventricles communicating by a large ventricular septal defect or whether there is a common ventricle (Fig. 47). If there has been a previous right heart catheterization, pressure measurements, oximetry or the course taken by the catheter will usually resolve this issue. If there has not been a previous right heart catheterization, or if it has failed to establish whether there are two or a single ventricle, then it is very important to employ the left anterior oblique projection for the left ventriculographic investigation of a possible ventricular septal defect.

In occasional cases, however, particularly when there is right ventricular hypertrophy, the ventricular septum is in the coronal plane and will therefore be best demonstrated in the true lateral projection. If, therefore, the left anterior oblique projection angiocardiography has shown a left-to-right shunt but has not demonstrated whether there are one or two ventricles, a further angiographic injection in the left lateral projection should be made.

Cine-angiocardiography with its simultaneous tele-viewing diagnostic facility is much preferred; full-sized film angiography is less satisfactory.

In every patient with a left-to-right ventricular shunt, an additional aortic arch angiographic injection may be made in order to investigate the possibility of an associated patent ductus. The association of a patent ductus and ventricular septal defect is a frequent one in infants in heart failure. Before subjecting the patient to open heart surgery, it is essential to exclude the possibility of a patent ductus: the aortic injection must therefore never be omitted.

An important exception to the last statement is in very small infants in whom the diagnosis of a left to right shunt is generally made by right heart catheterization and angiography. During this investigation it is usually not possible to exclude a patent ductus (if there are more proximal left to right shunts). In the authors' clinic, the present treatment for infants severely incapacitated by a left to right shunt is to band the pulmonary artery. During the surgical exposure for this, a patent ductus is searched for, and if it be present, it is ligated and divided. We do not therefore consider that, in these small infants (often no more than birth weight), left heart catheterization and pre-operative exclusion of a patent ductus is a necessary investigation (Grainger, Taylor and Verel, 1966).

An occasional complication of ventricular septal defect is *aortic incompetence* sometimes associated with a *prolapsed aortic cusp* (Figs. 53, 54). This is an important association, for the aortic incompetence may prevent satisfactory retrograde aortic perfusion during the period of cardiac arrest and by-pass. The possibility of aortic valve incompetence can be investigated by an angiocardiographic injection into the ascending aorta with radiography in the lateral position (p. 118). This injection will also serve to investigate the possibility of a patent ductus but it must be appreciated that neither the site of the injection nor the radiographic projection is ideal for the demonstration of a small patent ductus.

Left ventricular to right atrial shunt (Gerbode shunt)

This is a rather unusual shunt through a defect in the extreme upper part of the interventricular septum (in fact, at this point, the septum separates the left ventricle from the right atrium). The diagnosis is best made by an angiographic injection into the left ventricle. The optimal radiological projection is the A.P., for in this view, the opacification of the right atrium is best observed. Unless the A.P. projection is employed, the condition may be mis-diagnosed as a ventricular septal defect.

The combination of a high ventricular septal defect (with left to right shunt) and marked tricuspid incompetence will produce angiographic and oximetry findings identical to those of the Gerbode shunt. With this combination, the contrast medium passes from left ventricle to the inflow tract of the right ventricle and then immediately refluxes through the cleft tricuspid valve into the right atrium. The actual deformity will be demonstrated at open heart surgery and no harm should result from the lack of the exact anatomical diagnosis on the pre-operative studies.

In the Gerbode defect the shunt is directly from left ventricle to right atrium. This should be differentiated from an ostium primum defect in which the combination of mitral incompetence and an atrial septal defect may provide a diagnostic angiocardiographic sequence following left ventriculography. The left atrium opacifies from the left ventricle, and this is followed by right atrial visualization. In some cases of ostium primum defect, however, there is *no* opacification of the left atrium as there is a direct L.V.→R.A. shunt (pp. 129 and 163, Fig. 46).

Ostium primum or cushion defect

In this abnormality there is a large low atrial septal defect associated with a deficiency of the atrio-ventricular cushions. The more serious lesions include a common atrio-ventricular canal. A common feature of these defective atrioventricular cushions is mitral incompetence due to a cleft septal leaflet of the mitral valve.

Ostium primum defect can usually be diagnosed clinically, being suggested by the presence of left axis deviation on E.C.G. in a patient with signs of an atrial septal defect. If the issue is not settled by right heart catheterization, and if the surgeon requests a pre-operative distinction between ostium primum, ostium secundum defect and the Gerbode shunt, then retrograde left ventriculography will be helpful. If mitral incompetence is demonstrated, it is likely that the atrial septal defect is of the primum variety.

In some patients with ostium primum defect, the contrast medium may pass from the left ventricle through the cleft mitral valve leaflet directly into the *right atrium* (Fig. 46). This is because the contrast medium refluxing through the incompetent mitral valve is propelled directly towards the defect in the lower part of the interatrial septum. The regurgitant stream passes through this defect to opacify the right atrium without prior opacification of the left atrium and a Gerbode shunt may be simulated. The right border of the left ventricle is abnormal and irregularly concave (Goose neck deformity) in ostium primum. This is well seen on left ventriculography in the antero-posterior view (Fig. 46).

The catheterization is performed in the usual manner from the femoral artery and the left ventricle is entered and injected as previously described for the study of rheumatic mitral incompetence. The angiocardiographic technique is identical. The left lateral or the right anterior oblique projections are the most satisfactory for demonstration of mitral incompetence. The supine A.P. projection is advised for demonstration of the atrial septal defect.

In ostium primum defect, a marked deficiency of the atrio-ventricular cushion may permit the catheter tip to pass from the left ventricle into the left atrium or into the right heart chambers. Should this occur, advantage should be taken by making pressure recordings and blood samplings for oxygenation from each chamber entered. If considered advisable, additional angiocardiographic injections can be made into these chambers.

LEFT HEART OBSTRUCTIONS

The most frequent obstructive lesions on the left side of the heart are mitral stenosis and aortic valve stenosis. Considerably less frequent are coarctation of aorta, obstructive cardiomyopathy, sub- and supra-valvar aortic stenosis (in descending order of incidence).

Mitral stenosis cannot be adequately assessed by retrograde left heart catheterization, but of course any associated mitral incompetence can be investigated by this method. With the above exception, all of the other obstructive lesions of the left heart can be demonstrated by retrograde catheterization of the left heart.

Aortic valve stenosis

Stenosis at the aortic valve may be congenital or acquired. Aortic incompetence is more likely to be associated with the latter variety.

If the aortic valve is tightly stenosed, it is unlikely that the operator will be able to introduce the catheter retrogradely through the valve into the left ventricle. There are various manoeuvres which can be adopted to encourage traverse of the valve. The use of a soft pliable polythene catheter (P.E. 240 or 280) is helpful. If the first catheter does not traverse the valve, it is always worthwhile changing the catheter after re-introduction of the

guide wire (p. 81) to another soft polythene catheter with a more sharply curved end or an S bend. The tight distal curve may then traverse the aortic valve. Pig-tail polyurethane catheters are also very useful to traverse the normal or stenotic aortic valve.

It is occasionally helpful to use the tip of the guide wire to find the orifice of the aortic valve. The most useful guide wires for this purpose are the plastic-coated flexible wires or a coiled spring wire with a J-tip and adjustable central core. A 'standard' coil spring wire can be used for catheter introduction and if difficulty in traversing the aortic valve is experienced, the guide wire can be changed to a more flexible one. Approximately 5 to 8 cm of the new wire can be passed through the catheter tip and 'played' over the aortic valve as previously described (p. 102). It is important not to expose the protruding wire in the blood stream for more than 1 or 2 minutes, for blood clot may form on its surface and may be scraped off as the wire is pulled back through the catheter (p. 102).

Some investigators find a catheter approach from the axillary or brachial artery to be more successful than from the femoral artery in traversing a stenotic aortic valve.

If the aortic valve is traversed, an angiocardiographic injection into the left ventricle is made, usually 40 to 60 ml of CardioConray or Urografin 76. The full-sized radiographic films or cine-radiography will demonstrate the rigidity or doming of the aortic valve. Cine-radiography will provide better visualization of valve-cusp movement and of any calcification which may be present, but doming may be better seen on the large films. In general, cine-angiography is preferred.

The supine projection is satisfactory but not ideal, as the outflow tract of the left ventricle is somewhat foreshortened in this position (Fig. 15.1B). The true lateral position is also not ideal for even more foreshortening of the left ventricular outflow is likely and the aortic valve plane is not generally parallel to the X-ray beam and film (Fig. 15.1A). Because of the 'tilt' of the aortic valve in the lateral projection, it is possible to produce an appearance of spurious 'doming' of the normal aortic cusps on the radiographs, which may simulate valve stenosis. The other features of valve stenosis (p. 64), e.g. jet, post-stenotic dilatation, reduced mobility of abnormal cusps, calcification and thickening will not be seen and the experienced investigator should not be misled by the spurious doming.

A very useful projection for the angiographic investigation of aortic valve stenosis is a left lateral tube position with the patient lying supine on the table-top but rotated on a vertical axis so that the head moves 20° to the patient's left and the feet 20° to the right (Fig. 15.1C). In this projection, the outflow tract of the left ventricle lies perpendicular to the lateral X-ray beam and the aortic

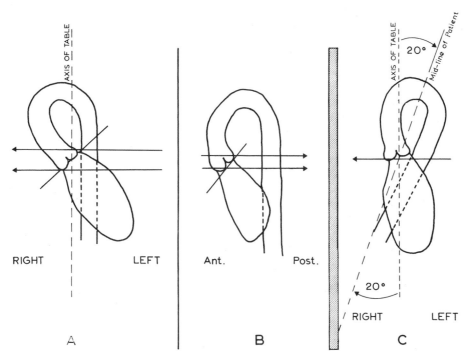

FIG. 15.1   *The Obliquity of the Aortic Valve*

A. As viewed from above supine patient. The arrows indicate the X-ray beam in the lateral projection. The aortic valve ring is projected as shown, very obliquely, with its left border well above the right border.

B. As viewed from the side of supine patient. The arrows indicate the X-ray beam in the A.P. projection. The aortic valve ring is projected as shown, very obliquely, with its anterior border well below the posterior border.

C. As viewed from above. The patient is supine but is rotated on a vertical axis so that the head is displaced 20° to the left (i.e. Fig. A rotated 20°). A lateral X-ray beam now projects the aortic valve tangentially so that its structure can be better appreciated. This rotated position (C) is a very useful projection for visualizing the aortic valve in profile. (Shaded area is the table top for Fig. 15.1B.)

valve plane will then be seen tangentially on the lateral films.

Unfortunately, in many types of installation of the X-ray equipment, it may be impossible to arrange for this rotation of the patient because of the fixity of some of the apparatus. The use of cranio-caudal tilt on the parallelogram U arm can also provide this projection.

A programme of 4 to 6 films per s for 3 or 4 seconds is usually satisfactory for full-size films, or 6 seconds of cine-recording.

After the angiocardiographic injection, the intra-ventricular pressure is recorded through the catheter and a withdrawal trace through the aortic valve is obtained, ending with an aortic tracing (Fig. 14.3). Any pressure gradient is thereby recorded; in the absence of a gradient, aortic valve stenosis can be excluded. It is important that the pressure waves caused by the extrasystoles as the catheter traverses the left ventricular outflow, be ignored in determining the valve gradient (p. 118).

During the fluoroscopic manipulation of the catheter, the aortic valve region must be carefully assessed for the presence of valve calcification which is much more readily visible on the television image than on conventional fluoroscopy. A permanent recording of the calcification should always be obtained with a few seconds cine run.

As previously described (p. 120), an angiocardiographic injection should then be made into the ascending aorta in order to assess any accompanying aortic incompetence. The optimum projection is the left lateral. Cine-angiography is much preferred. Some surgeons may require detail of the coronary arteries before operating on the aortic valve. Coronary arteriography may then be considered an additional necessary pre-operative investigation.

Coarctation of aorta

In many patients with aortic coarctation, the femoral arteries can be palpated and they may be catheterized percutaneously without undue difficulty. However, if the coarctation is a severe one, it is unlikely that the catheter will pass retrogradely through the constriction into the aortic arch. There is usually a sharp forward kink of the aorta at the site of the coarctation and it is often the kink rather than the narrowing which prevents the successful passage of the catheter (Fig. 90).

Another difficulty with retrograde aortic catheterization is that the catheter may pass into a large vertical intercostal artery behind the aortic arch. This will not be appreciated on A.P. or P.A. fluoroscopy and a test injection is essential to prevent the angiographic injection being made into the collateral artery which may be dangerous.

Femoral artery catheterization and retrograde aortography will therefore often demonstrate only the lower limit of the coarctation segment and the aorta below this. This is useful information for there are often abnormalities such as post-stenotic dilatation of the aorta and aneurysms of the intercostal arteries below the coarctation about which the surgeon wishes to be informed. However, the main object of aortography is to demonstrate the anatomy of the coarctation and of the aortic arch as well as the descending aorta. It may be important to obtain a pressure gradient. As this information will generally not be obtained by retrograde catheterization from the femoral artery, it is strongly recommended that the aortographic injection be made proximal to the coarctation. This implies either axillary artery catheterization (p. 80) or catheterization of the left heart by the modified Ross technique after atrial transseptal puncture (Chapter 11).

In children and infants, it is usually possible to obtain perfectly satisfactory visualization of the coarctation during right heart catheterization (Fig. 88). If the foramen ovale be patent, then the catheter should be passed into the left atrium, and the angiographic injection made into this chamber (Fig. 90) (or the left ventricle). In children, a septal defect often complicates a coarctation of aorta; in these cases advantage should be taken during right heart catheterization of making the angiographic injection into the left heart (Fig. 91). Even if it is not possible to enter the left heart chambers through a septal defect, a large angiographic injection into the main pulmonary artery of a child will generally produce very adequate demonstration of the aortic coarctation on the late films (Fig. 88).

In adults, the right axillary artery route may be preferred for the catheterization using 240 polythene catheter; the catheter tip should be sited in the middle of the ascending aorta (Fig. 89) before making the angiocardiographic injection. Films will be needed for 5 to 8 seconds and if full-sized angiography is used, the rate should be 3 per s for 3 s and then slower.

If the injection is made more proximally into the left heart chambers, then the films must be exposed over a longer period of time, say 8 to 10 seconds. If a right heart injection is being utilized, then the aorta will usually fill at about 6 to 10 seconds and the films should be taken for

10 to 14 seconds. For these intracardiac injections, rapid films are *not* necessary as the aorta will be opacified for rather longer and a rate of 2 films per s should be adequate.

Full-sized radiographs are superior to cine-radiography for the demonstration of the anatomical detail of the coarctation. The optimum projection will depend on the exact obliquity of the aortic arch. In the supine projection, a dilated ascending aorta may be directly in front of the coarctation region. An opacified left atrial appendage or pulmonary artery may also lie directly in front of the coarctation. In the lateral projection it may be difficult to secure a good view of the aortic arch as the shoulders tend to obscure the area. In most patients, an A.P. projection with the patient supine and then rotated 15° to his right (i.e. 15° L.A.O.) will nearly always present a satisfactory view of the coarctation and the related arteries. In this projection the ascending aorta is seen to the right of the spine and 'uncovers' the upper descending thoracic aorta (Fig. 87). An alternative projection is 45° L.A.O. Photographic subtraction is very useful in eliminating bone detail which may obscure the coarctation (Fig. 113).

Aortic valve stenosis is not uncommon in aortic coarctation, and if axillary artery catheterization is being employed, then it is advisable to pass the catheter through the ascending aorta, across the aortic valve into the left ventricle where a second angiocardiographic injection may be made. A pressure withdrawal trace across the aortic valve is then obtained so that the presence of aortic stenosis may be assessed.

A pressure tracing should be taken from the aorta above the coarctation. It is advisable, if the aortic narrowing is not gross, to take a simultaneous pressure recording below the coarctation so that the haemodynamic significance of the lesion may be assessed. The pressure in the lower segment is best obtained by needle puncture of the femoral artery—a procedure which is possible in the majority of patients with coarctations of all but the most severe degree. Sometimes the catheter introduced from above (e.g. via the axillary artery) may be manipulated through the coarctation into the lower segment, so permitting the pressure gradient to be taken. If the obstruction at the coarctation is of gross degree, then there is little purpose (other than academic) of measuring the pressure gradient pre-operatively.

Supravalvar aortic stenosis

This is a rare condition in which there is a severe constriction in the ascending aorta just above the aortic valve. There is a well-recognized syndrome in which the aortic lesion is associated with a peculiar ugly facies and an impaired intellect. There is considerable evidence that this syndrome is the aftermath of 'infantile hypercalcaemia with failure to thrive'.

There is usually a good femoral pulse and femoral artery catheterization is practical. The catheter is passed retrogradely round the aortic arch into the ascending aorta where it will generally traverse the narrowing and pass through the aortic valve into the left ventricle. Unlike coarctation, there is no kink to obstruct the catheterization. The angiocardiographic injection is best made into the left ventricle, as there may be an inadequate gap between the supra-valvar constriction and the aortic valve in which to position the catheter tip (Fig. 87).

The A.P. or P.A. projection with the supine patient rotated 15° to the right (15° L.A.O.) will project the ascending aorta clear of the dorsal spine. A 'lateral' projection will provide additional simultaneous information of the anatomy.

Either full-sized radiography or cine-recording will be satisfactory.

A pressure tracing is obtained as the catheter is withdrawn from the left ventricle into the aortic arch. There is no gradient at the aortic valve but, just above it, there will be a drop in pressure as the supravalvar constriction is negotiated.

The syndrome of supravalvar aortic stenosis referred to above may be associated with other arterial stenosis, e.g. at the aortic arch, above the renal arteries or the renal arteries themselves. These areas should be visualized during the same aortic catheterization. Pulmonary artery stenosis also may be present but this will require right heart catheterization for visualization.

Obstructive cardiomyopathy

Obstructive hypertrophic cardiomyopathy is a condition in which marked irregular hypertrophy of the myocardium embarrasses the action, and obstructs the outlet and often the inlet of the ventricles. The left ventricle is usually affected more than the right. The disordered function and anatomy of the left ventricle can be well demonstrated by retrograde cine left ventriculography.

The catheterization is conducted in the usual way from the femoral artery. There is no difficulty in traversing the aortic valve which is normal. The catheter can usually be placed without difficulty, deep into the left ventricular cavity.

Angiocardiographic injection into the left ventricle is made in the usual way (p. 117). The optimum projections are the A.P. or P.A. and the 'rotated' lateral view (previously described p. 131, Fig. 15.1) taken simultaneously, but as it may not be possible to position the patient in this way, standard A.P. or P.A. and lateral projections taken simultaneously will usually demonstrate the disordered anatomy (Figs. 111B, 112). The interventricular septum is often the site of the most marked muscle hypertrophy and an additional left anterior oblique projection will demonstrate this to better advantage.

G

Both cine-recording and full-sized films are valuable, for the former technique will best show the disordered mechanism of left ventricular contraction, whilst the latter method will best illustrate the disordered anatomy.

It is very important to take a pressure recording deeply within the left ventricular cavity for there are usually significant intraventricular pressure gradients due to obstructive changes consequent on the myocardial hypertrophy. The catheter tip should be manipulated into the left ventricular inflow and towards the apex of the chamber. Pressure measurements should be taken at these sites and a continuous recording should be obtained as the catheter is slowly withdrawn through the left ventricular outflow, through the aortic valve into the ascending aorta. The position of the aortic valve is readily identified by the sharp elevation of the diastolic pressure in the left ventricle (usually 0 to 10 mmHg) to aortic diastolic readings (usually 60 to 90 mmHg). The gradient in obstructive cardiomyopathy is systolic and occurs *within* the ventricular cavity before the aortic valve is reached. In this condition, the intraventricular pressure gradient can be greatly modified by drugs, e.g. isoprenaline, amyl nitrite, propranolol. The aortic pressure trace presents a typical sharp vertical rise at the onset of ventricular systole, compared to the slow rising anacrotic wave form of aortic valve stenosis.

Mitral-valve incompetence frequently occurs with hypertrophic obstructive cardiomyopathy, and will be observed, particularly if cine films are taken during left ventriculography.

SELECTIVE RIGHT ANGIOCARDIOGRAPHY

Congenital heart disease

LEFT TO RIGHT SHUNTS

Patients with suspected systemic-pulmonary shunts may be referred for cardiac catheterization in order to localize the cardiac defect and to assess the haemodynamic state and the pulmonary vascular resistance.

Selective angiocardiography is very valuable for shunt localization and in this clinic it has been found more reliable than oximetry. The shunt may occur at atrial level (atrial septal defect or anomalous pulmonary venous drainage), ventricular level (ventricular septal defect), or at aortic level (patent ductus arteriosus). There are several other possibilities which are far less common (e.g. Gerbode shunt left ventricle to right atrium; aorto-pulmonary window; coronary artery-pulmonary artery fistula).

The catheterization is usually best performed from the leg veins as an atrial septal defect is far easier to traverse from below than from the arm (p. 88). If the catheter can be manipulated through a defect into the left heart chambers, the site of the shunt may be confirmed by making an angiocardiographic injection into the *first* left heart chamber which is entered. The shunt is recognized by opacification of the right heart chambers by contrast medium which has been injected into the left chamber (Figs. 44, 46).

Atrial septal defect

The catheter can usually be manipulated from the leg veins (or, with experience, from the arm veins) through the right atrium across the atrial septum into the left atrium (p. 88). The catheter position may be confirmed by oximetry. An angiocardiographic injection is made into the left atrium (Fig. 44); a large volume (up to 60 ml in an adult) must be injected rapidly through a large bore catheter if a large shunt is suspected. The best radiographic projection is A.P. or P.A., for opacification of right atrium can readily be recognized in this view. If bi-plane radiographs are being taken, A.P. or P.A. and lateral projections are used. Another useful projection is 45° left anterior oblique, in which view the atrial septum may be tangential. Cine recording is preferable to full-sized films; 3 films per s for 4 seconds followed by 1 film per s for another 4 seconds is a useful programme if large films are being used.

If the catheter has passed across a *patent foramen ovale*, and if the angiographic injection is delivered into the left atrium, there will be *no* opacification of the right atrium as a left to right shunt cannot normally flow through the flap valve covering the foramen ovale (Figs. 29, 30, 31). In some patients however, the catheter may so deform the foramen ovale flap, that a left to right shunt may occur during the angiography: this is usually a small shunt. If there is an *atrial septal defect* (ostium primum or secundum), the right atrium will be seen to opacify from the left atrium (Fig. 44).

After the injection, a withdrawal trace is taken across the atrial septum; a significant gradient suggests a patent foramen ovale.

Aberrant pulmonary veins

Individual pulmonary veins may enter the right atrium separately (Figs. 38, 39) or they may all drain into a major vein such as a left superior vena cava which may enter the left innominate vein and thus return oxygenated pulmonary venous blood into the superior vena cava and right atrium (Figs. 41, 42). Occasionally the pulmonary veins pass downwards through the diaphragm to enter the hepatic or portal veins (Fig. 43).

If a pulmonary vein is entered from the right atrium, the catheter will be seen on fluoroscopy to enter the lung fields outside the cardiac silhouette and fully oxygenated blood will be withdrawn. It is not possible to decide merely from the course of the catheter whether the pulmonary vein has been entered directly from the right atrium, or whether the catheter has passed from the right atrium into the left atrium and thence into a normal draining pulmonary vein (Fig. 3). Confirmation of the anatomy is obtained by injecting (in an adult) 20 ml of contrast medium into the pulmonary vein and taking either a single radiograph or a 3-second series of films or cine-recording in the A.P. or P.A. projection (Fig. 39).

In some patients with anomalous pulmonary venous drainage, the catheter course may occasionally be very suggestive of the diagnosis. The catheter may pass from the right atrium into the coronary sinus into the left pulmonary veins, or from a left superior vena cava into a pulmonary vein. A small injection of contrast medium into the abnormal veins will confirm the diagnosis.

In suspected total anomalous pulmonary venous return, angiographic confirmation is best obtained by making a large injection into the main pulmonary artery, taking a *long* series of films to demonstrate the pathway of the pulmonary venous return (Figs. 41, 42, 43). The optimal projections are both A.P. (or P.A.) and true lateral.

The A.P. projection will demonstrate the detail of the confluence of the pulmonary veins (Figs. 41, 42). The lateral films are particularly helpful if the A.P. or P.A. films are not diagnostic, e.g. due to poor radiographic contrast. On the lateral films the left innominate vein is seen *end-on* and if it is returning opacified pulmonary venous blood to the right superior vena cava (as in the cottage loaf heart), it can readily be identified lying anterior to and above the aortic arch.

Cine-radiography will also demonstrate a major anomaly of pulmonary venous return, but will probably not detect the anomalous drainage of a single pulmonary vein. In fact, it may be impossible both with cine or full-sized film angiography to confirm the drainage of one or two pulmonary veins into the right atrium compared with an atrial septal defect with left to right shunt.

Ventricular septal defect

If the defect is traversed by the catheter, an angiocardiographic injection may be made into the left ventricle (p. 117). The ventricular septal defect is best visualized on the 45° left anterior oblique film and the shunt is confirmed by the opacification of the right ventricle. A lateral projection is also useful but may not demonstrate the actual septal defect; it will however confirm opacification of the anteriorly situated right ventricle. In the A.P. or P.A. and lateral projections, it may be quite impossible to distinguish a large ventricular septal defect from a single ventricle: a left anterior oblique projection will decide (p. 128 and Fig. 47).

Either cine-recording or full-sized films may be used. Radiography for 6 seconds is adequate, using 3 or 4 films per s for the first 3 seconds. Cine-recording is preferable.

If the ventricular septal defect is not traversed by the catheter, the technique of a large angiographic injection into the main pulmonary artery with an extended sequence of films should be diagnostic (p. 123). Cine-radiography is preferable, but full-size films are also satisfactory. The left anterior oblique projection is advised but in this view an A.S.D. may be undetected. If A.S.D. is a possibility, then an A.P. (or P.A.) projection may be necessary (p. 134).

Patent ductus arteriosus

The catheter can often be manipulated from the pulmonary artery through the patent ductus into the descending aorta. The course of the catheter is diagnostic (Fig. 11) but the tip of the catheter must be passed down the aorta to reach *below* the diaphragm—if this is not performed, a very similar catheter course may be found if the catheter has entered the posterior basal segmental pulmonary artery of the left lower lobe.

It is important not to make a pressure injection into the ductus itself—a cautious hand injection of contrast medium should always be made to exclude this possibility.

If the ductus has been traversed, the angiographic injection is best made with the catheter tip sited beyond the aortic entry of the ductus, just as the catheter enters the aorta. If there is a left to right shunt, the pulmonary artery will be opacified.

The ductus itself is best seen in the 45° L.A.O. or lateral (Figs. 49, 50) projection but faint pulmonary artery opacification is best confirmed on the A.P. film. A.P. and lateral bi-plane full-sized films are taken at a rate of 3 or 4 per s for seconds. Cine-radiography is preferred. The details of the injection are given on page 127.

If the ductus is not traversed by the catheter, the diagnosis may still be made angiographically by making a large injection into the main pulmonary artery and taking a long sequence of radiographs (p. 123), following the contrast medium into the left heart and aorta.

The less common left to right shunts

Gerbode shunt transmits a flow of blood from the left ventricle to the right atrium. The catheter may pass from the right atrium through the defect high in the ventricular septum into the left ventricle where the angiocardiographic injection should be delivered. The best projection is antero-posterior: cine or big films may be used, 3 or 4 films per s for 3 seconds followed by 1 film per s for 6 seconds. If the catheter does not pass from the right atrium to the left ventricle, then a retrograde left ventriculogram will confirm the diagnosis.

Aorto-pulmonary window is best demonstrated by retrograde aortography (p. 122 and Fig. 52), but during right heart catheterization, the window may be traversed by the catheter from the pulmonary artery and an injection of contrast medium into the origin of the ascending aorta will reveal the anatomy.

Coronary artery shunts. An aberrant coronary artery may transmit arterial blood from the aorta to the pulmonary artery, right ventricle or right atrium. The angiographic investigation is best conducted by retrograde aortography (p. 122) and selective coronary arteriography using cine. Further detail may be obtained by selective coronary angiography. (See Chap. 13.)

RIGHT HEART INJECTIONS FOR LEFT TO RIGHT SHUNTS
It is preferable to investigate left to right shunts by injection of contrast medium into the left heart chamber from which the shunt emerges, as previously described (p. 134). If this chamber cannot be entered by the catheter, an angiocardiographic diagnosis may still be achieved by a large angiographic injection into the main pulmonary artery (or less valuable right ventricle).

The principle of this technique is that the bolus of contrast medium passes through the lungs, is collected into the pulmonary veins and then passed into the left atrium, left ventricle and aorta. By the time the left atrium has opacified, the pulmonary artery will have cleared of contrast medium and the whole of the right heart should be free of contrast. If there is a left to right shunt, there will occur at this stage, opacification of the right heart chamber which receives the shunt.

In order to perform this technique satisfactorily, a *large bolus* of contrast medium must be delivered *rapidly* into the pulmonary artery. This necessitates *as large a bore catheter* as can be manipulated into position. If the catheter cannot be passed into the pulmonary artery, the injection may be delivered into the outflow tract of the right ventricle but the results are not as good. In the adult, 40 to 70 ml of contrast medium should be rapidly injected.

In order to detect recirculation it is essential to be certain that the pulmonary artery (and/or right ventricle) is clear of contrast medium before the left atrium opacifies, and that the film sequence covers the complete filling of the left heart and aorta. A useful programme is 3 films per s for 2 seconds (to visualize the pulmonary arteries) followed by 2 films per s for a further 8 to 14 seconds depending on the circulation time. Cine-recording is also satisfactory and must be taken for up to 15 s depending on the circulation time.

The optimum projections for this technique are true A.P. (or P.A.) and lateral. The radiographic exposure must be carefully controlled for it is most important not to over-expose the anterior portion of the heart shadow on the lateral film. This region is sometimes 'blacked out' when the exposure is ideal for the opacification of the left heart chambers: this must be avoided. Opacification of the right ventricle (via a V.S.D.) may be very faint. A slightly underexposed lateral radiographic technique and the use of a bright spotlight to illuminate the dark right ventricular area for faint opacification are essential.

Faint opacification of the right atrium (via A.S.D.) is

best recognized on a correctly exposed A.P. film, on which the right lateral and inferior borders of the right atrium can be identified if opacification occurs (Fig. 45). Reflux down the inferior vena cava or hepatic veins is diagnostic of right atrial opacification.

Faint opacification of the right ventricle (via V.S.D.) is best identified on the lateral radiograph as described above. The A.P. or P.A. film may give *no* suggestion of faint opacification of this chamber although the lateral film may be quite diagnostic.

Faint opacification of the main pulmonary artery (via P.D.A.) is best recognized on the A.P. or P.A. radiograph.

Both A.P. or P.A. and lateral films should be available which show the right heart and main pulmonary artery to be clear of contrast medium *before* opacification of the left heart occurs. These two films are then carefully compared with later films to assess any subsequent opacification of the right heart chambers. The *most proximal* right heart chamber to be opacified identifies the site of the left to right shunt.

In this unit, this technique has been repeatedly proven to be more accurate than oximetry in shunt detection. A left to right shunt ratio of 1·2 can almost always be detected with confidence by the above angiographic method.

One disadvantage of the method is that only the proximal of two or more left to right shunts will be detected. If more than one shunt is suspected, then retrograde aortography and left ventriculography (pp. 126–130) will be necessary to complete the diagnosis.

The failure to detect the more distal of two left to right shunts is based on simple haemodynamic principles. If there is both a V.S.D. and a patent ductus (both transmitting a left to right shunt) and if the pulmonary artery injection follow through technique (p. 135) is being used, the right ventricle will opacify via the V.S.D. when the left ventricle receives the contrast medium. The right ventricle will then expel its opacified blood into the pulmonary artery which will be seen to opacify on the radiographs. At this stage, the aorta will pass opacified blood through the ductus into the pulmonary artery, but as the latter vessel is already opacified, the newly arrived contrast medium from the ductus cannot be recognized with any degree of confidence. The angiographic diagnosis will then be 'V.S.D. but patent ductus cannot be excluded'. In fact, with the pulmonary artery injection follow through technique, once any left to right shunt has been identified, a more distal shunt can *never* be excluded. If there is any clinical, oximetric or angiographic suggestion of a second shunt, then retrograde aortography and left ventriculography (pp. 126–130) will investigate this possibility.

PULMONARY STENOSIS

Obstruction may be situated at the pulmonary valve, in the infundibulum of the right ventricle or in the pulmonary artery itself—in descending order of frequency. Infundibular obstruction may be fixed and fibrotic, or variable and muscular. Stenosis of the pulmonary artery may be congenital or acquired by surgical banding (for left to right shunts) (Fig. 59). Eisenmenger Reaction is a condition in which there is a high peripheral resistance in the pulmonary arteriolar bed—i.e. obstruction of the pulmonary artery outflow.

The angiocardiographic injection for all these lesions is best made into the right ventricle as described on page 123. Full-sized radiographs are preferred for investigating these stenotic lesions, using A.P. or P.A. and lateral projections, at 3 to 5 films per s for 3 seconds followed by 1 film per s for the next 8 to 10 seconds in order to visualize the left heart (and possibly a shunt into the right heart).

The pulmonary valve is best seen on the lateral projections (Figs. 57 and 58): the right ventricular infundibulum is also best seen in this projection. A spurious infundibular constriction may be caused by placing the catheter and delivering the angiographic injection just below the pulmonary valve. An angiographic distinction is generally possible between the mobile muscular hypertrophy of the right ventricle outflow induced by a pulmonary valve stenosis (Fig. 57) and the fixed fibrotic obstruction of the right ventricular outflow which is usually accompanied by a ventricular septal defect (Fig. 60).

Obstruction of the main pulmonary artery is best visualized on the lateral projection (Fig. 59) but stenosis of its branches are best seen on the postero-anterior films.

Whenever a severe obstruction is found on the right side of the heart or in the pulmonary artery, the films must be examined carefully for evidence of premature opacification of the left heart chambers via a right to left shunt. This will indicate a potentially cyanotic circulatory abnormality.

The most reliable angiographic method of identifying a very small right to left shunt on large films is by examining serial A.P. or P.A. radiographs for faint opacification of the descending thoracic aorta or carotid or subclavian arteries. With cine-recording, the small jets of shunt may be identifiable entering the left heart.

CYANOTIC CONGENITAL HEART DISEASE

With the exceptions of transposition and common atria or ventricles, there are always at least two abnormalities in cyanotic congenital heart disease: (1) an obstruction in the right side of the heart or pulmonary artery and (2) a more proximal communication between the two sides of the heart. The objectives of cardiac catheterization and angiocardiography are to identify these two abnormalities and to assess the size and capacity of the main pulmonary arteries and their branches.

During the right heart catheterization, the site of the obstruction is often identified by a pressure gradient or by inability to pass the catheter into the various right heart chambers. The angiocardiographic injection should be delivered into the mid-cavity of the chamber proximal to the obstruction. The details of the injection are discussed on page 123.

The optimal projections are A.P. or P.A. and lateral: full-sized radiographs may be preferred to cine. A useful programme is 3 to 5 films per s for 4 seconds followed by 1 film per s for 4 to 8 seconds.

The most frequent obstruction in cyanotic congenital heart disease is at the outflow of the right ventricle—either pulmonary valve or infundibulum, or both. The anatomy is best seen on the lateral films. This obstruction is commonly associated with a ventricular septal defect and this also is easily diagnosed on the lateral film. *Fallot's tetralogy* is the most frequent cause of cyanotic congenital heart disease after the first year of life, but *transposition* of the great vessels is a more frequent anomaly than cyanotic Fallot in the first few months (Grainger, Taylor and Verel, 1966).

Tricuspid atresia is best identified on the A.P. or P.A. films by angiographic injection into the right atrium when an absent (or non-functional) right ventricle will be noted and the contrast medium will pass directly from the right atrium to the left atrium (Fig. 75).

Eisenmenger Reaction is best identified by an injection into the main pulmonary artery when the abnormal peripheral pulmonary arterial bed will be recognized. If the right to left shunt is through the ductus, this will be demonstrated by aortic filling (Fig. 67). A more proximal shunt will probably be identified by catheter exploration or by a more proximal injection of contrast medium. It must be remembered however that right heart angiography in Eisenmenger Reaction carries a major risk, particularly in adults (p. 145).

Transposition of the great vessels poses a separate problem in cardiac catheterization. There are several anatomical variants but the most frequent pattern of uncorrected transposition is that the aorta rises anteriorly from the anterior (right) ventricle, whilst the pulmonary artery arises posteriorly from the posterior (left) ventricle. This relationship is best visualized on the lateral radiographs (Figs. 70–74). Two shunts (right to left and left to right) of equal volume must be present. These shunts may occur through a single or two septal defects or patent ductus. Pulmonary valve stenosis is a frequent accompaniment.

The first angiographic injection in suspected transposition is best made into the anterior ventricle. Full-sized films, A.P. or P.A. and lateral bi-plane, are recommended at 3 to 4 per s for 3 seconds followed by 1 per s for 6 seconds.

Further injections will probably be required to identify all of the anatomical defects. The sites of injections will depend on the chambers entered by the catheter. An angiographic injection into the right atrium is very useful as it is fundamental to determine the path of systemic venous blood. If it passes from the right atrium to the right ventricle to the anteriorly displaced aorta, the diagnosis is *uncorrected* transposition (Figs. 70–74). If the route of systemic venous blood is right atrium, inverted left ventricle to a posteriorly displaced pulmonary artery, the diagnosis is *corrected* transposition of the great vessels (Fig. 68), (Grainger, 1970).

Cine-recording will also be effective in establishing the diagnosis, but the greater detail obtained on either full-size films or miniature photofluorograms is a real advantage.

In all varieties of congenital heart disease, more than one abnormality is often present. Obstructions tend to be single; shunts tend to be multiple, e.g. combined A.S.D., V.S.D., and P.D.A. is a frequently occurring pattern of congenital heart disease in the infant. As the heart is being explored by the catheter, the anatomical abnormalities are successively encountered. The operator must be prepared to modify his basic plan of campaign at any stage and he must take advantage of and explore any chamber which the catheter enters. More than one angiocardiographic injection may be required: two is a frequent number, but occasionally three or four injections may be needed to reveal all the cardiac defects. Multiple injections are facilitated by pumps which permit multiple injections from one loading of the syringe. Cine-recording and/or miniature photofluorography also facilitate multiple injections as they save the considerable labour and expense of repeated loading of the large film cassette. After each injection, the information gained must be assessed and assimilated before proceeding to the next stage of the catheterization. Video-tape is most helpful in allowing immediate play-back of the cine view.

Acquired heart disease

MITRAL HEART DISEASE

Selective right heart catheterization may be indicated in patients with mitral valve disease in order to measure the pulmonary artery pressure and peripheral resistance, to measure left atrial pressure and in order to visualize the mitral valve.

Pulmonary angiography is rarely indicated in mitral valve disease except in the investigation of pulmonary emboli. In patients with mitral valve disease and severe pulmonary hypertension, we have found pulmonary angiography to be an unsafe procedure which may rarely be fatal (p. 145).

The mitral valve is best visualized angiographically by an injection of contrast medium into the left atrium. This chamber is best entered by the Ross technique of atrial transseptal catheterization—or one of its modifications

(p. 95); 30 to 50 ml of contrast medium is used. The optimum projection is the 45° right anterior oblique (right shoulder forward) when the mitral cusps may be seen in profile, but normal cusps are very difficult to see with certainty. Cine-angiography is preferred to full-size films as one obtains a clearer impression of left atrial action and valve motion.

PULMONARY DISEASE

Pulmonary angiography is occasionally indicated for the elucidation of pulmonary pathology of uncertain nature. Pulmonary arterio-venous malformations are confirmed angiographically. Congenital absence of a pulmonary artery can only be diagnosed with certainty by pulmonary angiography (Fig. 61).

Pulmonary emboli may be investigated by angiography. The larger emboli are well demonstrated as intra-luminal filling defects, often rather angular in shape, in the major pulmonary arteries. Smaller pulmonary emboli may be visualized by angiographic injection into the specific lobar or segmental artery; the use of fine focus X-ray tube, magnification technique and single full-size 'spot' films are helpful in the diagnosis of small peripheral pulmonary emboli.

Pulmonary artery aneurysms and arteriovenous fistulae are occasional causes of haemoptysis. They may be single or multiple, unilocular or multilocular: their anatomy and vascular connections are well demonstrated by pulmonary angiography (Fig. 101).

Primary broncho-pulmonary disease, particularly carcinoma of the bronchus may obstruct or distort a major pulmonary artery or vein, or a vena cava. Right heart catheterization and angiography is occasionally useful in these circumstances.

The technique of pulmonary angiography is described on p. 123. Full-sized radiographs should be used and the programme should include rapid films in the arterial phase e.g. 2 to 4 films per s for 3 seconds followed by 1 film per s for 5 seconds. The A.P. (or P.A.) projection is the most useful but other views may be necessary depending on the location of pulmonary disease.

Cine-recording is unlikely to provide the detail required, particularly when searching for small pulmonary emboli, where the emphasis is on maximum detail rather than dynamic movement.

References

BARON, M. G., WOLF, B. S., STEINFELD, L. & GORDON, A. J. (1963). Left ventricular angiocardiography in the study of ventricular septal defects. *Radiology* **81**, 223–235.

BARON, M. G., WOLF, B. S., STEINFELD, L. & VAN MIEROP, L. H. S. (1964). Endocardial cushion defects. Specific diagnosis by angiocardiography. *Am. J. Cardiol.* **13**, 162–175.

BRAUNWALD, E., MORROW, A. & COOPER, T. (1959). Left ventriculography in the diagnosis of persistent atrio-ventricular canal and related anomalies. *Am. J. Cardiol.* **4**, 802.

DEMANY, M. A., KAY, E. B. & ZIMMERMAN, H. A. (1966). An Angiocardiographic sign for the evaluation of the stenotic mitral valve. *Am. J. Cardiol.* **18**, 843.

EDWARDS, J. E. (1961). *An Atlas of Acquired Diseases of the Heart and Great Vessels.* Vol. II. Philadelphia & London: Saunders.

FIGLEY, M. M. (1964). Angiocardiography in valvular heart disease: morphologic and volumetric considerations. *Radiol. Clinics N. Am.* **2**, 409.

GRAINGER, R. G., TAYLOR, D. G. & VEREL, D. (1966). Cardiac catheterization and selective angiocardiography in congenital heart disease presenting in the neonate. *Clin. Radiol.* **17**, 12.

GYEPES, M. T. and VINCENT, W. R. (1974). Cardiac Catheterization and Angiocardiography in Severe Neonatal Heart Disease. Charles C. Thomas, Springfield, Illinois, U.S.A.

HYNES, D. & GRAINGER, R. G. (1969). The angiographic investigation of coarctation of aorta and similar abnormalities. *Clin. Radiol.*

KJELLBERG, S. R., NORDENSTROM, B., RUDHE, U., BJORK, V. O. & MALMSTROM, G. (1961). Cardioangiographic studies of the mitral and aortic valves. *Acta Radiol. Suppl.* 204.

LIPCHIK, E. O., SHREINER, B. F., MURPHY, G. W. & DE WEESE, J. A. (1966). Angiocardiography evaluation of mitral valve stenosis. *Radiology.* **86**, 839–842.

NAGLE, R. E., WALKER, D. & GRAINGER, R. G. (1968). The angiographic assessment of mitral incompetence. *Clin. Radiol.* **19**, 154.

RAPHAEL, M. J. & ALLWORK, S. P. (1974). Angiographic anatomy of the left ventricle. *Clinical Radiology* **22**, 95–105.

SWAN, H. J. C., BURCHELL, H. B. & WOOD, E. H. (1953). Differential diagnosis at cardiac catheterization of anomalous pulmonary venous drainage related to atrial septal defects or abnormal venous connections. *Proc. Mayo Clin.* **28**, 452.

VEREL, D., GRAINGER, R. G. & TIN, S. (1973). A comparison of oximetry and angiocardiography in the localisation and assessment of intracardiac shunts. *Zeitschrift für Kardiologie* **62**, 149.

16. Anaesthesia for Cardiac Catheterization

Pre-medication

The pre-medication of patients for cardiac catheterization is a matter which requires considerable judgement. A wide variety of substances has been used and here it may be sufficient to describe our current practice; this has been in use for some ten years.

In small debilitated infants, particularly those with cyanosis, no pre-medication of any kind is needed. The fasting infant is given a teat moistened with honey (some centres use brandy or sherry) to suck and all investigations are performed under local anaesthesia with 1 per cent procaine or lignocaine without added adrenaline. General anaesthetics have not been used either for catheterization or angiography.

In children weighing up to 50 lb (25 kg) we have used chloral hydrate in the form of syrup of chloral in a dose of 60 mg chloral per kg of body weight, given 30 minutes before the catheterization begins (60 mg/kg). This has proved an entirely satisfactory pre-medication in the vast majority (over 95 per cent) of children and can be reinforced if necessary at the beginning of the catheterization by a further dose of approximately half the primary dose of chloral. It results in the child who sleeps quietly but wakes at once if any pain is inflicted. This has seemed a very desirable feature as it leads to deft and gentle manipulation of the catheter and of the patient. Again no general anaesthetic has been administered for angiography and no complications of this regime have been encountered. A few infants have required a general anaesthetic if they have been unusually wakeful, or have been mentally sub-normal and therefore difficult to control when fully conscious.

In larger children and adults the usual practice has been to use Omnopon in a dose varying from 1/12 to 1/6 grain (5 to 10 mg) for children of about 60 lb (30 kg), to $\frac{1}{3}$ to $\frac{1}{2}$ grain (20 to 30 mg) for adults. The only exception to this has been made in the case of adult patients suffering from rheumatic heart disease who are orthopnoeic. These have been catheterized head up on a tilting table with a pre-medication consisting of a small dose of Sodium Amytal (1 to 3 grain or 60 to 180 mg).

A variety of 'tranquillizers' has been tried with varying success. Of these, diazepam has proved the most useful.

Various mixtures which have been advocated, including versions of 'lytic cocktail', have been tried in our department, but have been abandoned as it has seemed likely that they have been responsible for considerable respiratory depression in some cases, particularly with severely cyanosed children, in some of whom serious collapse requiring much resuscitation, developed. These drugs have proved less certain in their effects than chloral administered in the manner described and the analgesic action has not seemed to us a desirable feature. There has been a noticeable reduction in the incidence of cardiac irregularities during cardiac catheterization since their use was abandoned.

The extent to which premedication and local anaesthesia can be used in children is a complex matter of the child's confidence in adults and the operator's rapport with the patient. We have performed many percutaneous transseptal punctures and arterial Seldinger catheterization, in children under ten years of age under local anaesthesia. With the assistance of skilled and sympathetic nurses. On the other hand, right heart catheterizations have needed general aneasthesia in children who were frightened by their surroundings and lacked confidence in adults.

General anaesthesia

General anaesthesia is employed in some children (under 14 years) for percutaneous arterial catheterization; for all axillary artery catheterizations; for some transeptal procedures in children, and for the very exceptional, highly nervous patient. All other investigations including those with children, are performed under local anaesthesia.

Premedication is usually morphine (1 mg/7 kg) with atropine 0·3 to 0·6 mg given 1 h before induction. Scopolamine is substituted for atropine if the latter is definitely contra-indicated.

General anaesthesia is induced by either thiopentone or nitrous oxide, oxygen and Halothane. An endotracheal tube is preferred in children, using topical prilocaine 4 per cent to the larynx aided by intravenous suxamethonium. Intubation enables improved control of the airway and allows the anaesthetist to withdraw from the (X-ray) beam.

The endotracheal tube must not be too long for it may pass beyond the carina into (usually) the right main bronchus depriving the left main bronchus of its oxygen supply. This has resulted in temporary collapse of the left lung on a few occasions. This complication should be detected during fluoroscopy before commencing the intracardiac catheter manipulation.

The objective is to produce a steady state of the cardio-vascular and respiratory systems in which blood-gas analyses and the haemodynamics are not altered; 25 to 30 per cent oxygen probably induces less disturbance of oximetry than higher percentages of oxygen.

References

THORNTON, J. A., THOMPSON, I. & VEREL, D. (1964). The use of chloral hydrate as a hypnotic agent during cardiac catheterization of infants and small children. *Acta Cardiol.* **19**, 90.

17. Complications of Cardiac Catheterization

Even in skilled hands, cardiac catheterization carries a risk which is acceptable only when it is related to the clinical state of the patient subjected to investigation. The mortality reported varies greatly in different series, and depends on the clinical condition of patients investigated. For example, any unit which makes routine investigations in severely ill infants who are under three months old, will encounter a mortality higher than it would do if such cases were not catheterized until they were older. Necessarily, in the latter case, many patients will die uninvestigated. The indications for investigation must, therefore, include the consideration of possible therapy. It is our opinion that no investigation involving catheterization should be undertaken in an infant or child unless a decision relating to treatment depends upon the outcome of the investigation. In most cases this implies a decision on whether or not cardiac surgery could improve the patient's condition.

Complications of cardiac catheterization are uncommon but important, as the minor complications such as vascular thrombosis may be a cause of disability, and major ones such as embolism or ventricular fibrillation may be fatal. Complications may conveniently be considered as those due to manipulation of the catheter in peripheral vessels. those associated with manipulations in the heart, those peculiar to the Seldinger wire technique, and those which may accompany angiocardiographic injections.

Peripheral vascular complications

In a relaxed patient it is uncommon to encounter *venous spasm*. This curious phenomenon can be a cause of great difficulty. The vein in an anxious patient may grip a catheter so tightly that it can neither be advanced nor withdrawn. The operator must continually be on the watch for the onset of this complication. When the catheter is firmly gripped, it is sometimes possible to relax the vein by injecting Papavarine or other vasodilator into the vein alongside the catheter, but this is rarely successful since the area in spasm is commonly far out of reach. Radiological contrast media are vasodilators and a few ml injected through the catheter may relax the venous spasm. A general anaesthetic will sometimes relax spasm; more commonly it passes off after some minutes or hours and the catheter can then be withdrawn.

If the onset of venous spasm is noted (the catheter becoming difficult to manoeuvre in or out), the catheter should be quickly withdrawn and the investigation continued with a catheter of smaller diameter. Usually one size F smaller is successful.

Arterial spasm is common after puncture of the brachial artery but rare at other sites. In occasional cases, usually children, prolonged femoral artery spasm may follow catheterization and may lead to thrombosis in a few patients. This can be a cause of troublesome claudication. Similarly, brachial artery occlusion is sometimes followed by ischaemic symptoms in the forearm if a continuous activity such as knitting, piano playing or heavy work with a spanner is undertaken. In such a forearm, a low blood flow response to exercise with a reduced resting flow may be found years after the incident.

Arterial occlusion after catheterization may be due to pre-existing disease of the arterial wall with consequent lifting of an atheromatous plaque by the needle or catheter. Arterial occlusion may however occur in a previously normal vessel and the mechanism is probably that suggested (with much experimental evidence) by Jacobsson (1969).

Platelets and other formed elements of the blood aggregate on the *outer* side of the catheter whilst it is in the blood stream. When the catheter is removed from the artery, its outer surface is scraped clean by the muscular wall of the artery as the catheter is pulled through the small arterial puncture hole. The platelet aggregate forms a plug inside the arterial lumen and may occlude it. The outside of the withdrawn catheter is reassuringly clean, but it has left behind a potential major complication. It is apparent therefore that the complication will vary according to the surface area of the catheter which has been exposed to the blood stream—i.e. catheter diameter, length, multiple catheter exchanges. The surface texture and material of the catheter are also important, and heparin-bonded catheters have been recently tried with success in an attempt to reduce the incidence of this important complication of thrombosis inside or outside the catheter.

Deliberate compression of the arterial puncture site is essential for haemostasis (p. 83). It is again stressed that firm pressure may need to be applied for up to 30 minutes but the pressure should not be so firm as to occlude the vessel completely for more than a minute at a time.

Manipulations in the heart

There are a number of hazards due to *loops* or *knots* forming in the catheter which require complex manipulation and a clear mental picture of the catheter's position to enable them to be undone. An overhand knot can be tied in the catheter. This is best undone by pulling the catheter back into a narrower vein in which the knot will jam; the catheter is then advanced again and with luck the knot will become a loose loop which can be manipulated so that it is undone. As a last resort it may be necessary to remove the knotted catheter surgically after having withdrawn the catheter as far as possible. There is one account of an overhand knot being tied round one of the cordi tendini. This required open heart surgery for its removal. The main safeguard against these hazards is good quality screening and a fluoroscopy screen large enough to include the whole heart, so that loops and twists cannot form without the operator immediately being aware of them (Figs. 1–16).

Knots can also be tied in guide wires and in polythene catheters. When tied in a guide wire the knot should be drawn back to as near to the site of insertion as possible. A loose fitting radio-opaque catheter should then be passed up the wire to the knot under fluoroscopic control. A 7F Ross needle introducer (U.S.C.I. 7410) is suitable. The knot is then worked forwards and backwards in the vessel while the catheter is pressed against the tied section of wire. A loose knot can be untied in about 15 seconds by this technique. Care should be exercised not to tighten the knot. A catheter complicated by a tight knot should be removed through a small incision in the vessel.

A knot in a non-opaque polythene catheter may be difficult to detect if it is tightened and so occludes the catheter. If it is evident when the catheter is filled with contrast that it is knotted, the catheter is easily removed by steadily pulling it out: the knot tightens and pulls out through the skin. If the access to the vessel is still needed for further investigation, the withdrawal should be halted when the knot has appeared, the catheter cut off between the knot and the skin and a fresh guide wire inserted using the cut end of the catheter as an introducer. Anyone doing this must hold the catheter *firmly* as the cut end has no flange and can readily be pushed into the vessel by the wire and so be lost.

A less obvious hazard is *cracking* of the plastic of the catheter wall. In a catheter with the conventional woven nylon lining, this can be difficult to see if the screening quality is not good, but the appearances are quite typical if a good view can be obtained. It is noticed that on manipulation the catheter develops an acute angle quite unlike the usual smooth curve. This is sometimes associated with a tight twist which should be carefully undone

and the catheter withdrawn immediately and discarded. There is considerable danger of causing damage to the interior of the heart and great vessels with the sharp edges of such a broken catheter.

Perforation of the heart may well be commoner than is generally realized. The site is usually atrial, and, because of the absence of pressure gradient between atrium and pericardial sac, haemopericardium is rare. The pressure tracing from the pericardial sac usually shows only respiratory variations, and the catheter yields either *no* sample, or, on occasion, pericardial fluid. Injection of a *small* quantity of dilute contrast medium by hand provides a dramatic confirmation of the accident.

Arrhythmias are common during catheterization. The commonest are induced by the catheter tip in the outflow tracts of the ventricles, where multiple ventricular *extrasystoles* may be stimulated. Less commonly, the catheter may provoke abnormal beats from sites elsewhere in the ventricle or occasionally in the atrium. *Asystole* may occur at any time, particularly in small infants. It usually responds immediately to a firm thump on the lower third of the sternum. Occasionally, external cardiac massage is needed to maintain the circulation. In the authors' experience, the heart rarely needs any other stimulus to restore normal rhythm.

Ventricular fibrillation is also seen occasionally (Fig. 17.1). It has usually occurred without warning in worrying infants or children and has usually reverted to sinus rhythm following a blow on the chest or during external cardiac massage. If this does not succeed, then defibrillation with a direct current defibrillator, is almost always successful.

Other abnormalities are uncommon, but various degrees of *heart block, auricular fibrillation* and *auricular flutter* and other tachycardias may be seen. The heart block is usually transient, lasting moments or hours. Persisting flutter and fibrillation respond to D.C. countershock. These arrhythmias are probably due in most cases to traumatic stimulation by catheter. Rarely there has been clear evidence of a relation to other factors. In one child, 2:1 block occurred during skin cleaning before the catheterization commenced and was attributed to the pre-medication with 'lytic cocktail'.

The *management* of a patient developing an arrhythmia depends on circumstances. Complete block is best treated by withdrawing the catheter to the atrium and observing the electrocardiogram. If it lasts only a few seconds it may be feasible to proceed cautiously. If it persists, it is probably best to abandon the catheterization.

Tachycardia rarely seriously interferes with the catheterization unless it produces a fall in cardiac output to under 50 per cent of normal. If the patient is aware of uncomfortable symptoms, the catheterization is best abandoned unless the tachycardia responds to medication. Digoxin, Procaine amide, Propranolol and D.C.

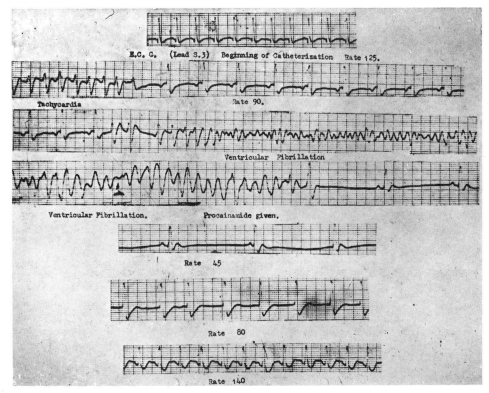

FIG. 17.1 An attack of ventricular fibrillation in the course of a cardiac catheterization. The top line shows the E.C.G. at the beginning of the investigation. The remaining strips of record are a continuous tracing cut for mounting. An episode of tachycardia is followed by a nodal rate of 90, then after three or four rapid beats, ventricular fibrillation occurs. External cardiac massage was instituted and an assistant injected procaine amide through the catheter. Slow sinus rhythm is restored and, after 9 beats at 80 per minute which are probably of nodal origin, sinus rhythm at 140 per minute returns, the myocardial ischaemia causing marked S-T depression. The investigation was abandoned. A few days later the investigation was successfully repeated without incident.

countershock provide the most effective measures for treatment.

Thrombophlebitis in the vein used for catheterization has been rare since routine ligation of these veins was abandoned in 1948. Except in small infants and patients with very high venous pressures (where the vein is ligated with absorbable catgut), all veins are left to bleed freely at the end of the cardiac catheterization. The closure of the skin incision by vertical mattress sutures is enough to provide haemostasis. In many cases it is possible to use the vein again if further catheterization is needed.

Antibiotics are occasionally given for two or three days after catheterization. In view of the risk of contamination with *B. coli*, Streptomycin is sometimes given in addition to small babies for three days after catheterization.

The *transseptal technique* is subject to a host of complications ranging from major disasters such as perforation of the aorta by the transseptal needle, to relatively trivial mishaps such as the plugging at the end of the Ross needle on one occasion by a core of tissue from

(?) the ventricular septum. Most of these have been described in the chapter on left atrial catheterization. One further potentially dangerous hazard should be mentioned. The Brockenborough catheters supplied by the U.S.C.I. are made of teflon. Using these, we have sometimes found that in the course of catheterization, blood may clot in the tip of the catheter beyond the proximal hole of the five holes bored in the end of these catheters. This clot is usually not displaced by a flat wound Seldinger wire, but may be forced out as an embolus if angiocardiography is performed through this catheter. Before angiocardiography, we now replace the Brockenborough catheter with a fresh one to avoid this possible complication.

Seldinger wire complications

The use of guide wires is associated with a wide range of minor and major complications. With experience most of these are avoidable, but even in the most experienced hands, accidents may occur.

During introduction of the guide wire into an atheromatous artery, a plaque of atheroma may be dislodged. In one such case the plaque turned down like a hinged valve and completely occluded the femoral artery. Emergency surgery was undertaken to re-establish the arterial lumen.

If the wire is introduced when the introducing needle is not free in the vessel lumen, the wire may become *acutely flexed*. This bend in the wire may not permit the catheter to pass over it. Similarly, it may be impossible to withdraw the bent wire through the introducer, particularly if a needle such as the Sutton needle has been used instead of a cannula to introduce the wire. Attempts to pull the wire back through the introducer in these circumstances may result in the wire shearing. The introducer should be drawn back along the wire and the wire gently manipulated out. If it is so badly distorted that it will not come easily out of the artery, a small arteriotomy should be made to free it. This procedure is however, rarely necessary. It has been done twice in more than 15,000 investigations.

In passing the wire up the vessels, a variety of *false passages* may be made. We have had very little trouble in venous catheterization apart from those associated with the transseptal left atrial technique. In arterial catheterization, however, there have been occasional accidents. These have included the passage of the wire from the abdominal aorta to the inferior vena cava in one patient without any complications. The aorta in this patient was very tortuous. In another patient, a large retroperitoneal haemorrhage occurred—again a patient with an atheromatous aorta. In both these patients the wire was withdrawn without difficulty after the false passage. In a younger patient with rheumatic aortic incompetence, the wire perforated the aortic arch and stuck. When an attempt to withdraw it was made, the spiral of the wire unwound. The spiral wire was cut off at the skin (the intact core was retrieved as it was soldered to the operator's end). The detached spiral wire fragment was removed through a thoracotomy. Safety wires with a fine central wire soldered to both ends of the wire spiral should prevent this hazard.

A rare and dangerous complication may occur when a guide wire is passed through from the hub end of angiographic catheters such as the Gensini catheter, to guide the tip in a desired direction. This manoeuvre is commonly used either to stiffen a soft catheter or to lead the tip through an orifice, e.g. the aortic valve during retrograde ventriculography (see pp. 102 and 130). The accident consists of the passage of the tip of the wire through one of the side holes near the tip of the catheter. In this use of the guide wire, the flexible tip of the wire is threaded up first. This consists of a simple spring with no core wire. If the side holes at the tip of the catheter are bored out on the convex aspect of the terminal bend of the catheter, the flexible end of the guide wire may pass out through a side

hole, instead of passing out through the end hole. If this happens, the flexible coiled tip may catch in the edge of the side hole and jam. Any attempt to withdraw the wire may fail as the spiral of the spring inside the catheter merely unwinds if strong traction is applied. If this accident occurs, the catheter with its wire should be gently withdrawn until the tip reaches near to the site of insertion. The vessel is then exposed by dissection and snared to control possible haemorrhage. The arterial needle puncture is enlarged longitudinally with a fine pointed scalpel until the catheter with the protruding wire can be withdrawn. Bleeding is controlled with the snares and the incision closed with longitudinal stitches using 00000 silk on an atraumatic needle. In this way the incision is converted into a transverse scar. Under no circumstances should the catheter with the wire protruding through a side hole be dragged out through the puncture made by the Seldinger needle as this may avulse the vessel. If the fit of the catheter in the vessel is too tight to allow the catheter with the protruding wire to be drawn back to the puncture site, an arteriotomy will be needed to retrieve the situation. This may have to be made in the thorax or abdomen, and entail surgical assistance. Since this danger has been recognized, some angiographic catheters used in the Seldinger technique have been made with side holes smaller than the diameter of the guide wire which, therefore, cannot readily make this false passage.

Guide wires rarely break when new. Repeated use, however, carries a risk of corrosion of any steel wire however 'stainless', as its resistance to human tissues depends upon a film of surface oxide. This can be penetrated by damage of any sort and in certain circumstances the sweat off the hands of the technician handling the wire after use may begin this process. The usual fracture is of the *spring*, not the core, and in our experience it is most common at the point where the inner core terminates and the soft tip begins. A kink in the guide wire at this point is occasionally produced during the introduction of the wire through the Seldinger cannula. This happens usually when the cannula is introduced into an artery at a steep angle with the cannula tip close to the distal wall. The tip of the guide wire slides in the vessel lumen but the stiffer part with the central core impacts into the arterial wall, producing a sharp angle in the wire at this point. A wire bent in this fashion should be cautiously withdrawn through the cannula and discarded. The angle between the vessel and the cannula should be reduced by lowering the cannula hub to lie parallel with the vessel, the cannula should be threaded a few mm up the vessel and a fresh wire inserted.

Rarely a wire may fracture in the spiral which covers the core wire. If the core wire is of the sliding type or is not held tightly by the coiled spring covering, a break in this position is a potential hazard. It is most usually encountered when the wire is being manipulated in a catheter. Good fluoroscopy is necessary to appreciate that the wire protruding from the catheter tip is capable of extrusion but does not move when the guide is withdrawn. In these circumstances the catheter and wire should be withdrawn together and usually the broken end will emerge from the puncture and be withdrawn. Very rarely a guide wire breaks in a vessel and it is not possible to retrieve it. In these circumstances, an arteriotomy must be made to remove it. Broken wires have a disconcerting capacity for unpredictable movement, and a radiograph should be taken to confirm the position immediately before exploration. Detached fragments of catheter or guide wire have been occasionally removed by Fogarty catheters or a loop of nylon thread passed up another catheter used as a snare.

The use of *safety* wires is strongly recommended. These wires have a fine central wire soldered to *both* ends of the Seldinger wire.

Complications of angiocardiography
CONTRAST MEDIUM REACTIONS
Modern radiological contrast media are much less toxic than those used twenty years ago. Contrast media suitable for angiocardiography are discussed on page 60, Chapter 6.

Ventricular fibrillation
Experimentally, ventricular fibrillation can be produced regularly by injecting radiological contrast media in large doses into the coronary arteries. The ease with which fibrillation can be so induced depends to a considerable extent on the sodium content of the contrast medium. It is therefore advisable to use a contrast medium with low sodium content for left heart or ascending aortic injections—such media are Triosil 370, Hypaque 65 or 85, Urografin 76 (Verel *et al.,* 1975). The optimal sodium ionic concentration is about the same as in plasma (140 mEq/1). Contrast media completely free of sodium ions cause an increased risk of ventricular fibrillation during coronary arteriography (Paulin and Adams, 1971), (see pp. 60 and 107).

Cerebral symptoms or toxic encephalopathy may rarely be caused when a large volume of concentrated contrast medium reaches the brain. The cause is very probably cerebral oedema resulting from an increased permeability of the cerebral capillaries. An epileptic fit followed by disturbed consciousness are the usual symptoms. This complication is most likely to arise during repeated injections for arch aortography or left ventriculography, but it may also occur after right ventriculography in a patient with a large right to left shunt as in Fallot's tetralogy or uncorrected transposition of the great vessels. There is some evidence to suggest that the sodium salts of contrast media are more likely to cause toxic encephalopathy than meglumine salts and therefore the same types of

contrast media mentioned in the preceding paragraph are probably safer.

Blood pressure changes may follow angiocardiography and, as all contrast media are potent vasodilators, *hypotension* is much the more frequent complication. It is difficult to determine the mechanism of the hypotension for there are many other factors which might be involved —e.g. prolonged recumbency in a patient in heart failure, psychological upset and fear, reactions to catheters, saline and any other drugs which have been used. Very occasionally, a *hypertensive* reaction may follow angiocardiography.

Pulmonary oedema may develop during catheterization of the heart. It is usually due to the failure of the left heart to clear the venous return from the lungs, as in a patient with severe mitral and/or aortic valve disease, who is being catheterized in the horizontal position. A large volume of contrast media will cause significant hypervolaemia because of the strong osmotic effect, and may therefore be an important factor contributing to the pulmonary oedema. The development of pulmonary oedema may be first detected by the radiologist on the television monitor by observing clouding or veiling of the lung fields. This sign may occur before clinical evidence and in the absence of any auscultatory finding. Once the development of pulmonary oedema has been noted, it is advisable to discontinue the catheterization and to tip the patient head up. This usually suffices to clear the lungs but more aggressive treatment of the heart failure may be needed, including intravenous diuretic (e.g. Lasix).

Acute pulmonary hypertension may complicate right heart injections of contrast media in patients with increased pulmonary arteriolar resistance. It is probably due to erythrocyte aggregation, sludging and cell deformity increasing the viscosity of the blood. Such injections must be avoided if possible when there is significant pulmonary hypertension.

Tamponade may follow intrapericardial injections of contrast media if the injection is made through a catheter which has entered the pericardial sac. This may occur in an attempted transseptal catheterization in which case the fluid should be aspirated through the catheter (Popper *et al.,* 1967).

Intramural injections
The pressurized injection of contrast medium into the heart occasionally results in some of the medium being deposited beneath the endocardium in the heart wall. The complication can be immediately recognized on the radiograph by a dense blob of contrast medium persisting in the heart wall instead of being rapidly mixed with the blood within the heart chambers. The intramural pool of contrast medium may spread out along the myocardial bundles in a striate pattern and often causes early filling of the coronary veins (Figs. 115, 116). Pulsus alter-

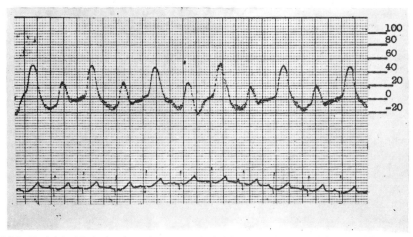

FIG. 17.2   Right Ventricle. Marked pulsus alternans recorded from the right ventricle in an infant after intramural injection of contrast medium. The negative diastolic pressure is an artefact due to the position of the pressure transducer some inches above the top of the catheter table.

nans or other arrhythmia may result (Fig. 17.2 and 17.3).

The accident occurs more frequently in the very small hearts of tiny infants. Most intramural injections are made into the ventricles, but damage to the heart wall may also occur during atrial injection—when the contrast medium may penetrate completely through the thin atrial wall into the pericardial sac.

The cause of intramural injections is basically the position of the catheter tip. If the tip is touching the endocardium at the onset of the injection, and if free recoil of the catheter is impeded by the papillary muscles or by the rigidity of the catheter, then the endocardium may be penetrated by the sharp flick induced in the catheter at the onset of the pressurized injection of contrast medium. A stiff, rigid catheter, a sharply pointed catheter tip, the absence of side holes in the catheter wall, a high pressure injection and a small heart chamber all increase the possibility of intramural injection. Every possible precaution must be taken. The catheter tip must be seen at fluoroscopy to move freely within the heart wall; the tip should be seen not to impinge on the heart wall; a test hand injection of contrast medium should be made before any pressurized intracardiac injection; an undamped pressure tracing should be obtained. Despite all these precautions, we recorded an incidence of about 1 to 2 per cent of deposition of a small pool of contrast medium in the heart wall (Grainger, 1965).

This incidence has been greatly reduced since we have used soft radiolucent polythene catheters or pig-tail catheters for left heart injections, and have taken intra-cardiac E.C.G. recordings through the cardiac catheter whenever a risk of intra-mural injection seemed likely. The details of the technique are described by Stentiford (1968). Sodium bicarbonate 5 per cent is injected as electrical conductor into the catheter lumen. The metal hub of the catheter or catheter holder is connected to the pectoral lead of the E.C.G. machine and the limb leads are used as the other electrode. When the catheter tip touches the endocardium, the ST segment is greatly elevated (Fig. 5.2): it immediately returns to the base line when the tip has been withdrawn from the endo-cardium into the lumen of the chamber. Using this preliminary precaution, we have not experienced any intra-mural deposition in several hundred injections.

The symptoms produced by intra-mural injections are very variable A small deposition may produce neither signs nor symptoms, but a larger pool may cause angina, ventricular tachycardia (Fig. 17.3), or pulsus alternans (Fig. 17.2) which usually subside spontaneously in a few minutes. Marked deviation of the ST segment of the E.C.G. may occur. We have not experienced ventricular fibrillation or massive cardiac rupture which have occasionally been mentioned in the literature.

Air embolism

Care must be taken throughout the catheterization to exclude the danger of air embolism, which is more likely to occur when the X-ray room is darkened to aid fluoro-scopy, and during the pressurized angiocardiographic injection. It is essential to exclude air from any syringe used to perfuse saline through the catheter and the operator should learn to hold the syringe vertically, nozzle down, to prevent any air bubbles entering the catheter. A rigid and strict technique is essential in filling the syringe of the pump. Some of the simpler syringe designs are difficult to load without the inclusion of a little air, and especial care must be taken if such equipment is being used. These pumps (e.g. Talley pump) should be mounted on a tilted ramp so that the piston end is uppermost and any bubble of air will remain in the syringe and catheter.

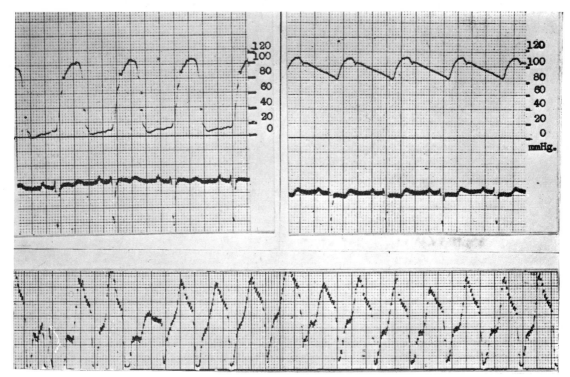

FIG. 17.3   *E.C.G. during Intramural Injection.* Intramural left ventricular injection. *Top left trace*—left ventricular pressure and E.C.G. trace before angiocardiographic injection. *Bottom trace*—Ventricular tachycardia immediately after an angiocardiographic injection, in which some contrast medium was injected into the *wall* of the left ventricle as in Fig. 114. *Top right trace*—Aortic pressure and E.C.G. ten minutes later. Note return to previous E.C.G. pattern and systolic pressure. (Reproduced with permission of the Editor of *The British Journal of Radiology.* Grainger, R. G. 1965, **38,** 201.)

The Talley syringe is best filled by injecting the contrast medium *into* it through its nozzle, by another syringe connected by tubing. Filling of the Talley syringe by applying negative pressure on its plunger usually results in a few bubbles of air entering the syringe. A few bubbles of intracardiac air are illustrated in Fig. 114).

MANAGEMENT OF COMPLICATIONS

Emergencies in the course of cardiac catheterization usually occur while the electrocardiograph is being monitored. This allows immediate recognition of the most untoward events. Since the attention of the operator is likely to be directed to the manipulation of the catheter, the technician responsible for monitoring must be familiar with the normal electrocardiographic pattern of the patient and the likely abnormalities. The technician must be accustomed to interrupting any procedure if an emergency occurs or appears to be impending.

The capacity to interrupt a catheterization requires confidence and nerve, qualities which are not found in all teenagers aspiring to work as electrocardiographic technicians. Technicians monitoring on our Unit, work in the catheterization room in close proximity to the remainder of the team. The technicians are expected to announce clearly the occurrence of any electrocardiographic abnormality, however minor. In this way the habit of speaking up is cultivated and the operator develops an almost subconscious attention to the sound of the technician's voice. The comment 'extras' becomes an indication that the catheter has reached the ventricle and 'atrial extras' a clear warning to draw the catheter back. Similarly 'S-T depression' invites a glance at the patient's face to make sure that increasing cyanosis is not present. Practised and audible commentary of this kind averts many unpleasant moments. Asystole is usually preceded by bradycardia, ventricular fibrillation by ventricular tachycardia (Fig. 17.1) or runs of extrasystoles which persist after the mechanical stimulation of the heart by the catheter has ceased. Audible warning of these events may allow the operator to avoid trouble.

Most emergencies respond to withdrawal of the catheter to a vessel outside the heart, the administration of oxygen and, if necessary, external cardiac massage. Rarely the abnormality persists—asystole, ventricular fibrillation, gross tachycardia or bradycardia or electrocardiographic evidence of damage, usually S-T deviation or splintering of the Q.R.S. complex. To cope with this, electronic equipment and drugs are needed. In addition to the oxygen already mentioned we have in readiness the following:

Apparatus	Defibrillator (Direct current)
	Pacemaker (Internal voltage)
	Suction apparatus
	Thoracotomy set
	Tracheotomy set
	Laryngoscope
	Endotracheal tubes
	Ventilator bag

Drugs	Acebutol HCl.
(all intravenous)	Adrenalin 1/10,000
	Isoprenalin
	Methylamphetamine
	Noradrenalin
	Atropine
	Digoxin
	Lignocaine
	Procaine Amide
	Propranolol
	Practolol
	Hydrocortisone
	Piriton
	Calcium Chloride
	Sodium Bicarbonate
	(8·4 per cent and 5 per cent)
	Saline/Dextrose

Excluding coronary angiography, in the course of well over 7,000 cardiac catheterizations, the defibrillator has been used twice, while the pacemaker, thoracotomy set and tracheotomy set have never been needed. Suction, however, is not infrequently life-saving in infants in heart failure. Most of the drugs mentioned have been used many times. Patients whose condition at the end of catheterization is not entirely satisfactory are returned to an Intensive Care Unit.

A comprehensive review of complications of cardiac catheterization and angiocardiography has been compiled by Braunwald and Swan (1968).

References

BAGGER, M. (1957). On methods and complications in catheterizations of the heart and large vessels with, and without, contrast injection. *Am. Heart J.* **54**, 766.

BAUNWALD, E. & SWAN, H. J. C. (Editors) (1968). Co-operative study on cardiac catheterization. *Circulation*, Suppl. 3, **37**.

BLOOMFIELD, D. A. (1971). Techniques of nonsurgical retrieval of iatrogenic foreign bodies from the heart. *Amer. J. Cardiol.* **27**, 538.

BOOKSTEIN, J. J. & SIGMANN, J. M. (1963). Intramural deposition of contrast agent during selective angiocardiography. *Radiology* **81**, 932.

CAMPION, B. C., FRYE, R. L., PLUTH, J. R., FAIRBAIRN, J. F. II & DAVIES, G. D. (1971). Arterial complications of retrograde brachial arterial catheterization: a prospective study. *Proc. Mayo Clin.* **46**, 589.

CHRISTIANSEN, I. & WENNEWOLD, A. (1966). Complications of 1,056 investigations of the heart. *Am. Heart J.* **71**, 601.

ESCHER, J. J., SHAPIRO, J. H., RUBINSTEIN, B. M., HURWITT, E. S. & SCHARTZ, S. P. (1958). Perforation of the heart during cardiac catheterization and selective angiocardiography. *Circulation* **18**, 418.

FISCHER, H. W. & CORNELL, S. H. (1965). The toxicity of the sodium and methylglucamine salts of diatrizoate, iothalanate and metrizoate. *Radiology* **85**, 1013.

FORMANEK, G., FRECH, R. S. & AMPLATZ, K. (1970). Arterial thrombus formation during clinical percutaneous catheterization. *Circulation* **41**, 833.

FRASER, R. S., MACAULAY, W. D. & RONALL, R. E. (1962). Arrhythmias induced during cardiac catheterization. *Am. Heart J.* **64**, 439.

GENSINI, G. G. & DI GIORGI, S. (1964). Myocardial toxicity of contrast agents in angiography. *Radiology* **82**, 24.

GLANCY, J. J., FISHBONE, G. & HEINZ, E. R. (1970). Nonthrombogenic arterial catheters. *Amer. J. Roentg. Radium Ther. & Nucl. Med.* **108**, 716.

GRAINGER, R. G. (1965) Complications of cardiovascular radiological investigations. *Br. J. Radiol.* **38**, 201.

HALPERN, M. (1964). Percutaneous transfemoral arteriography. An analysis of the complications in 1000 consecutive cases. *Am. J. Roentgen.* **92**, 918.

JACOBSSON, B. (1969). Platelet adhesion and aggregation following contact between blood and vascular catheters *in vitro. Scand. J. Haemat.* **6**, 216–220.

JACOBSSON, B., BERGENTZ, S. E. & LJUNGQVIST, U. (1969). Platelet adhesion and thrombus formation on vascular catheters in dogs. *Acta. Radiol. Diag.* **8**, 221–227.

JACOBSSON, B., PAULIN, S. & SCHLOSSMAN, D. (1969). Thromboembolism of leg following percutaneous catheterization of femoral artery for angiography. Symptoms and signs. *Acta Radiol. Diagn.* **8**, 97–107.

KLASTER, F. E., BRISTOW, J. D. & GRISWOLD, H. E. (1970). Femoral artery occlusion after percutaneous catheterization *Am. Heart J* **79**, 175.

MORTENSEN, J. D. (1967). Clinical sequelae from arterial needle puncture, cannulation and incision. *Circulation,* **35**, 1118.

NEJAD, M. S., KLAPER, M A., STEGGERDA, F. R. & GIANTURCO, C. (1968). Clotting on the outer surfaces of vascular catheters. *Radiology* **91**, 248.

PAULIN, S. O. & ADAMS, D. F. (1971). Increased ventricular fibrillation during coronary arteriography with a new contrast medium preparation. *Radiology* **107**, 45.

POPPER, R. W., SCHIEMACHER, D. & QUINN, C. H. (1967). Tamponade after pericardial injection of contrast. *Circulation* **35**, 933.

ROWE, R. D., VLAD, P. & KEITH, J. D. (1956). Selective angiocardiography in infants and children. *Radiology* **66**, 344.

SELDINGER, S. I. (1953). Catheter replacement of the needle in percutaneous angiography: a new technique. *Acta Radiologica* **39**, 368.

SILVERMAN, J. F. & WEXLER, L. (1976). Complications of percutaneous transfemoral coronary arteriography. *Clin. Radiol.* **27**, 317.

VEREL, D. & RICKARDS, D. F. (1973). Effect of the site of puncture of the femoral artery upon haemorrhage following aortic angiocardiography. *Clin. Radiol.* **24,** 62.

VEREL, D., WARD, C. & AMAN, M. (1975). Comparison of Triosil 370 with Urografin 76 and Hypaque 65 for coronary arteriography. *Br. Heart. J.* **37,** 1049.

VESTERMARK, S. (1964). Cardiac angiocardiography and catheterization in infants. An assessment of risk based on 711 cases. *Cardiologia* **45,** 91.

WENNEVOLD, A., CHRISTIANSEN, I. & LINDENEG, O. (1965). Complications in 4413 cardiac catheterizations of the right side of the heart. *Am. Heart J.* **69,** 173.

18. Assessment of Results

The assessment of results is a matter of the greatest importance in the management of congenital and acquired heart disease. The matter is a complex one and in this chapter some of the relative merits and pitfalls of methods described earlier will be considered. In reading this discussion it must be clearly borne in mind that the statements bearing on the value of the methods are expressions of opinion only and are not facts, although the facts on which the opinions are based will be presented as far as is possible.

The major difficulties which beset this diagnostic field arise from the risks involved in attempts at surgical repair of the heart lesion. For example, if the surgical risk of repair were nil, i.e. mortality and morbidity both zero, the risks in septal defects of such relatively infrequent complications as bacterial endocarditis and paradoxical embolism would themselves justify correction of any defect however small. Consequently, the diagnostic effort could be satisfactorily limited to the demonstration of the presence of a shunt through a defect as an adequate indication for surgery. Since, however, any surgical procedure carries a risk, the decision becomes the more difficult one of assessing relative risks of surgery and the clinical course of the patient treated and untreated.

Once this principle of balancing risks is accepted, the physician is placed in a much more complex situation where opinion is never likely to be uniform over the whole field, or constant in any one cardiological centre for any considerable period. This is illustrated by the attitude to the ligation of an uncomplicated patent ductus, or closure of a simple secundum type of atrial septal defect. In both cases the increasing expertise of the surgeons tackling these lesions has so reduced the risks of surgery that operation is advised in all patients from the age of a few months in the case of patent ductus and from the age of three years or so in the case of atrial septal defect. Clearly the introduction of new surgical techniques and further development of current ones is likely to widen the surgical field and reduce the risks of surgery so that the range of lesions offered surgery will increase in two directions—increasing safety of operation, leading to surgery on patients at present advised that their lesion is not sufficiently severe to merit operation: and a wider range of technique permitting safe surgery on lesions at present regarded as inoperable.

A further variable is the surgical resource available.

Thus, in a centre in which atrial septal defects are repaired using hypothermia at 30°C with no by-pass, it is vital to exclude all unusual or difficult cases such as ostium primum or sinus venosus defects. If, however, the by-pass technique is used routinely for all cases, this precision of diagnosis, while desirable, is not essential.

With this changing background in mind, the problem of assessing the diagnosis may be considered. Surgical experience showed very early that in advising on the suitability of surgery for any patient, there were a number of essential considerations. These may be regarded as primary and secondary:

Primary considerations
1. Presence of the abnormality.
2. Site of the abnormality.
3. Size of the abnormality.
4. Presence of associated abnormality.

Secondary considerations
1. Pressures in heart chambers and great vessels.
2. Vascular resistance in the lungs.
3. Direction of shunts.
4. Quantity of blood passing through defects.
5. The work done by the heart chambers.

In this classification it can be seen that the primary considerations are entirely anatomical, while the secondary considerations are dependent partly on the primary ones and partly on each other. They are capable of further subclassification in specific instances and the *relative* importance of the different factors in such a subdivision in making decisions about surgery cannot be exaggerated. This importance may be simply illustrated by considering the differential diagnosis in the following case:

A child presents with a history of increasing dyspnoea and, on exertion, the appearance of definite central cyanosis. The child is undersized, with slight cyanosis and doubtful clubbing.

This clinical presentation could be the result of a number of combinations of congenital heart defects and repair is clearly desirable, if possible. We may here consider some of these in tabular form (Table 18.1) from several points of view. There is first the question of the suitability of the lesion for surgical correction and, with this, the risk involved. In both aspects of this question it

TABLE 18.1

	Developing Eisenmenger reaction	Fallot tetralogy	Tight pulmonary stenosis	Ostium primum defect	Total anomalous pulmonary venous drainage	Primary pulmonary hypertension
Anatomical lesion in heart	A.S.D. V.S.D. or P.D.A.	V.S.D. and P.S.	P.S. Open foramen ovale	A.S.D. M.I.	A.S.D.	Nil
R.V.P. = L.V.P.	+	+	+ or R.V.P. > L.V.P.	±	−	often R.V.P. > L.V.P.
P.A.P. = Ao.P.	+	−	−	±	−	P.A.P. may exceed Ao.P.
R.V.P. = P.A.P.	+	−	−	+	+	+
Increased P.V.R.	+	−	−	(+)	(+)	+ +
Shunt L—R	(+)	−	−	+ +	+ +	−
Shunt R—L	(+)	+ +	+ +	±	+	−

A.S.D. — Atrial Septal Defect	P.S. — Pulmonary Stenosis
V.S.D. — Ventricular Septal Defect	M.I. — Mitral Incompetence
P.D.A. — Patent Ductus Arteriosus	Ao.P. — Aortic Pressure
R.V.P. — Right Ventricular Pressure	P.V.R. — Pulmonary Vascular Resistance
P.A.P. — Pulmonary Artery Pressure	L. — Left
L.V.P. — Left Ventricular Pressure	R. — Right.

is necessary to consider the evidence of primary and secondary order, separately and together.

An early stage of *Eisenmenger's reaction* can produce the clinical picture described. The outlook is uncertain, for while many patients die as children, others may survive with increasing disability until the fourth or fifth decade. Anatomical correction of the defect is simple in the case of uncomplicated patent ductus and a matter of only moderate difficulty in atrial septal defect or ventricular septal defect. However, the high pulmonary vascular resistance found in Eisenmenger's reaction imposes an operative mortality which most centres would regard as prohibitive. In this patient, surgery may be justified by the clinical deterioration if surgical policy is compatible with the very high risks involved. Referring back to our classification we may see that the mere demonstration of the presence of pulmonary hypertension with reversal of shunt renders the precise anatomical delineation of the site of the shunt of secondary importance. In other words, in this analysis, the primary evidence (the anatomy) is not the most important consideration. The vital consideration in this case is the pulmonary vascular resistance which may be considered as a tertiary phenomenon dependent on the pulmonary reaction to the shunt.

Somewhat different considerations apply to the second possible diagnosis. In *Fallot's tetralogy* the pulmonary vascular resistance is not raised and the risks of surgery are primarily related to the anatomy—the size of the pulmonary vessels, the size of the defect, the quality of the crista supraventricularis and the capacity of the left ventricle for work. Here the decision has to be made on the nature of the operation which will best confer benefit to the patient. The most useful evidence is that provided by angiocardiography while the records of pressure, oxygen saturation etc., are of secondary importance. The choice here is one of technique and timing of operation. A deteriorating infant may be treated at once by closed pulmonary valvotomy or infundibular resection, or anastomosis between the pulmonary artery and either aorta (Pott's, Waterson operation) or a subclavian artery (Blalock-Taussig operation). In older children there is in addition, the possibility of open pulmonary valvotomy or total repair in one or two stages. Many other factors modify the decision, the physical condition of the child, the resources of the surgeon, the previous experience with the available procedures, but, in the main, the vital factors here are the primary anatomical ones, not those of the secondary order.

In a child with tight *pulmonary stenosis* and open foramen ovale, the problem set is again one of age as a main factor determining the management. The stenosis in such children is usually valvar in situation and severe in grade. As age increases, the muscular hypertrophy of the right ventricle becomes greater, and an increasing degree of infundibular muscular stenosis occurs. What may be a low risk operation in a child of three or four years can become a procedure with considerable risk even three or four years later. Here the choice between open or closed operation and the timing of surgery is not easy.

A large *ostium primum defect* may present a very misleading picture. Here a large left to right shunt may co-exist with sufficient mixing of blood in the atria to permit a small right to left shunt with consequent arterial desaturation and slight finger clubbing. In such circumstances, the cyanosis increases on exercise if the pulmonary artery pressure be high and the appearances strongly suggest that the pulmonary vascular resistance is high and fixed, i.e. that Eisenmenger's reaction is present. In some of these cases, however, successful surgery is possible and the prompt fall in pulmonary artery pressure measured on the operating table at the end of surgery when the defect is closed, confirms that much of the pulmonary hypertension is a tonic response of the pulmonary vascular bed to the excessive pulmonary blood flow. The main difficulties may be the precise definition of the disordered anatomy and the interpretation of the estimates of pulmonary vascular resistance.

(A somewhat comparable difficulty in analysing data may occur in double defects; for example, in children with a patent ductus, a right to left shunt may be associated with either an atrial or ventricular septal defect at which a left to right shunt is present. Ligation of the duct in such cases may be followed either by a dramatic fall in pulmonary artery pressure or by reversal of the shunt at the remaining defect due to persistence of the pulmonary hypertension.)

Total anomalous pulmonary venous drainage is not common but may result in the presentation in childhood as described. In this condition the atrial septal defect is essential to continued survival. The diagnosis is suspected when all samples from the right side of the heart show high oxygen saturation and the samples taken from the left side do not show an increase in oxygen content. Diagnosis is confirmed by angiocardiography, an injection into the pulmonary artery being the most useful. There is a number of different types and the repair of the condition is a matter of great technical difficulty in some of these. The very gratifying results from successful surgery make the effort well worth while as the outlook in the absence of surgical treatment is poor. Here, the usefulness of the first and second order data is about equally balanced. It is important to appreciate that the lesion in the heart (atrial septal defect) is essential to survival. All the blood from the lungs and body returns to the right atrium and recirculates mainly through the lungs. Enough spills over to the systemic circulation by way of the atrial septal defect to maintain life. In a typical case the oxygen saturation in all chambers of the heart ranged from 87 per cent to 94 per cent, and calculation of the blood flow showed a systemic flow of 3 l. per minute, pulmonary flow 17 l. per minute. With such figures the calculations of output and resistance are grossly inaccurate.

Finally we may consider *primary pulmonary hypertension*. Here the presence of a forbidding degree of pulmonary hypertension may make the diagnosis somewhat academic, since surgery would not be contemplated at the time of writing, even if a defect were present. A firm diagnosis of *primary* pulmonary hypertension may be difficult to establish however. For example, in some patients with pulmonary hypertension there is an atrial septal defect: it may then be impossible to establish whether this is responsible for the hypertension.

The foregoing analysis has been presented to illustrate the ways in which evidence must be weighed in making a diagnosis. It is incomplete in several respects, for example, it takes insufficient account of the physical findings, electrocardiogram and phonocardiogram. It does show, however, that the value of the data obtained in different disorders varies both in its absolute worth and in its importance relative to the rest of the observations. Thus, in a patient with a ventricular septal defect and left to right shunt, the recordings of pressure from the right side of the heart, together with the oxygen analysis from the heart chambers is of first importance in deciding on surgery. If, however, the ventricular septal defect co-exists with an overriding aorta and pulmonary stenosis (Fallot's tetralogy), the advisability of surgery can be judged from the patient's history and the angiocardiographic findings without reference to either the pressure recordings or blood gas analysis.

This appreciation would have little point if the observations made during catheterization were always in agreement. However, it is not unusual to find ambiguities in the interpretation of data, or discrepancies between the pre-operative diagnosis and the operative findings. For this reason, it is necessary to proceed now to consider the absolute and relative worth of the data obtained at catheterization, bearing in mind the way in which they may be used to substantiate a diagnosis of disordered anatomy and function. The evidence may be considered under the following headings:

1. Evidence from the passage of the catheter.
2. Evidence from blood sampling from the catheter.
3. Evidence from pressure tracings.
4. Evidence from injection of tracer substances.
5. Evidence from angiocardiography.

1. Evidence from the passage of the catheter

The evidence obtained from the path taken by the catheter is often of diagnostic value. For example, if passed from the left arm it is a certain method of identifying a *left superior vena cava* since it takes a characteristic course to the right atrium by way of the coronary sinus (Fig. 6). This information is not entirely without point, for the presence of this anomaly may be embarrassing at open heart surgery, when large amounts of blood pour down the coronary sinus into the right atrium. In a number of varieties of anomalous pulmonary venous drainage too, the left superior vena cava is implicated.

In many other ways, the path of the catheter may be of assistance. If the inferior vena cava fails to form in the embryo, the infra-diaphragmatic venous drainage to the heart is by *persistent vena azygos*. Here a catheter passed from below pursues an odd course to reach the upper part of the right atrium in the mid-thoracic region, a situation which may give rise to confusion (Fig. 10.10). As in many similar perplexing sites, the injection of a small amount of contrast medium may bring enlightenment, particularly if the patient is screened in the lateral position when the characteristic forward curve of the azygos vein can be identified.

Within the heart, some caution is necessary in interpretating the catheter movements. In many subjects when viewed in the usual anteroposterior plane, the position of the catheter wedged in the *coronary sinus* resembles that of the catheter passed to the right ventricular outflow (Fig. 8), and, with an end hole catheter, the wedged coronary sinus pressure tracing may resemble a damped recording from the right ventricle (Fig. 18.2). Here the blood sample may be the most useful item in clarifying the situation, coronary sinus blood being usually very desaturated. Again, a cautious injection of 2 ml of contrast medium made by hand will show a characteristic pattern, as the coronary veins and sinus are outlined.

Passing the catheter to the left atrium through an *atrial septal defect* is most easily done from below, because the inter-atrial septum is inclined at about 45° to the sagittal plane and at about 80° to the horizontal plane, being orientated so that the right atrial side 'faces' downwards, forwards and laterally. Because of this inclination of the septum, it is not usually possible to say at what level a cardiac catheter passes through, and statements that the catheter passed through the atrial septum, 'low down' or 'high up' should be accepted with some caution. Some indication that the defect is large may be obtained if a loop of catheter can be swung through the defect, but inferences of size from the ease of passage can be very misleading. A large flap-like foramen ovale may be completely physiological and yet allow a catheter to pass repeatedly and easily from the right to the left atrium. Occasionally the presence of two defects creates a misleading effect. The author on one occasion inferred the presence of a very large atrial septal defect from the ease with which a large loop of catheter outlining both atria could be formed. At operation there proved to be a secundum effect in the upper part of the septum with a primum defect low down. The catheter had been looping in through one defect and out through the other.

The passage of a catheter into the veins of the right lung frequently appears to indicate *anomalous venous drainage* of that lung, but far more often it is a misleading appearance, the catheter in fact having traversed an atrial septal defect or foramen ovale and entered the left atrium

before entering the pulmonary veins (Fig. 3). The appearance of the catheter in the left lung veins (confirmed by pressure and oxygen saturation) may be evidence, not of an atrial septal defect, but merely of a *foramen ovale*. The presence of a foramen ovale rather than a defect may be inferred from pressure records across the septum showing a gradient. The pressure in the left atrium is normally some 5 to 10 mmHg higher than in the right atrium, and the normal left atrial pressure tracing shows much more definite A and V waves than is common on the right side. Withdrawal across the septum through the foramen ovale, therefore, usually shows an abrupt and clear-cut change in pressure and contour. Occasionally, however, a gradient may be found in a case with a small atrial septal defect, through which a large flow is occurring. In case of doubt, oxygen analysis may give good evidence of an atrial shunt, or alternatively a tracer curve using, e.g. ascorbic acid may demonstrate an atrial shunt. Finally in atrial septal defect, contrast medium injected into the pulmonary artery may be seen in the P.A. view to appear in the right atrium *after* passage through the lung (Fig. 45). This injection site may be preferable to the left atrial injection where a 'closed' septum occasionally shows a 'puff' of contrast coming through the foramen ovale if the catheter holds it open. (This is unusual.) Angiocardiography will often reveal how the catheter apparently in the left atrium in fact has its tip far down a pulmonary vein draining the posterior aspect of the lung. Judging when the tip of the catheter is in the cavity of the left atrium is not always easy.

The *atrial appendages* are a frequent source of confusion if they are long. In a long mobile appendage in an infant, it is sometimes possible to move the catheter in the right appendage over to the left of the mid-line. The same may occur in the left atrial appendage. Here again blood sampling or an injection of a few ml of contrast is helpful in clearing the confusion.

In the *ventricle*, the catheter position is usually not misleading, although in all varieties of transposition of the great vessels there may be difficulty in finding the outflow valves. This, however, is frustrating rather than confusing. Ready passage through a *ventricular septal defect* should raise a suspicion of corrected transposition, but, in Fallot's tetralogy, it is often possible to pass the catheter into the pulmonary artery or through the override to the aorta at will (Fig. 13). Undue ease in passing from one ventricle to the other and to the left atrium is very suggestive of an endocardial cushion defect.

In the pulmonary artery, the passage of the catheter through a *ductus* produces a characteristic appearance, the catheter running down near the mid line to below the diaphragm (Fig. 11). Occasionally in this manoeuvre the pressure tracing will reveal a coarctation. In occasional patients with patent ductus, the catheter will pass from the pulmonary artery up the arteries of the neck from the aortic arch instead of down the aorta, but this is uncommon and should raise the suspicion that an aorto-pulmonary window or aortic over-ride is present. Occasionally passage of the catheter down the pulmonary artery to the left lower lobe may look like the traversing of a ductus into the aorta; if it is in a pulmonary artery, the catheter will not pass below the diaphragm. In case of doubt a small hand injection of contrast medium is the most useful manoeuvre. This will show the blood is not passing down the aorta. Both the pressure and the blood oxygen saturation may be similar in the aorta and the pulmonary artery if Eisenmenger's reaction is present.

The evidence from the path taken by the catheter is, therefore, often entirely reliable, but equally may require cautious interpretation. It is particularly important to obtain all possible information as to the site if doubt arises, without moving the catheter tip; to record the pressure, obtain a blood sample (if possible), make a cautious test injection of contrast medium while screening and, if necessary, inject a tracer, record tracer curves and take a plain X-ray film as a record.

2. Evidence from blood sampling

Evidence obtained from blood sampling is likewise not without its difficulties. Some possible technical errors have been considered elsewhere. Here we are concerned with the possibility of *error from faulty inference*, the actual estimations being correct. The principle underlying the study of the oxygen saturation of the blood in the different heart chambers is, of course, a simple one—the identification of a shunt of arterial blood into the right side of the heart, or of venous blood into the left. In practice this may provide incontrovertible evidence in some cases, while in others it may be highly misleading. The possible sources of error cannot be dealt with exhaustively, but some that are common will be exemplified.

Various levels of oxygen saturation have been quoted as limits for normal venous blood. Few authors writing on this subject have mentioned the effects of temperature regulation upon the rate of blood flow. When the hands are warm, the venous blood returning from the extremities in the superficial veins is virtually indistinguishable from arterial blood. This is due to the rapid passage of blood through the palms of the hands and soles of the feet. Its effect is to cool the body by increasing skin temperature and thereby heat loss.

In subjects with cold extremities, however, the venous blood is desaturated because the rate of flow through the limbs is low. The effects of this variability in flow on the saturation of mixed venous blood appear to be considerable, a cold subject having a relatively low venous saturation, while in a warm one the saturation is high. The normal range is at least from 55 per cent to 85 per cent saturation for mixed venous blood (i.e. pulmonary

artery blood in subjects with no intracardiac shunt): a saturation of 90 per cent in the superior vena cava is occasionally encountered in normal subjects.

This variability of saturation has a secondary effect upon the ease with which a shunt can be detected by oximetry, particularly if the shunt be small. If the oxygen saturation in the venae cavae is in the range 60 to 65 per cent, a jet of oxygenated blood entering from the left side of the heart causes a greater change in oxygen saturation than it will do in the same patient when the blood in the venae cavae is 80 to 85 per cent saturated. This apparent paradox arises from a number of causes. Firstly, it is a consequence of the shape of the oxygen dissociation curve that small increments in oxygen tension produce relatively larger changes in saturation at 65 per cent saturation than at 80 per cent saturation. Secondly, since the blood coming through a shunt commonly 'streams' in the heart chambers (i.e. mixes relatively slowly), a small shunt will produce a more evident effect when it is picked up by multiple blood sampling if it contrasts markedly with the remaining blood in the right side of the heart. Finally, the technical errors of most methods of oxygen determination increase as the blood becomes more oxygenated (largely, once more, as a result of the shape of the oxygen dissociation curve of blood).

It might be thought that salvation from this difficulty might lie in a flight to the slide rule and calculation of the blood shunted. A brief consideration of the method of calculating cardiac output by the Fick equation, and the further calculations based on it will remove this illusion. Any method of oxygen estimation is subject to error, and in common with many laboratory procedures, it is not possible to get the accuracy of the final product (either the oxygen saturation or content) to much closer limits than $\pm 2\frac{1}{2}$ per cent. The calculation of cardiac output has been described elsewhere. On one occasion the author took two pulmonary artery samples for the estimation of cardiac output, one at the beginning and the other at the end of a 10 minute period, during which oxygen uptake was measured. The saturations of the samples measured by absorptiometry were 85 per cent and 81 per cent respectively. This difference is within the limits of experimental error. In calculating the Fick output the oxygen content of mixed venous blood is subtracted from the arterial content. In this case the 5 per cent difference between these samples is magnified by this process of subtraction to a 40 per cent difference in output ($4/81 \times 100 = 5$ per cent).

Data:
  Oxygen saturation of pulmonary artery blood
  Sample 1   81 per cent = 178 ml O_2/l.
  Sample 2   85 per cent = 187 ml O_2/l.
  Oxygen content of brachial artery blood
    211 ml O_2/l.

Oxygen uptake 160 ml/min
Cardiac output (sample 1) $= \dfrac{160}{211-178}$
$= 4\cdot8$ 1/min
Cardiac output (sample 2) $= \dfrac{160}{211-187}$
$= 6\cdot7$ 1/min

The process of subtraction in this calculation magnifies the original difference of 5 per cent (which separates 81 per cent and 85 per cent) to 40 per cent—the difference between $4\cdot8$ and $6\cdot7$ (or, of course, between $211-178 = 33$ ml and $211-187 = 24$ ml).

When the effects of the errors of measurement in arterial oxygen are considered, the range becomes even larger. In the foregoing sample the arterial oxygen saturation was 96 per cent, the figure found might have been 94 per cent or 98 per cent. Taking the extreme figures, the arteriovenous oxygen difference in this patient could have been 98 per cent to 81 per cent, or 94 per cent to 85 per cent, i.e. either 17 per cent or 9 per cent. These figures lead to estimates of cardiac output of $3\cdot8$ litres per min and $7\cdot9$ litres per min respectively. Thus an apparently trivial difference of measurement has lead to a situation where one estimate of cardiac output is more than double the other, the difference divided by the mean being 70 per cent. This error will affect not only the calculation of output by the Fick method, but all calculations based upon it, that is, the measurement of pulmonary and systemic blood flow in patients with intra-cardiac shunts, and the estimation of pulmonary and systemic vascular resistance. In this example the mean pulmonary artery pressure was 50 mmHg. The mean left atrial pressure measured by direct puncture was 15 mmHg. These figures give estimates of pulmonary vascular resistance of $8\cdot9$ and of $4\cdot4$ units respectively.

The 'natural' error of this estimation is less if the arteriovenous oxygen difference is larger. Thus, if in the above example the mixed venous saturations found had been 61 per cent and 65 per cent (a difference of $\pm3\cdot3$ per cent) instead of 81 per cent and 85 per cent, the maximum disparity in arteriovenous oxygen difference becomes:

1. 98 per cent to 61 per cent = 37 per cent
2. 96 per cent to 65 per cent = 31 per cent.

These figures result in a difference in cardiac output of 'only' $24\cdot2$ per cent instead of the 70 per cent difference found when the mean figure for mixed venous blood was 83 per cent saturated.

It is clear that the precise calculations of cardiac output and of vascular resistance, which depends on it, are *theoretically* simple and satisfactory. But *in practice*, the nature of the calculation demands a precision of measurement inapplicable to the type of biological phenomenon observed.

A possible solution to this dilemma is to take multiple samples to determine a mean figure. This sort of remedy is appropriate in certain situations, for example, a mean of six estimates of weight on a micro-balance is more accurate than a single measurement. However, in the biological situation created by cardiac catheterization there are so many variables—error of sampling, error in the measurement of oxygen uptake, change in output and arterial pressure, that it is probably realistic to accept that these measurements, although apparently precise, are in fact no more than crude approximations.

In patients in whom shunts are occurring, the calculations are still further complicated by the difficulty in deciding on the *saturation of mixed venous blood*. In the right atrium, the blood from the venae cavae meet and the sampling technique will usually miss the very desaturated coronary sinus blood which enters the atrium close to the tricuspid valve. Any figure is likely to be sufficiently erroneous to produce a sizable error and it must be accepted that calculations of this type based on catheterization data are of indifferent value. They may be regarded as giving a crude indication, but little more.

In assessing *congenital heart disease* it is probably misleading to calculate pulmonary vascular resistance and so derive an apparently precise figure which can have little meaning. It is more realistic to divide cases into those with low pulmonary arterial pressure, small L→R shunt; low pulmonary pressure, large shunt; high pressure, small shunt; high pressure, large shunt and those with high pulmonary artery pressure and reversed shunt.

If calculations *are* to be made, they should be kept as simple as possible with the minimum of variables. The simplest is probably the *ratio of pulmonary to systemic blood flow* in which the only parameters are saturations. Here errors due to measurement of metabolic rate and pressures are eliminated. This is shown earlier, see page 32. The equation may be written:

$$\frac{\text{Pulmonary B.F.}}{\text{Systemic B.F.}} = \frac{(\text{Arterial} - \text{R.A.}) \text{ per cent saturation}}{(\text{P.V.} - \text{P.A.}) \text{ per cent saturation}}$$

This calculation, which is no more inaccurate than any so far mentioned in this chapter, can, with a little practice, be readily done in the operator's head or while glancing at the catheterization data. Consider the following data by catheterization (oximetry by absorbtiometer).

	Pressure	Saturation per cent
S.V.C.	—	69
H.R.A.	—	67
M.R.A.	5/–1	66
L.R.A.	—	66

	Pressure	Saturation per cent
I.V.C.	—	71
L.R.V.	50/0	85
H.R.V.	50/0	81
P.A.	50/20	88
W.P.C.P.	7/–1	98
F.A.	140/80	96

The following is apparent by inspection:

1. Diagnosis: Ventricular Septal Defect

2. Shunt Ratio: $\dfrac{30}{10} = 3:1 \left(\text{i.e.} \dfrac{96\text{--}66}{98\text{--}88} \right)$

3. Vascular resistance only slightly increased.

4. Operative risk acceptable.

Errors of inference made from oximetry may arise from the *proximity of a shunt to a heart valve*. It is common to find no clear evidence of an atrial shunt of blood in cases in which there is a small ostium primum defect. Here the arterial blood enters the atrium close to the tricuspid valve and streams close to the septum to enter the right ventricle. A similar difficulty may mask a Gerbode lesion. The correct diagnosis may be suggested in either case by the clinical picture, by the pressure tracings obtained if the catheter traverses the lesion, and by angiography, particularly by selective injection into the left atrium and ventricle. The ascorbic acid tracer technique is probably more sensitive in picking up this stream of blood than oxygen analysis.

A similar error of inference may arise in the reverse direction if valves are incompetent. This is most commonly seen in patent ductus arteriosus with *pulmonary valve incompetence* due to pulmonary hypertension. The reflux of arterial blood from the pulmonary artery to the right ventricle during diastole may lead to a rise in oxygen saturation in the pulmonary outflow tract. This suggests a double lesion—patent ductus with ventricular septal defect and pulmonary hypertension. If this mistake is made, the simple lesion may be missed and curative ligation of the duct not attempted. As has already been mentioned, tracer techniques such as that employing ascorbic acid are likewise subject to erroneous inference by this phenomenon. Here aortography and left ventricular angiocardiography will usually reveal the error. In the same way a cleft or *incompetent tricuspid valve* may permit reflux in a case of ventricular septal defect and suggest the presence of an atrial septal defect. In such a case angiocardiography may again be very helpful in clarifying the anatomy.

Even in the presence of a gross lesion, the inferential diagnosis from oxygen saturation may prove misleading. An infant was catheterized before angiocardiographic equipment was installed. Blood taken from the right atrium was desaturated and the right ventricular samples suggested the presence of a ventricular septal defect. Total anomalous pulmonary venous drainage was subsequently found. The error had been due to sampling all three atrial specimens of blood from the lateral aspect of the atrium where the desaturated blood from the venae cavae was streaming. The saturated blood entering by the coronary sinus from the aberrant pulmonary veins and passing through an atrial septal defect to the left atrium was missed.

Heavy premedication may be a cause of marked anoxia if ventilation is impaired by depression of respiration. We have encountered this most frequently in adult patients premedicated with morphine or its derivatives. It is rare in children given chloral but not uncommon when 'triple mixture' is used. Hypoventilation may cause two important effects: arterial desaturation and pulmonary hypertension.

Arterial desaturation may be marked, especially if the pulmonary venous pressure is high, as under these conditions the gas transfer across the alveolar membrane may be further impaired by pulmonary oedema. The risks of morphine premedication in patients with mitral stenosis were recognized when, during catheterization, low oxygen saturations were found in the pulmonary vein blood. The lowest saturation measured in mitral valve disease was 64 per cent. In congenital heart disease an oxygenation level of 83 per cent has been encountered in the pulmonary venous blood. Administration of oxygen for five minutes restores the pulmonary vein blood saturation to normal in most cases when the cause of the desaturation is hypoventilation. If the reason for the desaturation is not appreciated, the presence of arterial desaturation may suggest a right to left shunt—and much time may be expended on fruitless investigation designed to identify its site.

The pulmonary hypertension induced by hypoventilation is very variable. It has been extensively investigated in anoxic lung disease and appears to be a complex response to the reduction in oxygen content as well as to the increase in carbon dioxide content in arterial blood. The degree of pulmonary hypertension resulting from the same stimulus varies from one individual to another. It may be sufficient in some people to be misleading in the assessment of the effects of heart disease—tending to make lesions appear more severe than they really are. Again, administration of oxygen reduces the pressure in the pulmonary artery towards its usual level.

Clearly, the combination of arterial desaturation and pulmonary hypertension, both induced by hypoventilation, may seriously confuse the assessment of septal defects or patent ductus by erroneously suggesting the presence of an Eisenmenger Reaction. This diagnostic error may be very serious as the mistake may well be responsible for denying curative surgery to a patient with a left to right shunt.

It would be inappropriate to leave this section without

a note on the *calculation of valve area*. This again is data of vital importance which is often in doubt. In 1951 Gorlin and Gorlin proposed a formula for calculating the area of the orifice in a stenosed mitral valve based on hydraulic considerations. The calculation requires some data which are difficult to estimate with any accuracy and some data which are assumed. It is based on a formula for calculating the area of a narrowing in a pipe, the fluid passing along the pipe being a homogeneous liquid exhibiting laminar flow. The application of this formula to turbulent flow of a non-homogeneous fluid (blood) through irregular constrictions in odd shaped membranes which partition the irregularly shaped heart chambers is clearly unjustifiable, but is a measure of the need for such a formula. It has proved very difficult to confirm or refute the value of this calculation. Not the least difficulty is the precise measurement of valve area *in vivo* by mechanical means to check the formula. The gloved finger of a surgeon is generally held to provide a very indifferent estimate.

3. Evidence from pressure tracings

Evidence from pressure tracings is, on the whole, reliable and errors are due more often to a faulty appreciation of the site of the catheter than from a misinterpretation of the recording. Some of the possible errors resulting from technical faults are discussed in the section dealing with technique: here we are concerned with errors of inference.

It is first desirable to emphasize again the effect of *damping* in making recordings. Only a pressure transducer mounted on the tip of a catheter is free from the distortions of the record associated with the oscillations of the catheter. These are least with narrow catheters (5F or 6F) and may be gross with wide bore catheters such as 9F or larger. In general, the larger the gauge of the catheter, the larger the recorded oscillations. Any harmonic of the catheter tube may be damped out by a suitable electrical circuit or mechanical device such as a length of capillary tubing, but the introduction of such damping will remove physiological oscillations having the same period. Troublesome artefacts are commonest with large catheters, and in such catheters the period of oscillation is relatively low. Since physiological oscillations are also of low frequency, it is inevitable that important detail may be obliterated by damping in circumstances in which damping is most often needed. If damping is used, therefore, the degree of damping applied should be noted, and a length of undamped tracing should be recorded. It is often possible to remove most of the undesirable oscillation in a tracing by a minor repositioning of the catheter. All damping systems should be tested to ensure that they do not reduce the amplitude of the response to pressure change.

Cardiac catheters may terminate with a simple end hole, or in a series of openings intended for angiocardio-

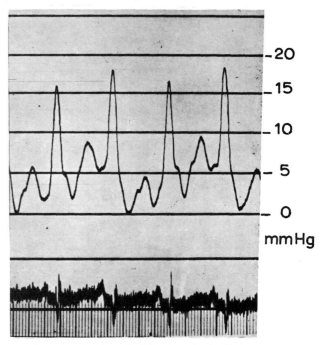

FIG. 18.1   A tracing from the left atrium obtained by a catheter passed by the Seldinger-Ross technique. This shows very high peaked A waves. These are due to the atrial contraction striking the catheter and producing an artificially high transient pressure. The true pressure in this atrium was about 12/0.

graphy. Somewhat different artefacts are associated with the two types. The *end hole catheter* is particularly liable to produce a tracing of the kind shown in Fig. 18.1. Here the catheter is in the left atrium near the mitral valve, and with each systole the membrane of the valve strikes the end of the catheter producing a false high pressure wave recognizable by its brief peaked appearance and its prompt disappearance when the catheter is moved into the cavity of the atrium. These artefacts may also occur when the catheter tip lies in the right atrium due to movements of the tricuspid valve. Similar artefacts are less common in the ventricle, but may sometimes be seen in pulmonary arterial tracings, particularly with a stiff wide bore catheter.

The unusual appearance of certain *wedge tracings* taken with an end hold catheter may also cause confusion. In the coronary sinus the wedge pressure usually resembles a damped ventricular tracing. When wedged in the coronary sinus, the catheter, viewed from in front may appear to lie in the right ventricular outflow tract. The trace may also suggest right ventricle as shown in Fig. 18.2. The position of the catheter in the coronary sinus was confirmed by blood sample and the injection of contrast medium. Another unusual coronary sinus tracing is shown in Fig. 18.3, here a saline infusion caused

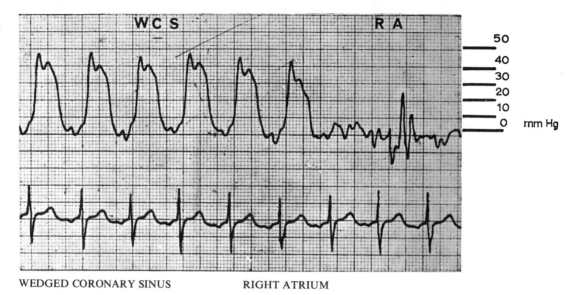

WEDGED CORONARY SINUS   RIGHT ATRIUM

FIG. 18.2   The wedged coronary sinus pressure closely resembling a right ventricular pressure. The position was confirmed by a hand injection of contrast medium and a blood sample showing the very low oxygen saturation of coronary sinus blood. The tracing also shows oscillations due to catheter movement caused by the beating heart, and a draw back to the right atrium.

a gross artefact. Similarly the pulmonary vein wedge pressure may closely resemble the pulmonary artery tracing, and in some cases a pulmonary vein wedge position obtained in atrial defect may be mistaken for a pulmonary arterial recording.

An unusual cause of confusion is the recording of a very *high ventricular pressure* with an end hole catheter.

This may happen if the catheter is pushed into the recesses among the papillary muscles. The tracing is usually rather featureless, like that seen in marked pulmonary stenosis and is due to the catheter being exposed to local pressure in the myocardium. Pressure above 300 mmHg has been recorded by the author in this way from a right ventricle with a cavity pressure of only 60 mmHg. The nature of

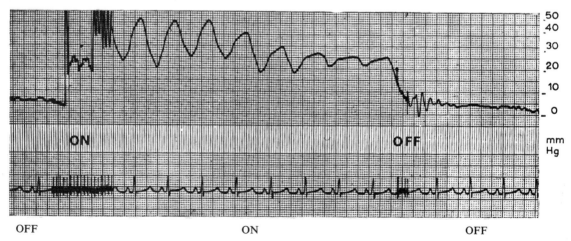

OFF   ON   OFF

FIG. 18.3   *Effect of saline infusion through pressure-head on recording of coronary sinus pressure.* An unusual effect of running saline infusions during catheterization. On the left of the tracing the normal coronary sinus pressure is 5 mmHg. The saline infusion was then turned on to clear the catheter, which had an end hole. A high pressure of 50/25 was recorded. The saline was then turned off and the pressure subsided to 5 mm once more. The wave form is occasionally recorded without any saline transfusion running, and may be mistaken for a right ventricular tracing. It is the form most usually seen in a wedged coronary vein. The coronary sinus recording shown on Fig. 18.2 is unusual.

the artefact was demonstrated by a cautious injection of 1 ml contrast medium which showed myocardial infiltration of the injected material. The pressure fell promptly when the catheter was dislodged back into the ventricular cavity.

A somewhat uncommon phenomenon of a different sort is occasionally seen when the end hole catheter is lying in the orifice of a stenosed pulmonary valve. If the fit of the catheter in the hole is suitable, a *negative pressure* may be recorded as the catheter is drawn back through the valve, as in Fig. 18.4. This is a simple *venturi effect*, the forces acting on the catheter tip being the same as those which suck scent into the nozzle of a scent spray or petrol through the jet of a carburettor. It does not necessarily follow that the negative pressure measured is present in the absence of the obstruction occasioned by the catheter.

Finally, the pulmonary artery pressure measured with a catheter may be to some extent determined by the *size of the catheter* passed through the pulmonary valve. In tight pulmonary stenosis the catheter may almost obstruct the orifice and lower the pressure measured beyond it. The most alarming example of this phenomenon recorded by the author occurred during a diagnostic investigation in which 8F Cournand catheter was manipulated into the pulmonary artery with complete disappearance of all oscillations in the tracing. The pressure fell to below the zero base line and the electrocardiogram showed S-T depression. The patient was found to have become deeply cyanosed. The catheter, which had presumably corked up the pulmonary valve, was withdrawn: the patient rapidly recovered. In such

circumstances the pressure measured is clearly of no value as a basis for calculations of pulmonary vascular resistance.

Angiocardiographic catheters are not liable to cause so much difficulty in interpretation as those with an end hole, as it is not possible to record a wedge pressure with them. Occasionally, however, a misleading recording may occur when the side holes in the catheter bridge a stenosed valve, for example, at a tightly stenosed pulmonary or aortic valve. The tracing here may be intermediate between that in the artery and ventricle and suggest the presence of an infundibular chamber. A curious example of this type of artefact is shown in Fig. 18.5. In this infant the angiographic catheter was passed from the right ventricle to the aorta. The pressure tracing was recorded while the catheter was slowly drawn back from the aorta into the right ventricle. As the side holes in the catheter enter the ventricle, the pressure recorded gradually rises to a higher level than in the aorta. Angiocardiography from the right ventricle in this infant showed a form of Fallot's tetralogy with severe pulmonary valve and infundibular obstruction, a small ventricular septal defect, and only slight right to left shunting through the V.S.D. Presumably, the unexpected high ventricular pressure was made possible by the size of the V.S.D. Note that the gradual transition from aortic pressure to right ventricular pressure in this tracing obscures the events occurring in the region of the aortic valve. It is not possible to say whether the catheter has passed directly from the right ventricle through the aortic valve as it can do in a typical Fallot's tetralogy where the aorta overrides the septal defect, or has passed

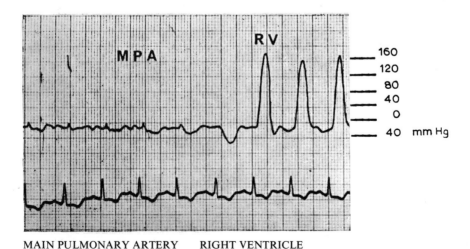

FIG. 18.4   An example of a venturi effect at the pulmonary valve. In this patient, with pulmonary valve stenosis, the pulmonary artery pressure was slightly below zero because the pressure head lay above the normal zero point. On drawing back the catheter, which has an open end and no side holes, a negative pressure of more than −40 mmHg was recorded before the ventricular cavity was entered. The ventricular pressure was 160 systolic. Note the typical rounded systolic forms of the pressure tracing in a ventricle with an obstructed outlet.

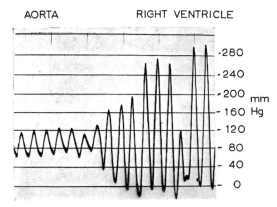

FIG. 18.5 A withdrawal trace taken with a 6F angiographic (NIH) catheter from aorta to right ventricle. The patient was an infant weighing 9 kg. Angiocardiography showed Fallot's tetralogy with a marked pulmonary stenosis and only a small right to left shunt. At operation, after a successful pulmonary valvotomy, balanced pressures in the aorta and right ventricle were found. Note in this tracing how the multiple end holes of the angiographic catheter produce a gradual transition from one pressure to another. An attempt to pass a Cournand catheter to the aorta in this child failed.

through to the left ventricle which in this case must be working on a much lower systolic pressure, or, if at the same pressure, be associated with aortic valve stenosis. In this case an attempt to pass a Cournand catheter to the aorta by the same route failed. The anatomical detail was clarified by an angiocardiography using full-sized films taken on a biplane AOT changer.

This is a convenient place to mention a phenomenon of some value associated with the characteristic pressure changes which accompany ventricular extrasystoles. In normal subjects, or those with a fixed obstruction to the ventricular outflow due to a valve stenosis or a diaphragm, the beat following an extrasystole has a higher ventricular systolic pressure and, in the artery beyond the valve, an increased pulse pressure. Brockenborough, Braunwald and Morrow (1961) have pointed out that when the outflow obstruction is muscular as in hypertrophic subaortic stenosis, the arterial pulse pressure behaves paradoxically. The increased intraventricular pressure of the beat following an extrasystole is accompanied by a *reduced* arterial pulse pressure. This observation is useful as an indication of the type of outflow obstruction present, but may occasionally be equivocal. In Figure 18.6 the aortic pressure was recorded by a catheter passed up from the groin to near to the aortic valve. The pressure in the left ventricle was recorded by a Brockenborough catheter passed transseptally and then through the mitral valve. Three large ventricular beats are shown which follow extrasystoles. The aortic pulse pressure is reduced doubtfully after the first, little changed after the second and slightly in-

creased after the third. The patient was a boy of nine years. Left ventricular angiocardiography showed a hypertrophic subaortic stenosis.

A tracing occasionally encountered in marked calcific aortic stenosis is shown in Figure 18.7. This was obtained by passing a fine polythene catheter through a needle into the left ventricle, and on through the aortic valve. The pressure was then recorded during the draw back to the ventricle. The tracing suggests the presence of a subvalvar chamber. At surgery no such chamber was present and the mechanism of this artefact is unexplained. The form of the pressure wave in the zone between the aortic trace and the ventricular trace, however, is unlike that seen in a case of subvalvar diaphragm in whom the withdrawal was recorded by a similar technique (Fig. 18.8.).

Misleading pressure tracings are commonly recorded from the atria. One often seen is the already mentioned apparent high transient systolic pressure due to the catheter tip impinging on the mitral or tricuspid valve leaflets as they are driven backwards at the beginning of systole (Fig. 18.1). Another also referred to earlier is a somewhat similar but longer lasting systolic rise in pressure which may be found in long atrial appendages (Fig. 11.6).

4. Evidence from tracer techniques

The evidence from tracer techniques can be conclusive on some occasions, while on others the quality of the curves obtained may be extremely poor (Fig. 18.9). It is not always possible to be sure of the causes of failure. The experience of the author has been that good curves are almost invariably achieved when the injections of contrast medium are made into the pulmonary artery. They

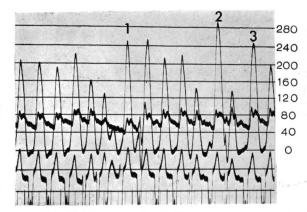

FIG. 18.6 Simultaneous record of pressure from the left ventricle recorded by transseptal catheter, and aorta recorded close to the aortic valve by a retrograde aortic catheter in a nine-year-old boy suffering from hypertrophic obstructive cardiomyopathy. Three beats which follow an increased filling time due to previous extrasystoles are indicated by the numbers 1 to 3. For explanation, see text.

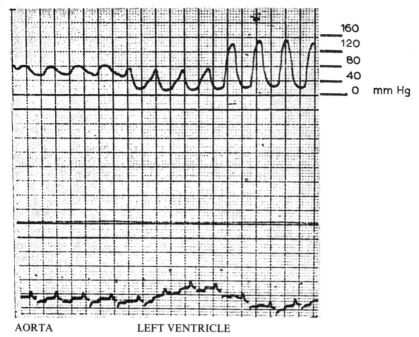

AORTA   LEFT VENTRICLE

FIG. 18.7   Withdrawal trace from aorta to left ventricle in a case of calcified aortic stenosis. The catheter through which the measurements were made was passed through a needle stabbed into the left ventricle. The tracing suggests the presence of a sub-valval stenosis. At surgery a simple valve lesion was present. A misleading tracing of this type has been encountered on several occasions, but its cause has not been determined with certainty. Cf. Fig. 18.8.

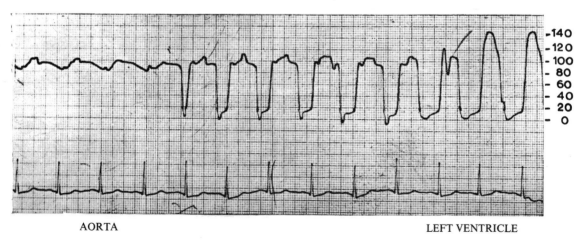

AORTA   LEFT VENTRICLE

FIG. 18.8   A tracing from a patient with a sub-valvar diaphragm in the left ventricle. This tracing was obtained by floating a polythene tube through the aortic valve from the cavity of the left ventricle. The slightly damped aortic pressure is seen on the left followed by a zone in which the systolic pressure is the same as at the aortic valve but the diastolic pressure is ventricular, and finally two beats in the ventricular cavity. There is a gradient of 40 mm at the diaphragm. Cine-angiography did not define the presence of a diaphragm. At surgery there was found to be only two centimetres between the diaphragm and the valve. Note the pressure marks and scratches on this tracing. This is a typical example of the spoiling of records that can easily occur when heat sensitive recording paper is carelessly handled.

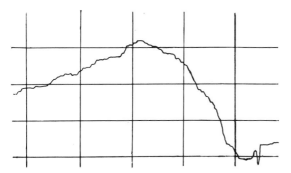

FIG. 18.9   A very poor dye dilution curve recorded in a patient with an atrial septal defect and large left to right shunt. The dye was injected into the right atrial appendage from which it cleared only slowly. This has resulted in a slow appearance time. Recording direction left to right.

tend to become progressively less certain in the ventricle and atrium. Quite worthless dilution curves may be recorded from the veins of the limbs, particularly if the extremities are cold. Some of the causes underlying this variability become apparent if injections of dye mixed with contrast medium are made under X-ray screening. Pulmonary artery injections are almost immediately swept off into the lung field. Injections into the ventricle, particularly if made at the apex, may linger for a few beats before being fully cleared into the pulmonary tree. Atrial injections, especially if they are placed in the atrial appendage, may persist for as many as six or seven beats before being moved completely out of the heart (Fig. 31). This variable rate of removal is seen in even more marked fashion if injections are made into the veins of the limbs. Dye may persist for minutes in small veins, and in many patients there is surprisingly little tendency for the dye to sweep quickly even up a major venous channel. The disappointing, rather formless curves which may be produced on some occasions are no doubt due in part to phenomena of this kind. Marked respiratory oscillations may also make interpretation difficult (Fig. 18.10).

With qualitative tracer techniques, such as hydrogen inhalation and ascorbic acid dilution curves, the limitations of the technique are largely similar to those using oxygen analysis which have been described earlier. Thus, they will fail to distinguish between valve incompetence and shunting in the same circumstances as does oxygen saturation, e.g. in the case of 'hypertensive' patent ductus where pulmonary incompetence allows a leak back to the right ventricle. The results can be interpreted as due to a high ventricular septal defect. Tracer curves do, however, have a useful place in the distinction between anomalous pulmonary venous drainage of one lung and atrial septal defect. Here injection of a tracer into the right pulmonary artery when the pulmonary veins of the right lung drain to the right atrium produces evidence of recirculation through the right side of the heart, while injection into the

left pulmonary artery produces a normal curve. In a surgical unit which has easy access to bypass, this pre-operative distinction is not, however, of great importance.

5. Evidence from angiocardiography

Selective angiocardiography provides the most direct, and probably the most reliable evidence of the anatomy of the living heart. As in any other sophisticated investigation, its value is directly related to the adequacy of its technical performance and to the reliability of its interpretation.

The manual dexterity of the doctor performing the catheterization is most important because, particularly in infants and small children, a high degree of skill is necessary. The radiological facilities must be suitable and the radiographic technique must be of high standard. Each catheterization must be based on an established routine pattern but must also be modified for the particular patient being investigated: this requires a detailed understanding of the individual clinical problem.

Even with a sound technique, angiocardiography, like any other method, has its limitations which may lead to errors both of commission or omission. Some of these are discussed below.

Difficulties may arise in the angiographic demonstration of *left to right shunts*. Atrial shunts may be demonstrated by the follow through technique described on p. 135, i.e. making the angiographic injection into the pulmonary artery, and recognizing on the late A.P. films (almost) simultaneous opacification of the right and left atria. The same angiographic findings are seen when one or more pulmonary veins drain aberrantly into the right

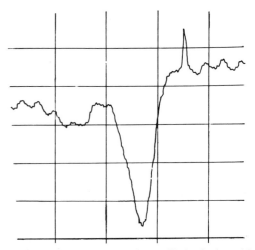

FIG. 18.10   This tracing shows a fine oscillation in time with the heart beat and a coarser oscillation possibly related to the respiratory cycle. Modern electronic systems will usually eliminate the pulse oscillations, but the coarser wave usually does not respond to adjustment of the ear oximeter or of the recorder controls. Recording direction right to left.

atrium. It is often impossible by this technique to identify the exact site of the pulmonary veins, for the atrial septum slopes obliquely backwards and to the right. The diagnostic error of mistaking aberrant pulmonary venous drainage for atrial septal defect should not cause a surgical problem, for the anatomy will be evident when the right atrium is opened. There are, however, angiographic techniques which will provide the correct diagnosis: the aberrant vein may be entered by the catheter from the right atrium and a small injection of contrast medium will confirm its drainage (Fig. 38), or a large injection of contrast medium can be delivered very rapidly into the right atrium and may produce reflux into aberrant pulmonary veins if the pulmonary circulation is slowed as by deliberately increasing the intra-bronchial pressure (Nordenstrom, 1960).

A left ventricle to right atrium (Gerbode type) shunt may be seen in *ostium primum defect* (Fig. 46). This has been seen at left ventriculography in at least four of our patients. It is due to marked mitral incompetence, permitting contrast medium to pass from the left ventricle through the cleft mitral septal leaflet. This leaflet lies immediately below the ostium primum defect. The direction of the regurgitant stream from the left ventricle may be such that the refluxing contrast medium passes backwards and to the right through the mitral valve, then through the septal defect into the *right* atrium instead of passing straight back into the left atrium. The true nature of the defect (ostium primum) can usually be recognized on the A.P. left ventriculogram as the mitral valve is misplaced to the left and narrows the left ventricular outflow to produce a swan-neck appearance of this outflow tract (Fig. 46).

A Gerbode shunt (left ventricle to right atrium) may be simulated (both at angiocardiography and oximetry) by a ventricular septal defect combined with tricuspid incompetence. Following a left ventricular injection, the contrast medium may be shunted into the right ventricle through a ventricular septal defect and may then leak retrogradely through an incompetent tricuspid valve to opacify the right atrium. In this way the right atrium opacifies after a left ventricular injection and a Gerbode defect is simulated.

The reverse situation may also occur. In a true Gerbode defect, the opacification of the right atrium (following left ventriculography) may be so fleeting as to be missed on the reading of the films. A ventricular septal defect is then likely to be diagnosed.

The angiographic diagnosis of a common atrioventricular canal may be very difficult, particularly if separate injections are not made into both left atrium and left ventricle followed by rapid or cineangiocardiography.

A patent ductus may not be demonstrated by an injection of contrast medium at the usual site because very occasionally (and usually in cyanotic congenital heart disease) the ductus arises from a very unusual site, e.g. the right subclavian artery (p. 127).

Multiple left to right shunts will probably not be demonstrated by the follow through technique as described on p. 135. The more proximal shunt will be detected but the distal one is likely to be missed as discussed on p. 136. The more distal defect will be detected by retrograde aortography or left ventriculography. Multiple left to right shunts are quite common in infants in cardiac failure; often atrial and ventricular septal defects coexist with a patent ductus. We have also encountered an aortopulmonary window 1·5 cm proximal to a patent ductus, the proximal lesion being missed at angiography.

The demonstration of the *ventricular septum* may be surprisingly difficult if there is a large shunt through a ventricular septal defect. Left ventriculography will opacify the right ventricle but the obliquity of the septum may prevent septal visualization on both antero-posterior and lateral films, so that a common ventricle may be suspected. (The absence of cyanosis does not vitiate the latter diagnosis as intra-ventricular streaming may permit surprisingly little mixing of blood.) The left anterior oblique projection is most likely to project the interventricular septum tangentially, but several different degrees of obliquity and cine-radiography may be required to differentiate angiographically between a large ventricular septal defect and a common ventricle.

Echocardiography is proving of increasing value in defining the interventricular septum.

In *cyanotic heart disease* an occluded right ventricular outflow may produce a very similar angiographic appearance to tricuspid atresia. If the angiographic injection is made into the right atrium, there may be no demonstrable opacification of the right ventricle in either condition. In the former anomaly, the right ventricle although sizeable, acts as a blind sac with little blood flow: in the latter condition the right ventricle is atretic or absent. A right ventricular injection is possible in the former anomaly and will demonstrate the correct anatomy.

In that variety of *persistent truncus arteriosus* in which a main pulmonary artery arises from one side of the truncus, it is sometimes possible to deliver the angiographic injection selectively into either the aortic or the pulmonary element (Fig. 82A). The correct diagnosis may not be made if this occurs. The reason may be that the catheter has been passed too far through the truncus into one of its major divisions, but it may also result from streaming following a correctly placed injection at the root of the truncus.

The *main pulmonary artery* often appears to be narrowed at its bifurcation in cyanotic congenital heart disease, and there may seem to be post-stenotic dilatation of its two branches. Whilst such narrowing is occasionally found at surgery to be haemodynamically significant, more often than not, the surgeon will report that no significant narrowing was found. Pressure measurements are unhelpful here. Pulmonary stenosis may so limit blood flow that no pressure gradient may exist across a significant pulmonary artery stenosis.

Short segments of a *narrowed vessel* may be obscured if they do not lie perpendicular to the X-ray beam. An example is narrowing of the aortic arch between the origins of the left carotid and subclavian arteries. This narrowing may be missed on the A.P. film because of its obliquity, and it may be obscured on the lateral projection by the radio-opaque shoulder joints. The only satisfactory projection is the left anterior oblique.

Angiocardiographic assessment of the *cardiac valves* may occasionally be misleading. This is usually due to faulty technique as when an *aortic injection* is delivered too high above the aortic valve and fails to demonstrate its incompetence.

A technically perfect retrograde aortogram may demonstrate an apparently normal aortic valve with no suggestion of aortic reflux, but the presence of an aortic diastolic murmur may still convince the clinician that a small aortic leak is, in fact, present.

Aortic valve stenosis causes doming of the aortic valve but this feature may not be well seen on either A.P. or lateral films because of the obliquity of the valve ring (p. 30, Fig. 15.1). Other features of aortic valve stenosis, e.g. jet or post-stenotic dilatation will be observed. Conversely, a normal aortic valve may very closely simulate aortic valve doming on the lateral angiogram films because of the obliquity of the valve (Fig. 15.1), but the other features of stenosis will not be present.

In the assessment of *mitral incompetence*, an injection delivered too close to the mitral valve may produce spurious incompetence. Occasionally even when the left ventricular injection is delivered at an optimal site, spurious mitral incompetence may be produced: cine films at 200 frames/s have shown that this may be due to the catheter being actually propelled into the mitral orifice during ventricular systole. Ventricular extrasystoles frequently cause spurious slight mitral incompetence as seen on cine film, but this can be recognized as due to the extrasystoles. The large film technique rarely demonstrates this (Nagle, Walker and Grainger, 1968). A soft catheter passing through the mitral valve (as in transseptal catheterization, p. 95) rarely causes significant spurious mitral incompetence.

Care must be taken not to confuse the border of the left atrium with the mitral valve leaflets, for the normal leaflets are very thin, curved, move rapidly and are rarely seen tangential to the X-ray beam.

The *pulmonary valve* is often not seen on the A.P. film because the right ventricular outflow tract may be directed antero-posteriorly. In the lateral projection, the pulmonary valve may be entirely obscured by an opacified right atrial appendage and visualization of the valve may therefore be completely inadequate if the catheter flicks back into the right atrium during a right ventricular injection.

Conclusions

The reader of the foregoing jeremiad may wonder if any touchstone is to be found on what appears to be a field beset by pitfalls. It is unlikely that any combination of techniques will completely eliminate occasional mistaken or incomplete diagnoses, but adherence to four principles will keep such errors to a minimum.

First, the diagnosis suggested by the catheterization data should be considered in the light of the clinical findings. Here the experience of the physician as a clinician and as an investigator is of critical importance when the clinical diagnosis is at odds with the catheter findings. Diagnosis then becomes a matter requiring great judgement since either some of the data (clinical or laboratory) is erroneous, or is being misinterpreted, or the diagnosis is incomplete. A simple example may clarify this concept: a young adult has a moderately enlarged heart with an obvious rough systolic precordial thrill and murmur, with a fixed split pulmonary second sound. Catheter data, including left atrial angiocardiogram, show an atrial septal defect with considerable left to right shunt and normal pressure in the pulmonary artery and right ventricle. Electrocardiogram is not diagnostic. Here the obvious thrill suggests that a simple atrial septal defect is not a sufficient diagnosis. A coincident pulmonary valve stenosis is excluded by the pressure findings, provided the withdrawal tracing from pulmonary artery to right atrium is reliable. However, in occasional cases the catheter may flick from an infundibular chamber directly to the right atrium in cases with pulmonary infundibular stenosis, and the zone of high pressure in the inflow of the ventricle may thereby be missed. Pressure measurement during passage of the catheter to the apex of the right ventricle should avoid this. The angiocardiogram from either atrium is likely to give a poor visualization of the right ventricular outflow tract as the right atrial appendage is opacified. Even an angiocardiogram placed in the right ventricle may be a poor guide, for example, in cases with a subvalvar diaphragm which is often very difficult to see. Another possible cause of the thrill in the case under discussion is a small ventricular septal defect. This is commonly undetectable even by left ventricular angiocardiography and tracer techniques in the presence of a large atrial septal defect. Alternatively the findings might be due to the coincidence of aortic valve or pulmonary artery stenosis, the presence of a Gerbode lesion or some other anomaly. Only careful analysis of the clinical and catheter findings will allow a reasonable diagnostic compromise to be reached—in general the aim should be to exclude the presence of conditions likely to compromise an attempt at surgical repair of the established lesion (in this case an atrial septal defect), while avoiding a possibly dangerous pursuit by further investigation of lesions which can be safely neglected.

The *second* principle in preoperative diagnosis is the attempt to establish the presence of a lesion at catheterization by at least two independent methods. In the previous example of a patient with an atrial septal defect, the presence of the lesion would be suggested by the analysis of oxygen in the blood from the venae cavae and right atrium showing the entry of arterial blood into the right atrium; by the passage of the catheter from the right to the left atrium; the absence of a pressure gradient between the atria; the angiocardiography and, perhaps a tracer technique. Of all these techniques, the left atrial angiocardiogram is the most reliable. A foramen ovale can be traversed by the catheter as mentioned earlier but rarely allows a significant passage of contrast from the left atrium. The oximetry findings in atrial septal defect and anomalous pulmonary venous drainage are indistinguishable (and the distinction unimportant if the possibility is recognized). A pressure gradient may occasionally be found across a small atrial septal defect.

A further common example of the need for corroborative data is seen in infants with Fallot's tetralogy. Here it is unusual to enter the pulmonary artery and so record a gradient, but the angiocardiographic findings must be supported by a high systolic pressure recording from the right ventricle consistent with the diagnosis. If both ventricles can be entered by catheter, their pressures are almost always identical in Fallot's tetralogy. Very rarely the pressure in the right ventricle considerably exceeds that in the left (Fig. 18.5 and p. 160).

It is evident that the degree of corroboration and cross checking of catheter data which is possible, varies with the lesion and the resources available. When the apparatus is all working well and the investigator fortunate, the accuracy of diagnosis is close to 100 per cent. On off-days for either, there may be a galling and frustrating diagnostic performance which leaves the investigator unsatisfied. In such circumstances a further diagnostic catheterization may be needed.

Thirdly, decisions involving surgical treatment should be reached after joint consideration of the clinical and catheterization data by the surgeon, physician and radiologist. For this to be effective, regular meetings at which the angiocardiograms and catheter data are displayed for criticism and discussion should take place. The value of such discussions depends greatly on a mutual understanding of the limitations of the diagnostic and surgical techniques, since the welfare of the patient depends upon reaching the optimal balance between the diagnostic assessment of the lesion and the possible

benefit from a surgical modification of the anatomy, along the lines described at the beginning of this chapter—see the discussion of Table 18.1. In the great majority of cases the diagnosis is clear, and the decision a matter of little difficulty. In a few cases, however, the extent of any further desirable investigation may need much discussion of the interpretation of the available findings and the yield likely to accrue from further diagnostic procedures. Here it is essential for all concerned to know the limitations of each other's techniques. A simple example may be quoted. Heart failure is commonly due in infancy to the presence of a large ventricular septal defect. This is readily and safely demonstrated by venous catheterization of the right side of the heart when oxygen analysis of the blood samples and an angiocardiogram performed from the pulmonary artery or the left atrium will both demonstrate the lesion. Both techniques, however, may fail to show a coincident patent ductus. In this situation an aortogram can be performed, but is a difficult investigation involving arteriotomy and a considerable risk of causing narrowing or obliteration of an artery likely to be needed for open heart surgery when the infant is older. It is better at this age to leave the question of the ductus to the surgeon who can inspect the ductus and ligate it, if necessary before proceeding to band the pulmonary artery.

In complete contrast, when the child is older and being considered for repair of ventricular septal defect by open heart surgery using cardiac bypass, a patent ductus *must* be excluded if there is the least possibility of its presence, since the bypass technique is unworkable if the ductus arteriosus is patent. Here an aortogram by the Seldinger technique is a relatively simple exercise. (It is relevant to mention here that we have on two occasions so far encountered coincident ventricular septal defect and patent ductus in children in whom the right heart pressures were normal, the pulmonary artery samples did not show the second shunt, and there was no characteristic murmur of a ductus. The first patient was diagnosed on commencing bypass, the second by angiocardiography.)

Finally, errors of judgement should be accepted as failures of a team and their origin identified. In this endeavour the services of a pathologist are often necessary, for the risks of cardiac surgery leave little margin for mistakes of any kind. We have been fortunate in our pathologist colleagues who have preserved specimens of hearts and lungs intact so that the venous and arterial connections can be examined, and in the many detailed and helpful expositions of congenital abnormalities which we can compare with the diagnoses made in life from the catheterization data. The most useful form of inquisition into mistakes is a retrospective presentation of all available data with a critical discussion of the available facts. If a pathological specimen is available, its demonstration by the surgeon or pathologist is usually most illuminating.

A discussion in such a case between the surgeon, physician, radiologist and pathologist is well calculated to remove any symptoms of megalomania and induce a valuable humility in each one's approach to the other's problems.

Examples of some problems may help the reader to accept the limitations and difficulties of his craft. We have found double valve lesions on the left side of the heart peculiarly difficult to assess in better than the crudest terms. When both the mitral and aortic valves are stenosed the output is reduced and assessing the relative parts played by the individual valves is in our experience virtually impossible. Similarly mitral incompetence in patients with aortic valve disease may be the result of organic damage to the valve or functional changes in the ventricle. In many cases it is likely that both factors operate but the clear differentiation in the nature of the mitral leak is in our hands a very uncertain business. Reliable facts about these valves are easy enough to gather from catheter data, but reliable inferences from these facts are very limited in their scope. We find the demonstration by X-ray screening of heavy calcification in the mitral and aortic valves is of more value in deciding on the nature of the surgery required than all the tracings of pressure. Similarly the patient's account of his symptoms and capacity to work remains the prime consideration in advising him as long as valve replacement remains a matter of inserting a gadget or homograft of uncertain performance.

The difficulties are multiplied when a valve prosthesis is inserted. A single replacement on the left side can be assessed with fair precision by retrograde aortography and simultaneous transseptal catheterization but with mitral and aortic prostheses in place only gross failures can be demonstrated. As most failures of this order are accompanied by dramatic physical signs the catheter demonstration is commonly superfluous. More commonly the problem is to demonstrate that some unexpected sign, for example a cardiac murmur, does *not* indicate failure. Here simple pressure measurement will often give reassuring figures if it does not provide an explanation.

Infants not infrequently present with multiple intra- and/or extra cardiac septal defects. A particularly intriguing combination is a ventricular septal defect with a large left to right shunt, pulmonary hypertension and a patent ductus arteriosus with a right to left shunt. As in these infants the systemic arterial saturation is usually normal in the head and neck and reduced below ductus level, the calculations of cardiac output and the resistance in the pulmonary and systemic circuits is an exercise of more than usual complexity. It is a nice question whether it is reasonable to regard them as having a dynamic pulmonary hypertension in view of the shunt at ventricular level, or an Eisenmenger reaction as they shunt into the systemic system at the ductus arteriosus. In practice it

does not matter. The surgeon ligates the ductus and then if the pulmonary artery pressure remains high, bands the pulmonary artery.

Two further examples may illustrate difficulties in the diagnosis of particular cases. A fit, active uncyanosed boy of ten years was found to have catheterization data suggesting a simple ventricular septal defect. Angiocardiograms were not of good quality as the catheter used was of too small a bore to give an adequate bolus of contrast medium. After an abortive operation, the surgeon averred that the child had a common ventricle, a statement accepted by the physician with some reservations as the catheter data, although not entirely satisfactory, were incompatible with such a diagnosis, and the complete absence of symptoms or cyanosis was also highly unlikely in such a case. Some years later the investigation was repeated. The chamber entered on the first catheterization and believed to be a right ventricle proved to be an infundibular chamber. It opened into the pulmonary artery from a common ventricle into which normal mitral and tricuspid valves discharged their arterial and venous blood. The little mixing that occurred was masked by the left to right shunt into the pulmonary circulation. This shunting was only slight as the lungs were protected by the infundibular narrowing. The distance from the tricuspid valve to the origin of the side chamber (in which the pressure was only 40 mmHg) was only a centimetre or two. The original catheterization made when the child was much smaller had failed to record the short zone of high pressure just distal to the tricuspid valve. Even with good quality angiocardiograms, the infundibular chamber could not be distinguished with certainty in this case as the contrast medium filled the common ventricle quickly and obscured the detail in the right ventricular outflow tract where the catheter could not be persuaded to remain for angiocardiography. Each time a selective right outflow injection was made the catheter whipped out into the main ventricular cavity as soon as the pressure in the catheter increased. Injection into the pulmonary artery did not of course, show the abnormality.

This experience demonstrated a number of valuable lessons. All concerned had made a correct but incomplete diagnosis. The relatively inexperienced investigator at the initial catheterization had omitted a routine measurement which would have pointed to the need for further investigation—the withdrawal tracing from ventricular apex to the right atrium. The same lack of experience had led him to attempt an angiocardiogram with too small a catheter, since the insertion of a larger one would have necessitated a further skin incision to expose a larger vein. Better technique has permitted the recognition of this anatomy on a number of subsequent occasions, and it is now suspected in any case of apparent ventricular septal defect or Tetralogy of Fallot in which the catheter can only be retained in the 'right ventricle' with difficulty. Careful catheter manipulation and placing of the angiocardiogram injections will usually permit a reasonably certain diagnosis, and demonstrate that the apparent 'right ventricle' is in fact a side chamber opening off a larger, common, ventricle.

A further example illustrates the difficulties of assessing the dynamic state of the heart. A man of 38 was referred with increasing breathlessness. Some years previously he had been investigated and an atrial septal defect diagnosed. He was referred to another centre for advice. It was there concluded that the high pulmonary artery pressure and small shunt indicated a fixed high pulmonary artery resistance. He was advised that surgery was not possible. Reinvestigation showed a further rise in pulmonary artery pressure but a persisting left to right shunt. The patient had not worked for some years and felt himself a burden on his family. He was game for any risk, and urged that something be done. Surgical closure of the defect was therefore undertaken. With the defect closed, a pulmonary artery pressure of 25 mmHg was recorded on the operating table—a fall of 50 mm from the catheter figure. The patient returned to work and at recatheterization 3 years later was found to have completely normal pressures throughout the right side of the heart with no residual shunt.

In this case a somewhat experimental operation had a successful outcome. It illustrates the fallibility of calculation based on catheter data, and the need for having a patient's confidence and cooperation. The risks of surgery must be frankly discussed with a patient and his relatives, and set against continuing the status quo. Surgery of this sort is not always successful or, equally important, patients may refuse surgery which would confer great benefit at little risk. The physician and surgeon need a robust philosophy to live with the paradox which this paragraph has indicated—which is the greater failure (and whose failure is it?)—the unsuccessful operation on a patient who has encouraged the doctor by a courageous decision to take a considered risk, or the patient whose confidence does not extend to taking a much lesser risk?

References

BYAR, D., FIDDIAN, R. V., QUEREAU, M., HOBBS, J. T. & EDWARDS, E. A. (1965). Fallacy of applying the Poiseuille equation to segmental arterial stenosis. *Am. Heart J.* **70,** 2.

CAREY, J. S., WILLIAMSON, M. & SCOT, C. R. (1971). Accuracy of cardiac output computers. *Annals of Surg.* **174,** 762.

CARLETON, R. (1971). Change in left ventricular volume during angiocardiography. *Am. J. Cardiol.* **27,** 460.

FEICHTMEIR, T. V. (1957). Uses of cardiac catheterization in acquired heart disease. *New Engl. J. Med.* **257,** 121.

FOWLER, N. O., MANNIX, E. P. & NOBLE, W. (1957). Difficulties in the interpretation of right heart catheterization data. *Am. Heart J.* **53,** 343.

KITLAK, W. (1966). Diagnostische Schwierifkeiten in der Abgrenzung eines offen Ductus Arteriosus Botalli von einem aorto-pulmonalen Septumdefect. *Z. Kreislaufforsch.* **55,** 557.

MEYER, P., MOORE, G., BROBMAN, G. F. & JACOBSON, E. D. (1970). Assessment of an electromagnetic catheter tip velocity meter. *Am. Heart J.* **80,** 846.

MORRIS, J., THOMSON, H. K., Jr., RACKLEY, C. E., WHALEN, R. E. & McINTOSH, H. D. (1966). Problems and complications with the use of side-hole catheters. *Am. Heart J.* **71,** 313.

NAGLE, R. E., WALKER, D. & GRAINGER, R. G. (1968). The angiographic assessment of mitral incompetence. *Clin. Radiol.* **19,** 154.

NORDENSTROM, B. (1960). Contrast examination of cardiovascular system during increased intrabronchial pressure. *Acta Radiol.,* Suppl. **200,** 1–110.

OLSSON, B., VANDERMOTEN, P., VARNAUSKAS, E. & WASSEN, R. (1970). Validity and reproducibility of determination of cardiac output by thermodilution. *Cardiology* **136,** 148.

RICHTER, H. S. (1963) Mitral valve area: measurement soon after catheterization. *Circulation* **28,** 451.

VEREL, D., GRAINGER, R. G. & TIN, S. (1973). A comparison of oximetry and angiocardiography in the localization and assessment of intracardiac shunts. *Zeitschr. f. Kardiologie* **62,** 149.

Atlas

KEY TO ILLUSTRATIONS IN THE ATLAS

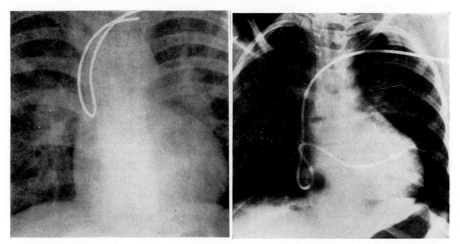

Fig. 1   Fig. 2

Fig. 1. An awkward situation which may follow an attempt to enter an atrial septal defect by looping the catheter in the atrium. The catheter descends via the innominate vein to the right atrium where it loops back up the innominate vein again. The loop will usually undo if the tip of the catheter is gently passed back to the right atrium by pushing more catheter into the vein at the operator's end. Occasionally this manoeuvre fails because the tip of the catheter does not move and pushing in more catheter merely enlarges the loop. In such a case, the loop has to be undone by passing the tip of the catheter into a neck vein, when withdrawing the catheter will then straighten out the loop.

Fig. 2. Another potentially dangerous situation. The tip of the catheter lies in the right ventricle and the catheter has a complex loop in the right atrium. A straight pull on this catheter results in the loop being tightened and drawn up into the superior vena cava. Pushing in more catheter enlarges the loop without undoing it. The catheter should be rotated gently one way and the other until it is apparent which way round the catheter is twisted. It can then be withdrawn after the appropriate rotation to loosen the loop has been applied.

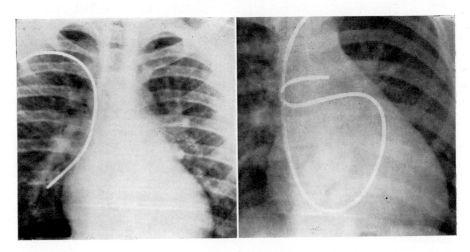

Fig. 3   Fig. 4

Fig. 3. Catheter passed to the right pulmonary veins by way of the right atrium, through an atrial septal defect into the left atrium. The appearance suggests an anomalous pulmonary vein draining into the *right* atrium, but an atrial septal defect was confirmed at operation. The obliquity of the atrial septum makes it *impossible* to determine whether the catheter has passed into the pulmonary vein from the right or the left atrium. A hand injection of contrast medium will usually confirm into which atrium the vein drains.

Fig. 4. An odd appearance which illustrates the limitations of the screening technique. The loop lies in the pulmonary artery. The appearance of a loop caught round the catheter in the right atrium is an illusion. Occasionally a catheter will not pass up the outflow tract of the ventricle tip first, but will enter the pulmonary artery while looped in this fashion. The loop is straightened by rotating the catheter slightly and withdrawing, when the tip can easily be persuaded to enter the left pulmonary artery.

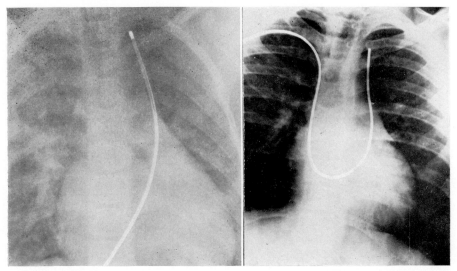

Fig. 5   Fig. 6

Fig. 5. The catheter tip lies in a left superior vena cava. The pressure measured at the tip is low; the oxygen saturation of the blood is usually fairly high. The catheter path in this case is inferior vena cava, right atrium, coronary sinus and left superior vena cava. Contrast medium injected by hand confirms the position, as it is seen under fluoroscopy to run back along the course of these veins until it is dispersed in the right atrium.

Fig. 6. Another catheter in a left superior vena cava. In this case and in Fig. 5, lateral screening shows the catheter passes behind the heart into the coronary sinus and thence into the left superior vena cava.

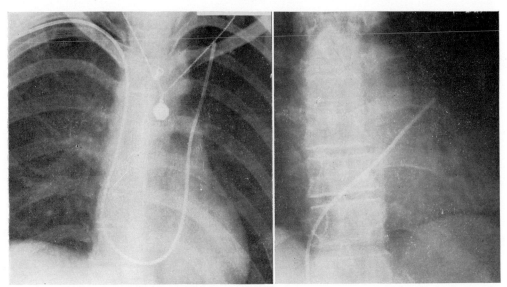

Fig. 7   Fig. 8

Fig. 7. The catheter lies in the left upper lobe branch of the pulmonary artery. If the catheter is wedged, the pressure tracing may resemble that found in a left superior vena cava. However, injected contrast medium outlines the pulmonary arteries and flows onwards. Withdrawal of the catheter while watching the pressure record, confirms the site in the pulmonary artery. (Note how closely Fig. 7 resembles Fig. 6.)

Fig. 8. The catheter in a coronary sinus. Note how it appears to lie in the right ventricular outflow tract. The wedge pressure in this site may resemble that of the right ventricle (Fig. 17.2). However, contrast medium injected by hand is seen to outline the coronary veins (Fig. 36 A/B) and flows back along the course of the catheter into the right atrium. Withdrawal shows low pressure once the catheter tip dis-impacts. If no left superior vena cava is present, the oxygen saturation is low (25 per cent or less). (A lateral film will show the catheter tip to lie posteriorly, not anteriorly as it would be were it in the right ventricle).

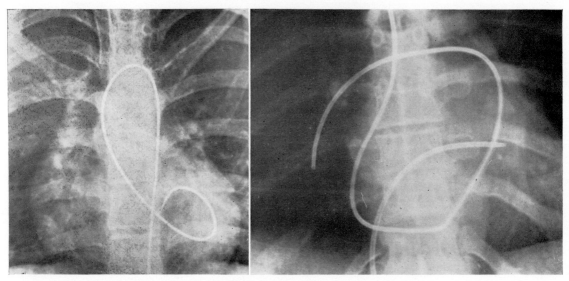

Fig. 9   Fig. 10

Fig. 9. Catheter passed from femoral artery and retrogradely through aorta and aortic valve into left ventricle.

Fig. 10. Catheter positions for simultaneous measurement of left atrial pressure and pulmonary wedge pressure (see Fig. 11.1). One catheter (Brockenborough transseptal) ascends the inferior vena cava to the right atrium and passes through the foramen ovale to the left atrium. The other catheter (Cournand) descends the superior vena cava to the right atrium, passes through the right ventricle to enter the pulmonary artery and wedges in the right lower zone.

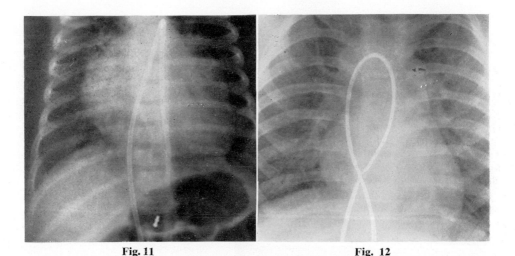

Fig. 11   Fig. 12

Fig. 11. Typical appearance of the passage of a catheter through a patent ductus arteriosus. The catheter passes up the inferior vena cava, then to the right atrium, right ventricle, pulmonary artery, through the ductus and down the aorta. Passage to the left lower lobe pulmonary artery may look very similar: the pressure and oxygen saturation may be no guide if Eisenmenger's Reaction is present. However, in the pulmonary artery, injected contrast medium is seen to flow to the pulmonary capillaries; if the catheter is in the aorta, the medium passes down the aorta. The passage of the catheter in this case to *below* the diaphragm confirms the aortic site.

Fig. 12. The catheter is passed from the leg veins through the inferior vena cava (on Rt. of mid-line), through right atrium, right ventricle, truncus arteriosus and round a right sided aortic arch to descend down a right descending aorta which crosses the mid-line at the diaphragm to descend as a left sided abdominal aorta. (This is the same 2 yr. old child whose angiograms are illustrated in Fig. 82A and B.)

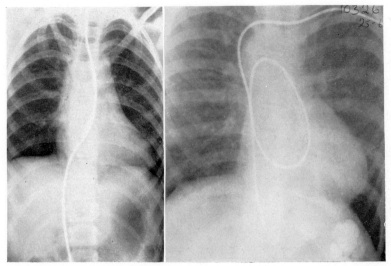

Fig. 13   Fig. 14

Fig. 13. Typical appearance of a catheter passed into an over-riding aorta in Fallot's tetralogy. The catheter passes up the inferior vena cava to the right atrium, the right ventricle and directly to the ascending aorta. A somewhat similar appearance is sometimes seen in patients with a ventricular septal defect when the progression of the catheter is right atrium, right ventricle, left ventricle and aorta.

Fig. 14. An unusual catheter position in a patient with an aorto-pulmonary window and right sided aorta. The progression here is left arm, superior vena cava, right atrium, thence to right ventricle, pulmonary artery, aorto-pulmonary window and right sided aorta. Again the aortic knuckle can be seen on the right—compare Fig. 12.

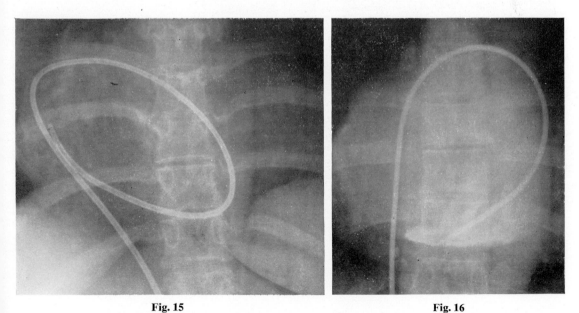

Fig. 15   Fig. 16

Fig. 15. Catheter looped in a large right atrium in a patient with tricuspid and mitral stenosis.

Fig. 16. Catheter looped in the left atrium in a patient with mitral stenosis. (Transseptal catheterization by Aldridge technique).

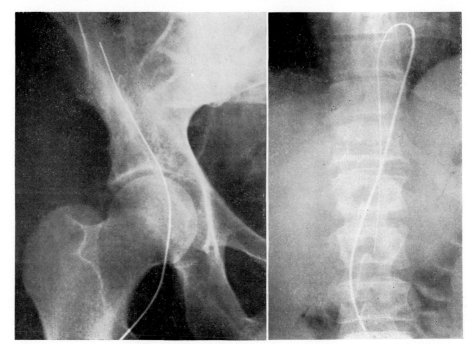

Fig. 17   Fig. 18

Fig. 17. Guide wire of Seldinger technique passed into right femoral artery: it travels laterally into the circumflex iliac artery instead of passing medially into the external iliac artery towards the aorta. See p. 101 for technique to correct this position.

Fig. 18. The guide wire from right femoral artery is looped so that its tip is pointed downwards instead of upwards. The catheter tip is sited at the apex of the curve but cannot be threaded on any further. (Guide wire was subsequently straightened by passing free tip into the left iliac artery—see Fig. 14.4).

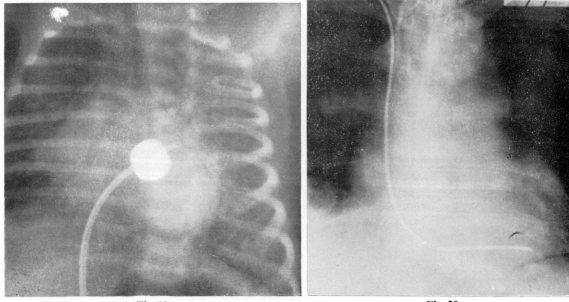

Fig. 19   Fig. 20

Fig. 19. Rashkind balloon catheter, fully inflated with 2 ml of contrast medium, lying in the left atrium of a 3 kg infant suffering from transposition of the great vessels. A number of previous withdrawals at lesser degrees of inflation had been made. The balloon should be withdrawn sharply into the right atrium and inferior vena cava until no resistance is felt as the atrial septum is traversed. In this manner, a large atrial septal defect is fashioned in order to permit mixing of blood.

Fig. 20. Bipolar endocardial pacemaking catheter in a stable position in the right ventricle.

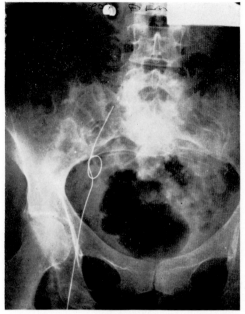

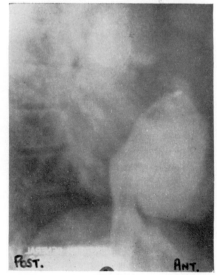

Fig. 21   Fig. 22

Fig. 21. Guide wire knotted in common iliac vein. This knot was tied during an apparently uneventful insertion of a Seldinger wire and revealed when the guide wire did not pass the catheter correctly. Before this film was taken, the catheter was removed from the guide wire. The knot was untied by the technique described in the text (page 142).

Fig. 22. Float catheterization in transposition of the great vessels. In this child an attempt to enter the pulmonary artery by a manipulation of the catheter failed. The catheter was withdrawn. A Brockenborough transseptal puncture was performed and the catheter is shown in the left ventricle, having traversed the atrial septum and the left atrium. A fine polythene catheter is then passed through the Brockenborough catheter and floated up into the pulmonary artery where a small hand injection of contrast medium confirms its position. This child weighed 12·5 kg at the time of catheterization.

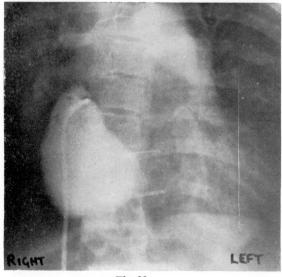

Fig. 23   Fig. 24

Normal Right Atrium

Catheter passed from saphenous vein through inferior vena cava into right atrium where the angiographic injection is delivered.

Fig. 23. Antero-posterior projection.
Fig. 24. Lateral projection. (N.B.—Dorsal spine on the Left.)

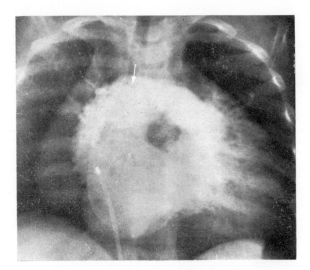

Fig. 25

Normal Right Atrium. Pericardial Effusion

Fig. 25. Right atrial injection demonstrating normal right atrium (with large appendage ↓) and right ventricle. 'Cardiac' shadow to right of atrium is due to pericardial effusion.

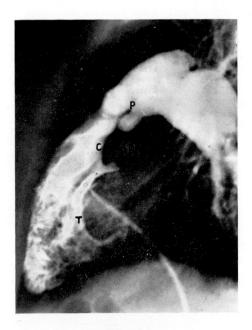 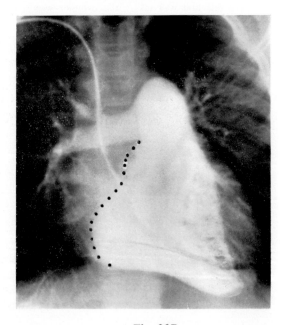

Fig. 26 A	**Fig. 26 B**
Normal Right Ventricle	**Normal Right Ventricle**

Fig. 26 A. Catheter passed through tricuspid valve (T) into right ventricle where the injection is delivered. The crista supraventricularis (C) separates the tricuspid valve from the pulmonary valve (P). This patient had pulmonary valve stenosis, and the jet of blood through the stenosed valve has caused the projecting nipple at the top of the pulmonary artery. (The dorsal spine is to the right of the photograph. This format is followed, with few exceptions, throughout this atlas.)

Fig. 26 B. Note triangular shape on antero-posterior projection, leading upwards into the pulmonary artery. Note that the right ventricle forms most of the diaphragmatic surface of the heart.

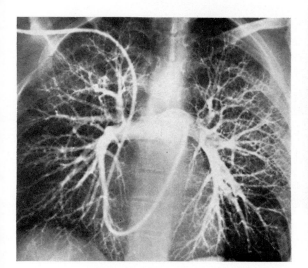

Fig. 27
Normal Pulmonary Artery

Fig. 28
Normal Left Heart (9 day infant)

Fig. 27. Injection delivered into main pulmonary artery. Even, gradual and delicate tapering of peripheral pulmonary arteries.

Fig. 28. Catheter passed from femoral vein through right atrium across patent foramen ovale into left atrium and then into the left ventricle where injection is delivered. Normal left ventricle, aorta, coronary, carotid, vertebral and subclavian arteries. Both carotid arteries and R. subclavian artery arise from a common origin. This occurs in about 7 per cent of normal people.

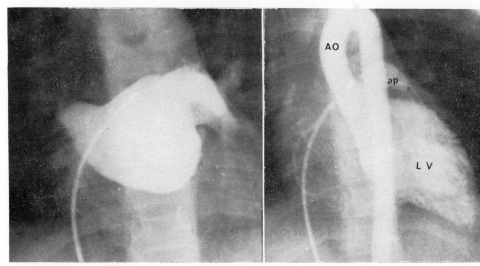

Fig. 29   Fig. 31

Normal Left Side of the Heart

Fig. 29. Catheter passed from leg veins into right atrium, through a patent foramen ovale into left atrium where the injection is delivered. Note prominent ear-shaped left atrial appendage forming midsection of left heart border. Mitral valve not yet opened.

Fig. 31. (Same patient 2 s later. Smaller magnification). Left atrium now clear of contrast medium except for appendage (ap) which is now much smaller. Normal left ventricle (LV) in diastole and aorta (AO).

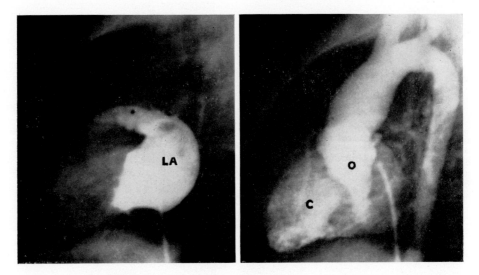

Fig. 30 A   **Fig. 30 B**

Normal Left Heart

A. Catheter passed from below through right atrium, foramen ovale into left atrium (LA). Note forward pointing atrial appendage.

B. The left atrium has now emptied into the left ventricle. Note the separation of the left ventricle into two distinct parts (1) the main cavity (C), and (2) the triangular outflow tract (O) leading up to the aorta.

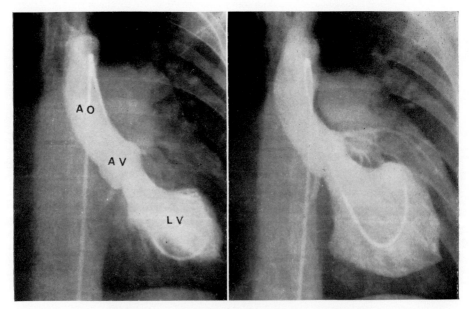

Fig. 32   **Fig. 33**

Normal Left Ventricle and Aorta

Retrograde passage of catheter from femoral artery through aortic valve into left ventricle.

Fig. 32.   Left ventricle (LV) in partial systole. AV—Aortic valve area. Coronary arteries beginning to opacify.

Fig. 33.   Left ventricle in diastole. Coronary arteries now well opacified.

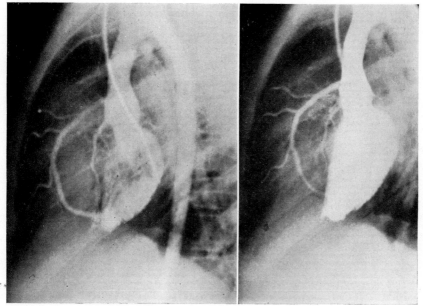

Fig. 34 A   Fig. 34 B

Normal Left Ventricle and Aorta

Catheter passed through arm veins into right atrium through foramen ovale into left atrium and thence into left ventricle where angiographic injection is delivered.

Fig. 34 A. Filling defect in mid left ventricle due to unopacified blood entering from left atrium.

Fig. 34 B. Ventricular septum seen tangentially in coronal plane, forming anterior border of left ventricle. This is unusual, as in normal heart the ventricular septum is 45° to coronal plane. Good aortic and coronary arterial visualization. Both frames are taken with ventricle in diastole. (Lateral projection.)

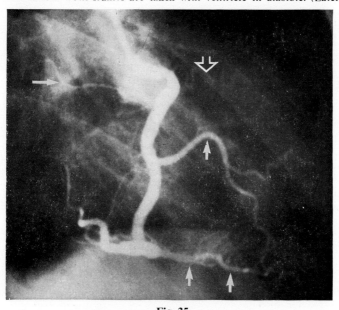

Fig. 35

Normal Right Coronary Arteriogram
Male aged 39 years
Right anterior oblique projection.
Judkins catheter.
Normal dominant right coronary artery.
(There was a localized stenosis of the left coronory artery). (Fig. 105.)

↑ Acute marginal branch.   ⇓ Conus branch.
↑ ↑ Posterior interventricular branch.   → Sino-atrial nodal branch.

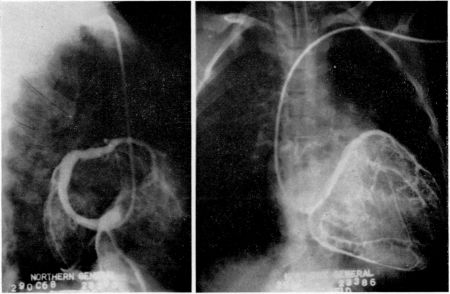

Fig. 36 A   Fig. 36 B
Normal Coronary Sinus

Fig. 36. Angiocardiographic demonstration of the coronary sinus system. These fine pictures of the venous system draining the myocardium were obtained when a catheter was passed to do a right ventricular angiocardiogram. The pressure tracings obtained were typical of the right ventricle, the catheter appeared to be in the right ventricular outflow tract, but no test injection was made to confirm the site of the catheter before angiocardiography. In fact the catheter was in the coronary sinus and the pressure tracing was a misleading one. No harm resulted from this unusual angiocardiographic investigation. (N.B. In Fig. 36A the dorsal spine is on the Left.)

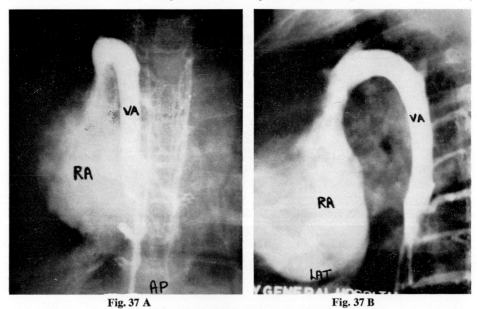

Fig. 37 A   Fig. 37 B
Vena Azygos Type of Venous Drainage
Girl aged 3 years

The venous drainage of the lower part of the body is conveyed by the azygos vein instead of by the inferior vena cava which is interrupted in the abdomen.

The vena azygos (V.A.) is greatly enlarged and arches over the right hilum to enter the posterior aspect of the junction of the superior vena cava and the right atrium (R.A.).

This venous anomaly is usually accompanied by intracardiac defects, frequently left to right shunts or malrotations. This patient had a large V.S.D.

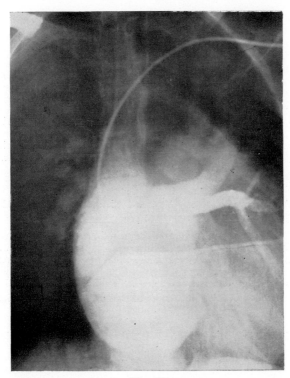

Fig. 38
Aberrant Pulmonary Vein (Left)

Fig. 38. Catheter passed from left arm vein into right atrium and then into the left upper lobe pulmonary veins which drains aberrantly into the right atrium. Injection into the L.U.L. vein confirms its drainage into right atrium.

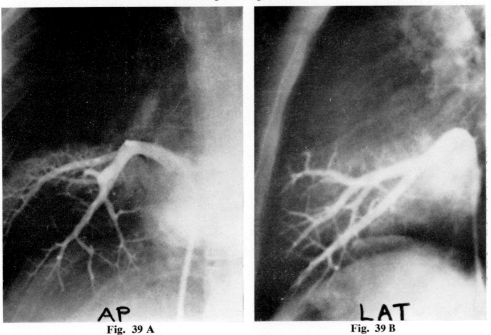

Fig. 39 A   **Fig. 39 B**
Partial Aberrant Pulmonary Venous Drainage
Male 24 years
The catheter has passed from the right atrium directly into the right middle lobe vein which conveys its oxygenated blood into the right instead of the left atrium.
This venous anomaly is often complicated by atrial septal defect, which this patient had.

Aberrant Pulmonary Vein (Scimitar)

Fig. 40. Scimitar vein drainage of the right lower lobe. In this patient a scimitar type vein drained the right lower lobe. A selective injection of contrast medium into this vein is shown. The vein is densely opacified by contrast medium which can also be seen in the right atrium. The scimitar vein drained into the inferior vena cava as is usual in these patients.

Total Anomalous Pulmonary Venous Drainage (Cottage Loaf Heart)
(Male 17 years)

Fig. 41. Catheter passed from right arm veins through right superior vena cava (R.S.V.C.) into right atrium (R.A.), and thence through right ventricle into main pulmonary artery where the angiographic injection is delivered. The illustration demonstrates the pattern of pulmonary venous drainage. The right main pulmonary veins (R.P.V.) pass behind the heart to join the left pulmonary veins (L.P.V.) to form the vertical vein (V.V.) which enters the left innominate vein (L.I.V.).

This crosses the mid-line to enter the right superior vena cava, which passes its blood into the right atrium.

This anomaly was completely corrected by fashioning an opening between the back of the left atrium and the junction of the pulmonary veins (R.P.V.), ligating the V.V. and closing the A.S.D.

Total Anomalous Pulmonary Venous Drainage (Obstructed)
(6 week old infant)

Fig. 42. Injection delivered into the main pulmonary artery. Right pulmonary veins (R.P.V.) join left pulmonary veins (L.P.V.) to form left superior vena cava (L.S.V.C. or vertical vein) which enters left innominate vein (L.I.V.). This vein is obstructed at ' O ' where there was a pressure gradient of 12 mmHg. The left innominate vein then enters the right superior vena cava which conveys blood back to the right atrium.

This infant presented in pulmonary oedema due to the obstructed pulmonary venous return. Autopsy confirmation: obstructing membrane found at ' O '.

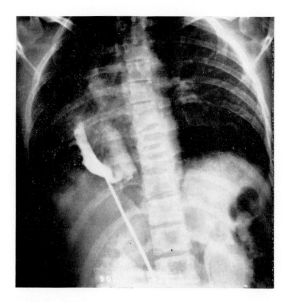

Fig. 40

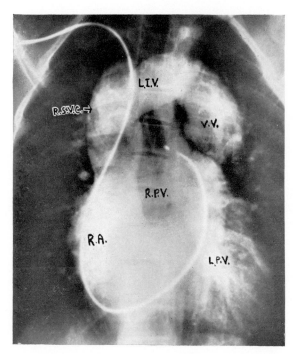

Fig. 41

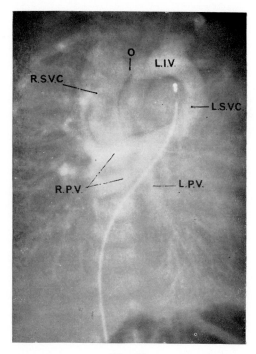

Fig. 42

Total Anomalous Pulmonary Venous Drainage. Infradiaphragmatic type

Fig. 43 A and B. Girl aged 2 months, presenting with pulmonary oedema. Death occurred in the next few weeks.

The catheter tip is in the pulmonary artery where the injection is delivered. The two illustrations demonstrate the pulmonary veins which join behind the heart to form a vertical vein (V.V.) which passes downwards, through the diaphragm to join the portal vein. This infradiaphragmatic type of aberrant venous drainage is almost always obstructed (either at the diaphragm or in the hepatic portal system), resulting in a severe rise in pulmonary venous pressure to cause pulmonary oedema, which is usually fatal. In Fig. 43 B the spine is on the left.

Atrial Septal Defect (Ostium Secundum)

Fig. 44. Catheter passed from arm veins through superior vena cava, through upper right corner of right atrium, across an atrial septal defect into the left atrium. The angiographic injection is delivered into the left atrium (L.A.) from which the contrast medium passes into right atrium (R.A.).

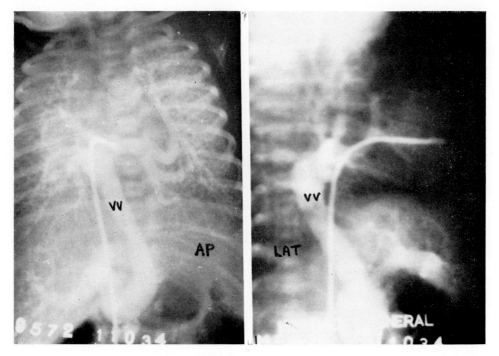

Fig. 43 A   Fig. 43 B

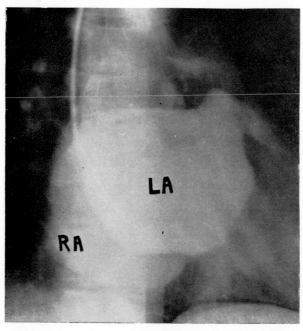

Fig. 44

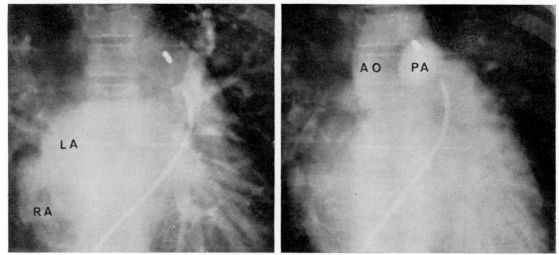

Fig. 45 A   Fig. 45 B

Atrial Septal Defect (Follow Through Angiogram)
Pulmonary artery injection in a patient with atrial septal defect

Fig. 45 A. The catheter tip can be seen in the pulmonary artery which is now empty of contrast medium. The left atrium (L.A.) has begun to fill, and already the right atrium (R.A.) shows early opacification through an atrial septal defect. This film was taken approximately three seconds after the pulmonary artery injection.

Fig. 45 B. A film taken 0·6 seconds later shows the right atrium completely opacified and the pulmonary artery (P.A.) now densely opacified by contrast medium. Both ventricles and aorta (AO) are also opacified by contrast medium. This series of angiocardiograms confirms the presence of atrial septal defect with a large left to right shunt, but does not eliminate the additional presence of ventricular septal defect or patent ductus.

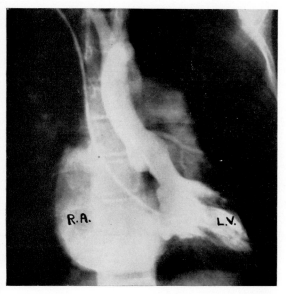

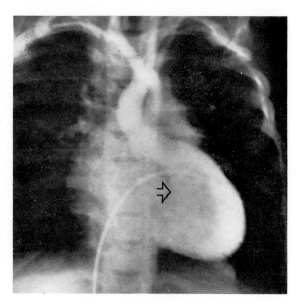

Fig. 46 A   Fig. 46 B

Atrial Septal Defect (Ostium Primum)

Fig. 46 A. Catheter passed from right arm veins through right atrium (R.A.) through atrial septal defect and left atrium into left ventricle (L.V.). Injection into left ventricle demonstrates large shunt directly into *right* atrium. The shunt actually passes through the incompetent mitral valve and then directly through the lower limit of the atrial septal defect into the *right* atrium. Despite the mitral incompetence, there is *no* opacification of the left atrium. See pages 129 and 163.

Atrium Septum Defect (Ostium Primum)

Fig. 46 B. Another patient. Injection into the left ventricle (catheter passed via right atrium and left atrium) demonstrates an abnormal concave right border of left ventricle which resembles a swan's neck in the AP view. This is due to the displaced mitral valve causing a deep concavity ($\Rightarrow$) of the right border of the left ventricle beginning immediately below the aortic valve. In this patient there is no mitral-valve incompetence.

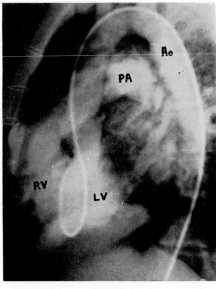

Fig. 47

Ventricular Septal Defect

Fig. 47. Catheter passed retrogradely round aortic arch into left ventricle (L.V.) where angiographic injection is delivered. There is a large shunt forwards into the right ventricle (R.V.) which ejects into pulmonary artery (P.A.). Note the interventricular septum is not seen in this lateral projection. See text, page 128.

This patient had previously had V.S.D. repair which broke down, as seen on this angiogram. Subsequent satisfactory V.S.D. repair at second operation.

Patent Ductus Arteriosus (4 year old girl)

Fig. 48 A. Catheter passed retrogradely round aortic arch into left ventricle where the injection is delivered. There is a faintly visible projection from the anterior wall of the upper end of the descending aorta. This is the patent ductus (↑) but there is very little flow through it.

Fig. 48 B. Same patient. The same catheter has now been manipulated from the descending aorta through the patent ductus, through the pulmonary artery into the right ventricle where the angiographic injection is delivered. No R to L shunt present. Catheter course confirms patency of ductus.

Patent Ductus Arteriosus (Before and After Ligation)

Fig. 49 A. Retrograde aortogram showing ductus ↑ (triangular in shape, base on aorta) leading to pulmonary artery anteriorly. Left to right shunt.

Fig. 49 B. Pulmonary angiogram (same patient) after operation of ductus ligation. Demonstrates an unusually long closed pulmonary stump of ductus ↓. No shunt.

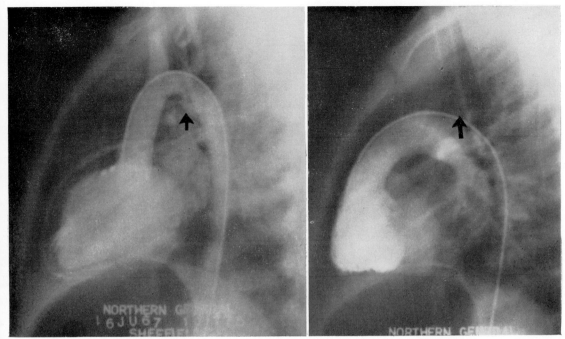

Fig. 48 A   Fig. 48 B

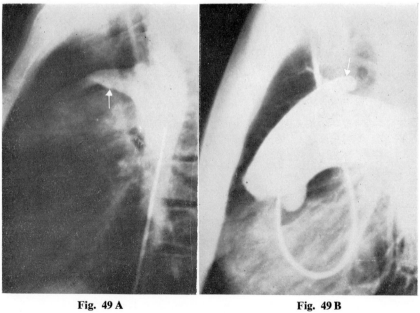

Fig. 49 A   Fig. 49 B

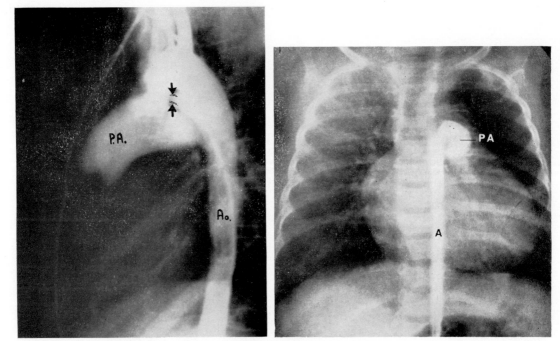

Fig. 50   Fig. 51

Patent Ductus Arteriosus (Young adult)

Fig. 50. Retrograde aortogram demonstrates descending aorta (Ao) from the upper end of which arises the patent ductus ↓ passing forwards to opacify the pulmonary artery (P.A.) which fills retro- ↑ gradely to the pulmonary valve.

Patent Ductus Arteriosus (4 week old infant)

Fig. 51. Retrograde aortogram demonstrates aorta (A) from upper aspect of which, the pulmonary artery (P.A.) opacifies through a patent ductus. Right heart angiogram demonstrated an associated atrial septal defect. Ductus ligatured at 9 months.

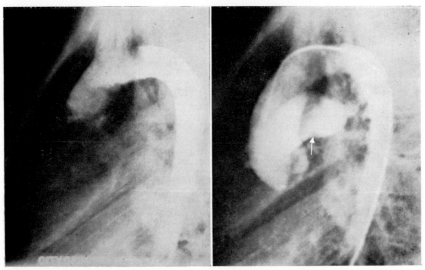

Fig. 52 A   Fig. 52 B

Aorto-pulmonary Window (Boy aged 11 years)

Fig. 52 A. Angiographic injection into aorta at usual ductus site. No shunt demonstrated and therefore patent ductus excluded.

Fig. 52 B. Catheter then advanced into ascending aorta where a second angiographic injection now opacifies pulmonary artery (↑). Indicating communication between *ascending* aorta and pulmonary artery.

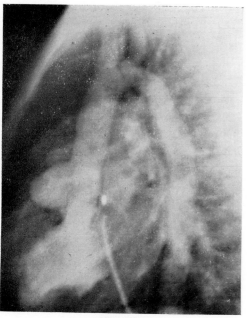

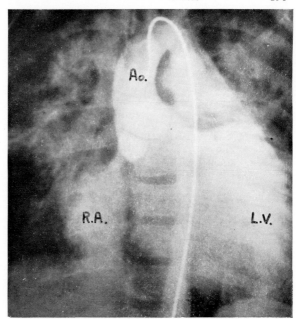

Fig. 53   Fig. 54

Prolapse of Anterior Sinus of Valsalva Aneurysm occluding Ventricular Septal Defect

Fig. 53. Catheter in left atrium. Angiocardiogram demonstrates aneurysm and an anterior prolapse of anterior aortic cusp. No shunt is seen at angiography but at operation the cusp was prolapsed into, and occluded a ventricular septal defect.

Prolapse of Anterior Sinus of Valsalva with Rupture into the Right Atrium
(Girl aged 4 years)

Fig. 54. Retrograde aortogram (Ao) demonstrates rupture of sinus of Valsalva with flow of contrast medium into right atrium (R.A.). There is also marked aortic incompetence (due to prolapse of aortic cusp) causing complete opacification of the left ventricle (L.V.).

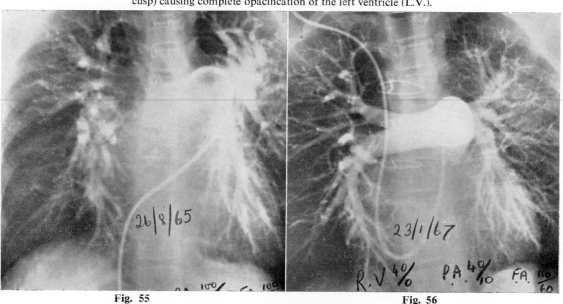

Fig. 55   Fig. 56

Closure of Ventricular Septal Defect
(Boy aged 12 years)

Fig. 55. Pulmonary angiogram demonstrates considerable pulmonary plethora. Equal systolic pressures in femoral artery and pulmonary artery (100 mmHg). Angiogram demonstrates left to right shunt (not seen here), but Eisenmenger Reaction is developing.

Fig. 56. Following surgical closure of ventricular septal defect, the pulmonary angiogram demonstrates normal pulmonary arteries. No shunt. Pulmonary artery pressure now reduced to almost normal level (40/0 mmHg). Marked clinical improvement.

Pulmonary Valve Stenosis

Fig. 57 A, B, C and D. Angiocardiographic injection delivered into right ventricle (R.V.) demonstrates jet (J) of contrast medium entering the dilated pulmonary artery (P.A.). The pulmonary valve cusps dome into the pulmonary artery during ventricular systole (A, C and D) indicating valve stenosis. The cusps are mobile as seen in diastolic phase (B). Note muscular contractions of infundibulum (INF) in systole (→ C): mobility of infundibulum is demonstrated by its relaxation in diastole (B). In D the contrast medium has already been entirely ejected from the right ventricle which now contains unopacified blood, which domes the stenotic pulmonary valve into the opacified pulmonary artery. Note eccentric dilatation of main pulmonary artery at point of impact of jet on upper border of pulmonary artery. A non-opaque jet can be seen (D). The radiographic contrast is now the reciprocal of (A).

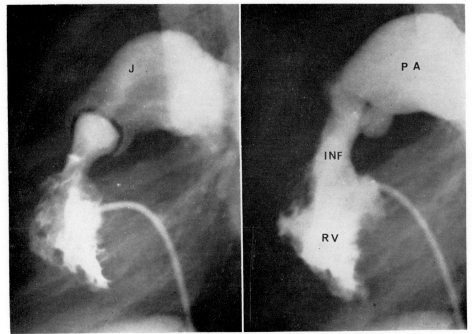

Fig. 57 A   Fig. 57 B

Pulmonary Valve Stenosis
(Adult)

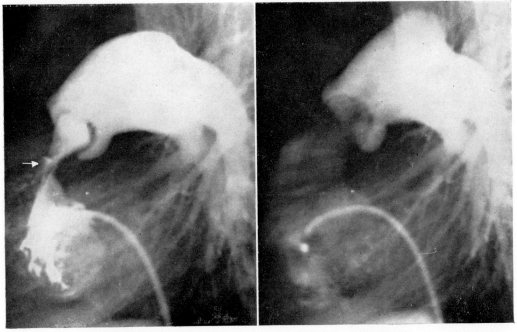

Fig. 57 C   Fig. 57 D

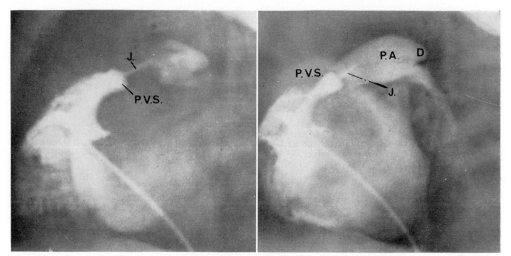

Fig. 58 A   Fig. 58 B

Pulmonary Valve Stenosis (Tight)

(6 weeks old)

Fig. 58 A and B. Injection delivered into right ventricle demonstrates 2 mm diameter jet (J) propelled through obstructing pulmonary valve (P.V.S.). Note variable narrowing of infundibulum of right ventricle below pulmonary valve. Dilated pulmonary artery (P.A.) presents a projection (D), which is the blind end of the ductus. Note that this projection (D) receives the jet emerging through the stenosed pulmonary valve as shown in Fig. 58 A. The infant died 1 day later, awaiting valvotomy.

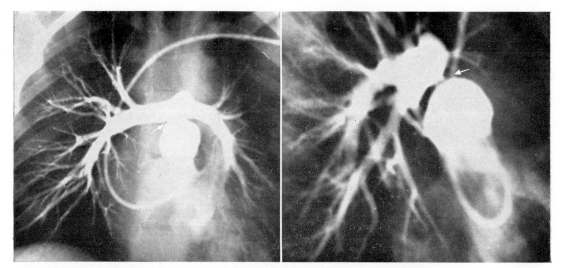

Fig. 59 A   Fig. 59 B

Banding of Pulmonary Artery for Ventricular Septal Defect

(Child now 3 years old)

Fig. 59 A and B. Two years previously the pulmonary artery was banded surgically to control a large left to right shunt through a ventricular septal defect. Note very tight constriction (→) of main pulmonary artery in A.P. (A) and lateral projection (B) due to the surgically applied band. There is now pulmonary oligaemia.

In Fig. 59 B the spine is on the left.

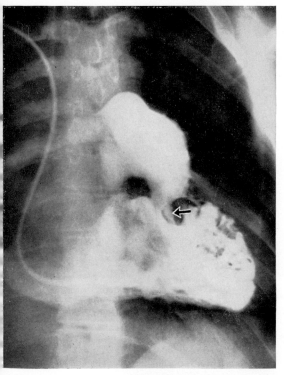

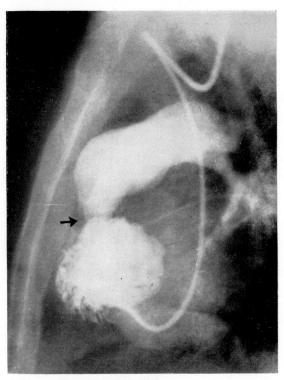

Fig. 60 A   **Fig. 60 B**

Fixed, Subvalvar Pulmonary Stenosis (Male aged 26 years)

Fig. 60 A and B. Marked narrowing of infundibular region of right ventricle (→), seen both on A.P. (A) and lateral projections. Right ventricular pressure of 140/0 mmHg.

At operation 5 G. of fibro-muscular tissue removed and a 3×4 cm teflon patch inserted in the right ventricular outflow. Post-operatively much improved. Post-operative angiogram **(C)** now shows normal outflow tract of right ventricle. Right ventricle pressure now only slightly raised—40/0 mmHg. No gradient at pulmonary valve.

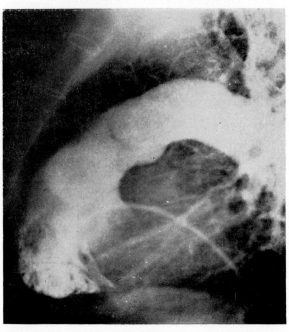

Fig. 60 C

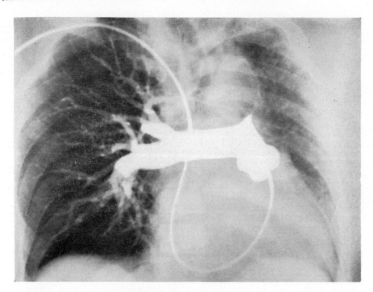

Fig. 61

Congenital Absence of Left Pulmonary Artery
(Male aged 30 years)

Fig. 61. Small left lung with no pulmonary arterial supply. This lung is perfused by hypertrophied bronchial arteries. This condition is better called 'Interruption of proximal left pulmonary artery' as the peripheral pulmonary tree may be present.

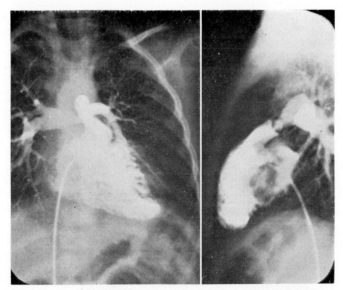

Fig. 62 A   **Fig. 62 B**

Fallot Tetralogy (Left Aortic Arch)

(Boy aged 3 years)

Fig. 62 A and B. Right ventricular injection demonstrates on the lateral film (B) a high, sub-cristal, ventricular septal defect, with opacification of the left (posterior) ventricle. The lateral film also demonstrates marked stenosis at and below the pulmonary valve. The antero-posterior film (A) illustrates moderate stenosis of the origin and distal post-stenotic dilatation of the right pulmonary artery. It also demonstrates premature opacification of the aortic arch and pulmonary oligaemia.

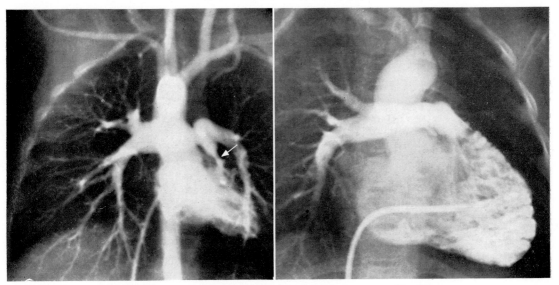

Fig. 63   Fig. 64

Fallot Tetralogy (Right Aortic Arch)

Fig. 63. Injection delivered into the right ventricle demonstrates very narrow irregular outflow tract (←). Aorta (right arch) filled because of right to left shunt at ventricular level. Left innominate artery with mirror image branching as is typical of right aortic arch in cyanotic congenital heart disease.

Fallot Tetralogy with absent Left Pulmonary Artery

Fig. 64. Angiographic injection delivered into right ventricle (enlarged and trabeculated)—pulmonary stenosis not well seen on this AP film. Absent left pulmonary artery. Left lung supplied by bronchial arteries which are not seen here. Marked right to left shunt demonstrated by opacification of aorta (left arch).

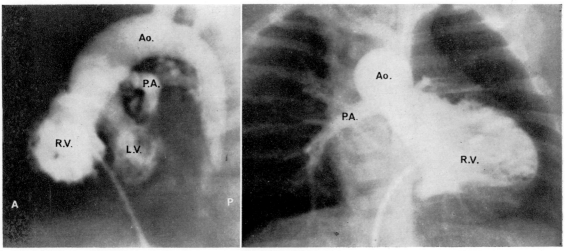

Fig. 65 A   Fig. 65 B

Severe Fallot Tetralogy
(2 months old infant)

Fig. 65 A and B. Angiographic injection delivered into right ventricle (R.V.) demonstrates right to left shunt into (posterior) ventricle (L.V.), small pulmonary artery (P.A.) and large aorta (Ao). The pulmonary artery and aorta arise in the same coronal plane, as seen on lateral radiograph (A). Severe pulmonary oligaemia.

C

Ventricular Septal Defect (Right to Left Shunt)

Fig. 66. Catheter passed from leg veins through right atrium into right ventricle (R.V.) where injection is delivered. Because of increased peripheral pulmonary arterial resistance (Eisenmenger Reaction), the right ventricular pressure is equal to left ventricular pressure. The ventricular septal defect ⥮ situated below the crista transmits a bi-directional shunt, the right to left component of which is shown here entering the left ventricle (L.V.).

Patent Ductus Arteriosus (Right to Left Shunt) (Eisenmenger Reaction)

(Child aged 2½ years)

Fig. 67. Angiographic injection delivered by catheter into the outflow of the right ventricle. Contrast medium opacifies the enlarged main pulmonary artery (P.A.) and its peripheral branches which are abnormally tortuous and of constant calibre instead of the normal tapering. This indicates pulmonary arterial hypertension. There is a right to left shunt through the patent ductus which is obscured in this radiograph by the main pulmonary artery. This shunt of contrast medium opacifies the descending aorta (Ao). Right and left ventricular pressure are equal at 110/0 mmHg.

Corrected Transposition of the Great Arteries

Fig. 68 A. Catheter placed in pulmonary artery which is displaced to the right to lie exactly in the mid-line.

Fig. 68 B. A few seconds later, the contrast medium has passed through the lungs and pulmonary veins to opacify the left atrium (L.A.). The contrast medium then passes through the anterior (right) ventricle to opacify the aorta. The ascending aorta arches *anti*-clockwise over the left hilum to become the descending aorta. The aortic origin is displaced to lie to the left of the pulmonary artery and in the same coronal plane. Despite the transposition of the great arteries, the circulation pathways are physiological, i.e. the pulmonary venous blood is distributed by the left atrium and right ventricle to the aorta. The transposition of the great arteries is 'corrected' by the inversion of the ventricles, i.e. the right atrium empties into the inverted left ventricle, and the left atrium empties into the inverted right ventricle. Unless complicated by other anomalies, patients with corrected transposition of the great arteries are *not* cyanosed.

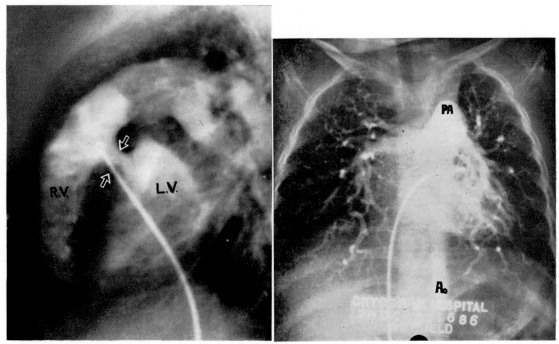

Fig. 66   Fig. 67

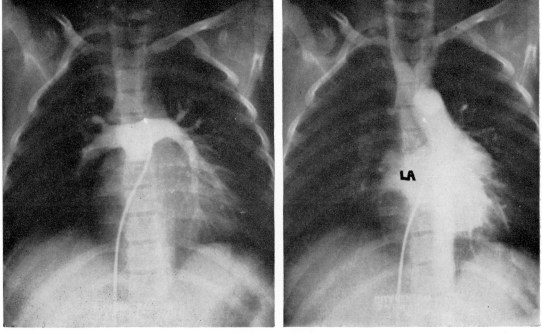

Fig. 68 A   Fig. 68 B

Corrected Transposition of the Great Vessels
Male aged 15 years

Fig. 69 A and B. (A) Lateral view and (B) Frontal view show anterior origin of transposed aorta. Note high position of aortic valve. Note anti-clockwise curve of aortic arch with the ascending aorta forming the upper left heart border in the frontal view. This is a characteristic feature of corrected transposition. Note abnormal origin of coronary arteries with anterior descending branch arising from the right (instead of the left) coronary artery. (Grainger, R. G. Transposition of the great arteries and veins. *Clinical Radiology,* 1970, **21,** 335—354.)

Transposition of Great Vessels (Uncorrected). Small Patent Ductus (7 days old)

Fig. 70 A. Anterior (right) ventricular (R.V.) injection opacifies the anteriorly transposed aorta (Ao) from which arises a small patent ductus (P.D.).

Fig. 70 B. Same patient. Posterior (left) ventricular (L.V.) injection opacifies posteriorly displaced pulmonary artery (P.A.). Intact interventricular septum.

S=sternum.

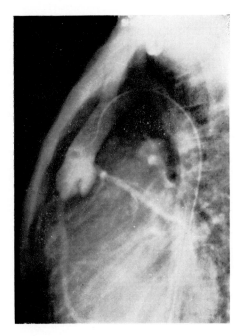
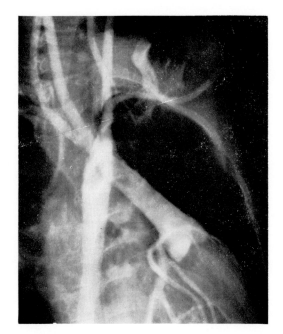

Fig. 69 A   Fig. 69 B

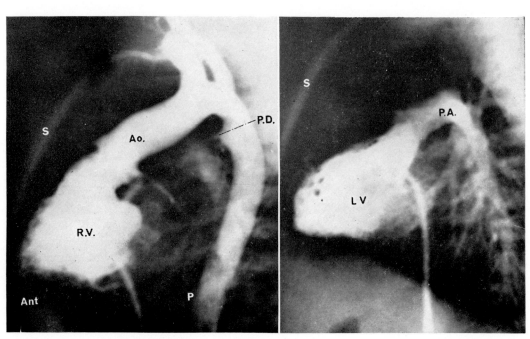

Fig. 70 A   Fig. 70 B

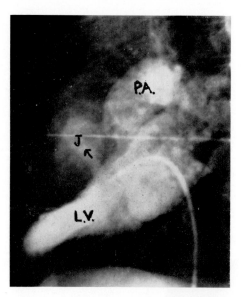

Fig. 71
Uncorrected Transposition of Great Arteries
Girl aged 4 years

Fig. 71. Catheter passed through left atrium into left ventricle where injection is delivered. Note the left ventricle (L.V.) empties into the posteriorly displaced (transposed) pulmonary artery (P.A.) Note jet (J) of contrast medium passing forwards through V.S.D. from left to right ventricle.

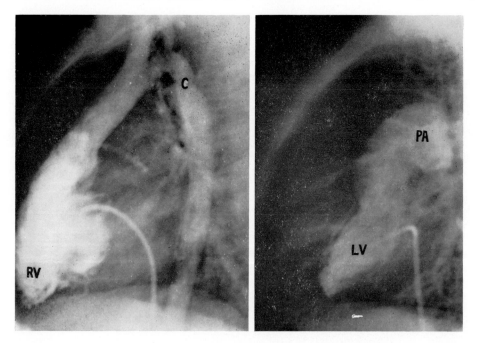

Fig. 72 A   **Fig. 72 B**
Transposition of Great Vessels (Uncorrected). Co-arctation of Aorta

Fig. 72 A. Boy aged 5 years. Right (anterior) ventricular (R.V.) injection demonstrates the anteriorly transposed ascending aorta. There is kinking and narrowing (coarctation, C) at the aortic isthmus due to coarctation.

Fig. 72 B. Left (posterior) ventricular (L.V.) injection demonstrates the posterior transposition of a large pulmonary artery (P.A.)

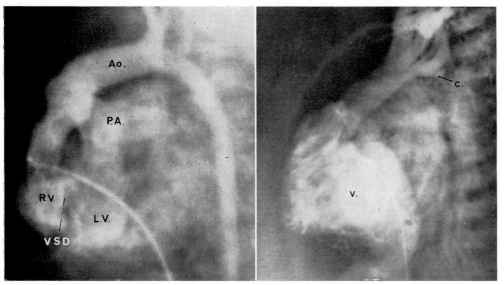

Fig. 73   Fig. 74

Transposition of Great Vessels (Uncorrected). Ventricular Septal Defect (3 weeks old)

Fig. 73. Right ventricular (R.V.) angiogram opacifies aorta (Ao), the origin of which is transposed forward to lie directly in front of the pulmonary artery (P.A.). Ventricular septal defect (V.S.D.) permits contrast medium to pass backwards into left ventricle (L.V.) which gives origin to posteriorly displaced pulmonary artery (P.A.). Note wide sweep of aortic arch and high position of aortic valve which lies above the pulmonary valve.

Transposition of Great Vessels (Uncorrected). Coarctation of Aorta (7 days old)

Fig. 74. Injection into common ventricle (V.) from which arises an anteriorly transposed aorta which is completely obstructed at coarctation (C). Faint pulmonary artery opacification behind ascending aorta.

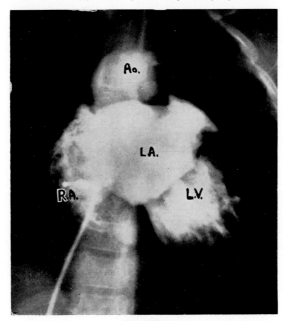

Fig. 75
Tricuspid Atresia

Fig. 75. Catheter tip touching right wall of right atrium (R.A.) into which the angiographic injection is delivered. There is no opacification of the right ventricle (note triangular gap between lower parts of right atrium and left ventricle). Instead of entering the right ventricle, the contrast medium has opacified a large left atrium (L.A.) which subsequently passes the medium into the left ventricle (L.V.) and aorta (Ao). Note no arteries are seen supplying the lungs. Later radiographs will show the lungs supplied either via V.S.D., P.D.A. or large bronchial arteries.

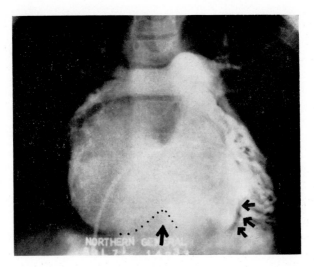

Fig. 76

Ebstein's Disease

Boy aged 10 years

Fig. 76. The right atrio-ventricular groove is indicated by ↑ . The displaced tricuspid valve is indicated by ←.

Between the two sets of arrows is the atrialized portion of the right ventricle.

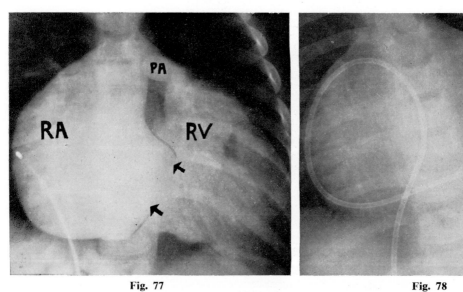

Fig. 77 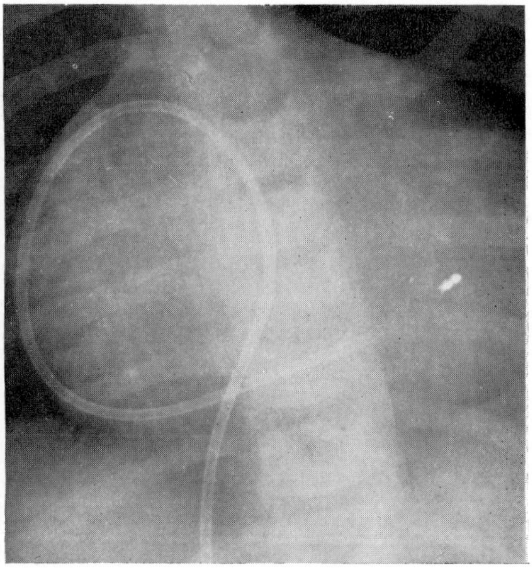   Fig. 78

Ebstein's Disease

Fig. 77. Large atrium (R.A.) with tricuspid valve (←) displaced to left, leading to a small deformed right ventricle (R.V.) which ejects the contrast medium into a tiny pulmonary artery (P.A.).

Fig. 78. The large catheter loop indicates the size of the right atrium. The catheter tip has just traversed the tricuspid valve.

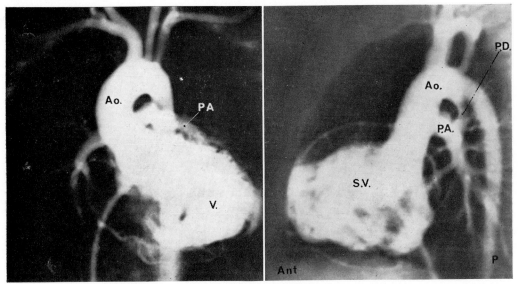

Fig. 79 A   Fig. 79 B

Atresia of Right Ventricular Outflow (Patent Ductus)

(4 days old infant)

Fig. 79 A and B. Injection into a single ventricle (S.V.) opacifies solitary outflow which is the aorta (Ao). There is no right ventricular outflow or proximal main pulmonary artery. A patent ductus (P.D.) passes contrast medium into peripheral pulmonary areteries (P.A.) — this is the mechanism of blood supply to the lungs which are oligaemic.

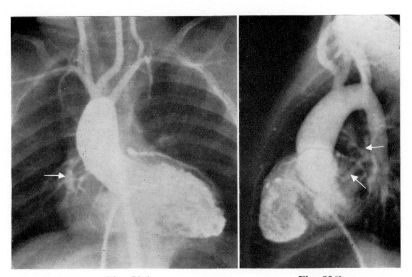

Fig. 80 A   Fig. 80 B

Pseudo-Truncus Arteriosus (or Type IV Truncus): Bronchial Arteries

(Child of 18 months)

Fig. 80 A and B. Injection delivered into the right (anterior) ventricle opacifies the left (posterior) ventricle via a high V.S.D. This is best seen on the lateral film which also demonstrates a solitary arterial outflow. This is the aorta or pseudo-truncus arising mainly from the left ventricle. The descending aorta supplies enlarged bronchial arteries (→) which provide the only blood flow to the lungs. Note absence of pulmonary arteries and the marked pulmonary oligaemia. Right aortic arch, which occurs in about 25 per cent of all truncus anomalies. If there is a diminutive R.V. outflow—the diagnosis is 'pseudo-truncus'.

Truncus Type IV: Very Large Bronchial Arteries
(Girl of 10 years)

Fig. 81 A. Catheter passed from leg veins, through common ventricle into aortic arch where injection demonstrates descending aorta (Ao) and many very large bronchial arteries (b), with stenoses (s) of two large right bronchial arteries.

Fig. 81 B. Catheter now in the functional common ventricle (C.V.) from which emerges a very large ascending aorta (Ao) or truncus. This narrows to a normal sized descending aorta after having supplied the large bronchial arteries. No pulmonary arteries are present, but there is a good blood flow to the lungs via the bronchial arteries. The aortic blood was found to have an oxygen saturation of 85 per cent.

Truncus Arteriosus (Type I)
(Boy aged 2 years)

Fig. 82 A. Catheter passed high into pulmonary artery where injection is delivered. Tortuous peripheral pulmonary arteries indicate Eisenmenger Reaction. Original film showed faint filling of a right descending aorta, indicating pulmonary-aortic arterial shunt, but the site was not visualized.

Fig. 82 B. Recatheterized from left arm. Injection delivered more proximally into the origin of the truncus arteriosus. Now there is opacification of both the aortic element (right sided arch) and the pulmonary artery arising from the left side of the truncus.

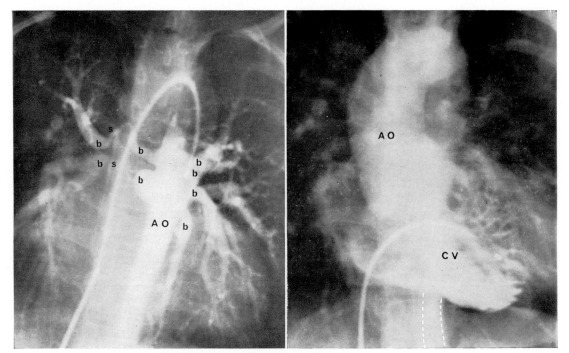

Fig. 81 A   Fig. 81 B

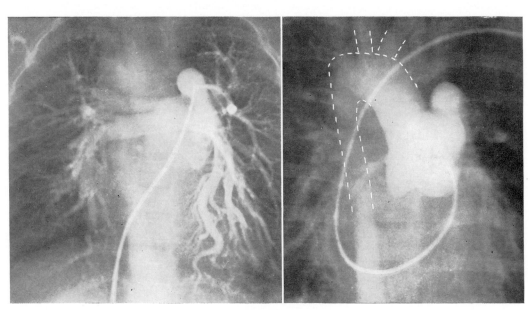

Fig. 82 A   Fig. 82 B

Hemi-Truncus with Pulmonary Stenosis
Left lung supplied by hemitruncus: Right lung supplied by miniature right pulmonary artery
(Girl aged 2 years)

Fig. 83 A. Catheter tip is placed in left ventricle. Angiographic injection into L.V. opacifies a truncus from which a large left pulmonary artery arises: the truncus continues into a right sided aortic arch. Note pulmonary valve stenosis (↑) with tiny pulmonary artery.

Fig. 83 B. The catheter is remanipulated into the small right ventricle, and through a stenotic pulmonary valve into a very small right pulmonary artery. The pulmonary valve stenosis can be seen on A to the left of the truncus. The left lung is therefore supplied by the left ventricle with a large quantity of oxygenated blood, but the right lung is perfused by a small quantity of blood from the small right ventricle.

[Fig. 83A and B are from the same catheterization session but the radiographs are reduced to different sizes for this illustration.]

Hemi-Truncus without Pulmonary Stenosis

Fig. 84 A and B. Girl aged 16 years. The right lung is supplied by a large pulmonary artery arising from the right ventricle. The left lung is supplied by a large pulmonary artery arising from the hemi-truncus. Note right aortic arch.

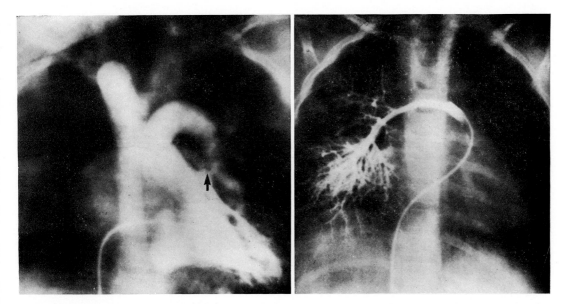

Fig. 83 A   Fig. 83 B

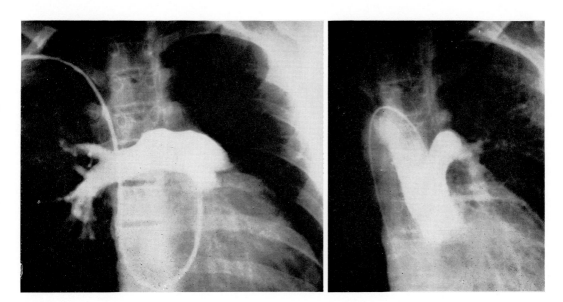

Fig. 84 A   Fig. 84 B

Congenital Aortic Valve Stenosis with Mobile Cusps (Girl aged 15 years)

Fig. 85 A. Aortic valve leaflets doming convexity upwards in ventricular systole indicating aortic valve stenosis. The cusps are adherent at their commissures and cannot separate. Considerable post-stenotic dilatation of ascending aorta affecting mostly the anterior aortic wall. Retrograde aortogram

Fig. 85 B. Same injection. Aortic valve cusps are now convex downwards in ventricular diastole. No aortic incompetence.

Acquired Aortic Valve Stenosis and Incompetence with Mobile Cusps (Adult female)

Fig. 86 A.   Aortic valve cusps now doming convexity upwards in ventricular systole—indicating valve stenosis.

Fig. 86 B. Injection delivered above aortic valve demonstrates moderate reflux into left ventricle (→). Valve cusps in diastolic position. Right coronary artery opacified.

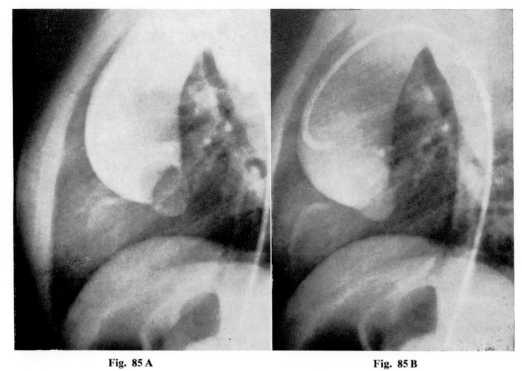

Fig. 85 A   Fig. 85 B

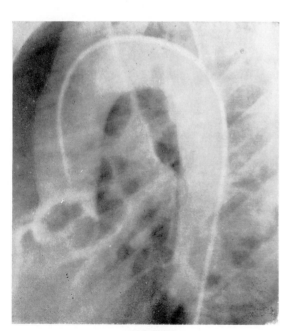
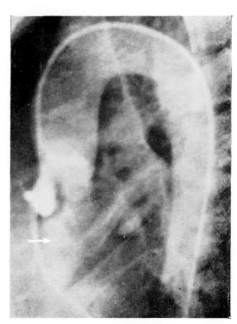

Fig. 86 A   Fig. 86 B

Supravalvar Aortic Stenosis

(Boy aged 7 years with characteristic facies)

Fig. 87. Well marked constriction of aorta immediately above the aortic sinuses which are dilated. Pressure in first part of aorta 160/80 mm. Pressure in aortic arch 120/80 mmHg.

Coarctation of Aorta (Long Segment)

(Girl aged 6 weeks)

Fig. 88. Right ventricular injection 8 seconds previously. Left atrium (L.A.), left ventricle (L.V.), ascending aorta (A.A.), coarctation (C.) and descending aorta (D.A.) are well opacified. Coarctation 8 mm long resected with end-to-end anastomosis.

Coarctation of Aorta with Aneurysms

(Male aged 23 years)

Fig. 89. Catheter (↑) introduced via right axillary artery into ascending aorta. Elongated coarctation demonstrated below origin of left common carotid artery. Multilocular aneurysms (An) distal to coarctation. Non-filling of left subclavian artery. Coarctation and aneurysms resected. Teflon graft.

Coarctation of Aorta with Sharp Forward Kink (Boy aged 3 years)

Fig. 90. Left atrial injection demonstrates left ventricle and aorta. Note very severe coarctation with tight ring stricture and marked forward kink. (N.B. posterior walls of aorta above and below narrowing show severity of kink.)

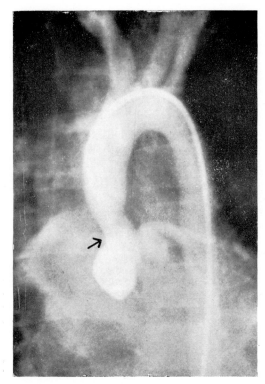

Fig. 87

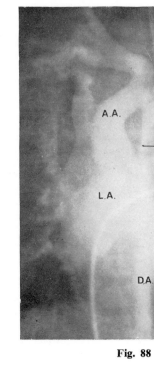

Fig. 88

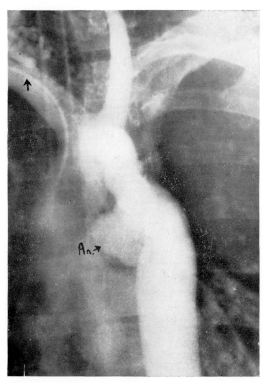

Fig. 89

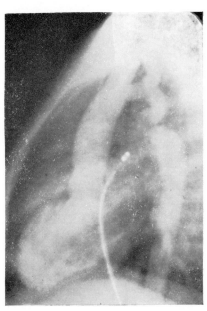

Fig. 90

D

Aortic Arch Hypoplasia

(Boy aged 10 days old)

Fig. 91. Left ventricular (L.V.) injection demonstrates normal ascending aorta (Ao) leading to a very narrow aortic arch (A), which proceeds to a normal descending aorta: (catheter passed through V.S.D.).

Pseudo-coarctation of Aorta with Sharp Kink (Girl aged 11 years. Left atrial injection)

Fig. 92. Sharp forward kink (K) of the descending limb of the aortic arch. No pressure gradient. No collateral circulation. Systolic murmur but no symptoms.

Pseudo-coarctation of Aorta

Fig. 93. Note high aortic arch, below which is the kink. The angiocardiographic injection is delivered into the rather large left atrium.

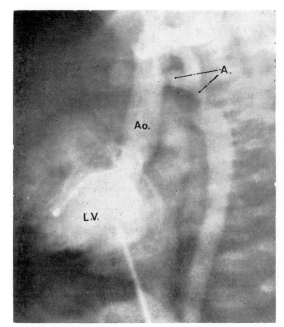

Fig. 91

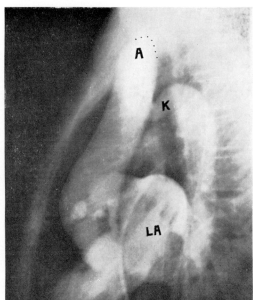

Fig. 92

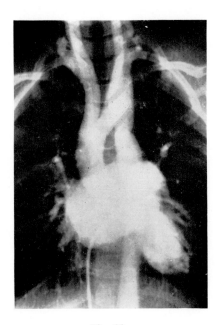

Fig. 93

Interruption of Aortic Arch

(Girl 1 month old. Right ventricular injection. Bi-directional shunt through V.S.D. opacifies the left ventricle)

Fig. 94. Complete obstruction of aortic arch beyond origin of left common carotid artery (←). No left subclavian artery opacification. 12 mm gap in distal aortic arch. The descending aorta opacifies later via a patent ductus which enters it distal to the atretic segment. The large P.A. obscures the atretic segment and the ductus.

Interruption of Aortic Arch (Post-stenotic Ductus)

(Boy 2 months old. Similar anatomy to Fig. 94)

Fig. 95. Pulmonary artery injection opacifies the descending aorta through a patent ductus transmitting a right to left shunt. The lower half of the body is supplied from the right ventricle as in the foetus. There was complete interruption of aortic arch as in Fig. 94.

Hypoplasia of Ascending Aorta. Coarctation. Patent Ductus with Aneurysm (Boy 3 weeks old)

Fig. 96 A and B. Angiographic injection delivered into right ventricle (R.V.). Pulmonary valve stenosis (P.V.S.), large pulmonary artery (P.A.) communicating by a patent ductus (P.D.) into descending aorta (Ao) which opacifies after a right ventricular injection. Aneurysm (A.) on patent ductus.
Very poorly developed hypoplastic ascending aorta (A.A.) which fills *retrogradely* from the ductus. Probably also a hypoplastic left ventricle.

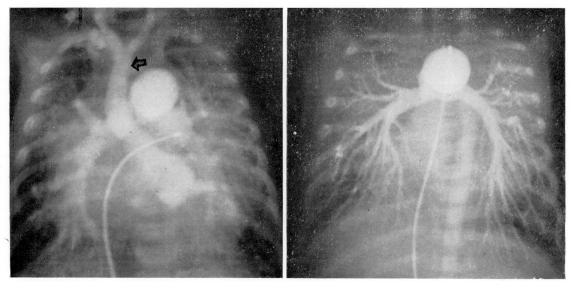

Fig. 94

Fig. 95

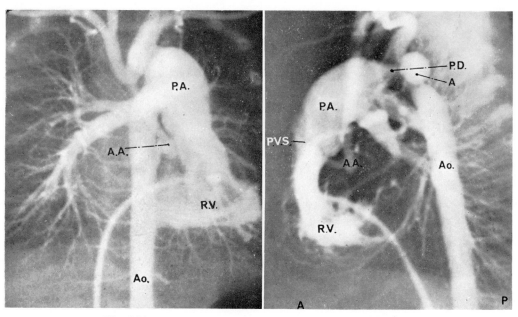

Fig. 96 A

Fig. 96 B

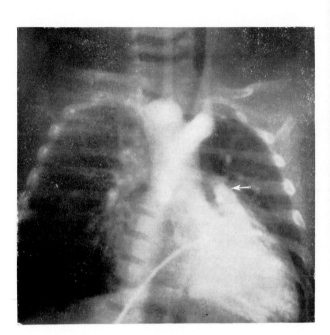

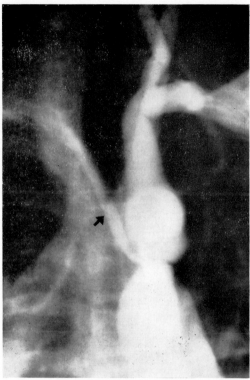

Fig. 97   Fig. 98

Double Aortic Arch or Aortic Ring in Patient with Fallot Tetralogy

Fig. 97. Angiographic injection delivered into right ventricle. Severe pulmonary outflow obstruction almost amounting to atresia (←). Large right to left shunt opacifies aorta which has a large right arch element and a smaller left arch element which join posteriorly to form a mid-line descending aorta. Each aortic arch supplies the carotid and subclavian arteries of its own side.

Coarctation of Aorta with Aberrant Right Subclavian Artery

Fig. 98. Note right subclavian artery (→) arising below the coarctation and passing upwards and to the right behind the oesophagus to reach the right axilla. This situation of the coarctation may cause notching of the left ribs but not of the right ribs.

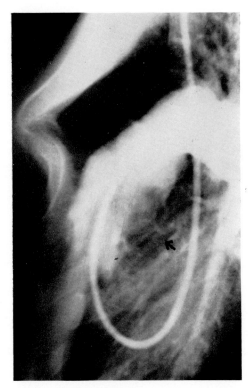

Fig. 99
Depressed Sternum

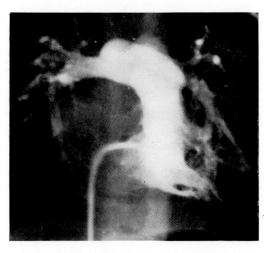

Fig. 100 A
Anomalous Left Pulmonary Artery
Girl aged 8 months

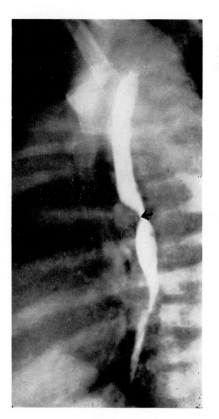

Fig. 100 B

Fig. 99. The right ventricular outflow is pressed backwards by the depressed sternum and is indented from behind by the unopacified ascending aorta (←).

Fig. 100 A and B. The left pulmonary artery arises to the right of the mid-line and winds round the right side of the trachea, then to the left between the trachea and oesophagus which it indents (→) as it passes to the left lung.

(Philip, T., Sumerling, M. D., Fleming, J. & Grainger, R. G. (1972). Aberrant left pulmonary artery. *Clinical Radiology*, **23,** 153.)

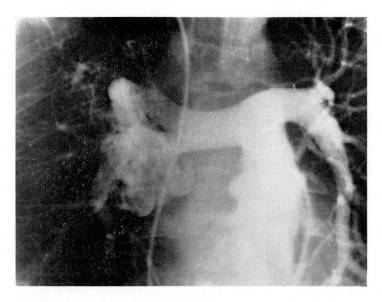

Fig. 101
Pulmonary Angioma
Adult male

Fig. 101. A large multi-locular aneurysm arising from the right upper lobar pulmonary artery.

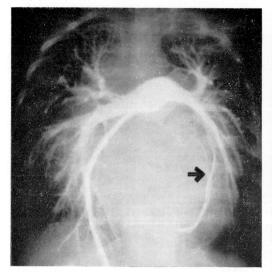 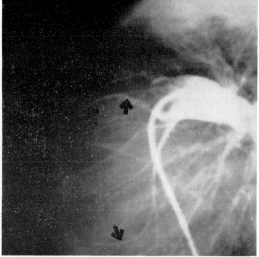

Fig. 102 A   **Fig. 102 B**

Anomalous Origin of Left Coronary Artery
Girl aged 1 week
Greatly enlarged heart, abnormal E.C.G.

Fig. 102 A and B. Pulmonary angiogram. The left coronary artery (→) including its anterior descending branch (↑) and obtuse marginal branch (↓) from the main pulmonary artery.
(Courtesy of J. Fleming.)

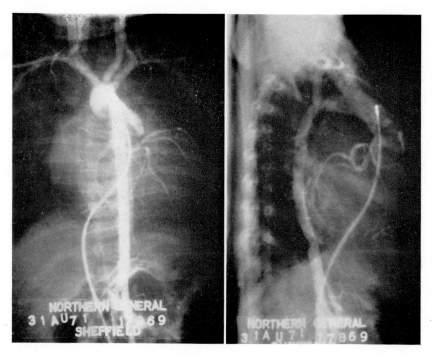

Fig. 103 A   Fig. 103 B

Single Coronary Artery

Fig. 103 A and B. Single origin of coronary artery in transposition of the great vessels. In this infant the angiocardiogram shows clear evidence of transposition with an anteriorly placed aortic origin. There is only a single (right) coronary artery. Rashkind balloon septostomy was carried out but the child did not survive more than a few days. The presence of a single coronary artery was confirmed by post mortem. In Fig. 103 B the dorsal spine is on the left.

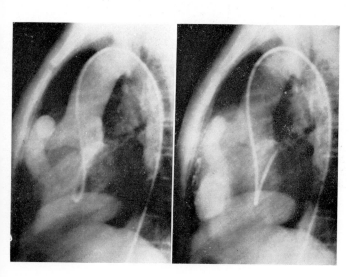

Congenital Right Coronary Arterial Fistula

Fig. 104. Girl with patent ductus arteriosus, previously ligatured. Persistent continuous murmur.

Injection into left ventricle demonstrates very large right coronary artery communicating with the right ventricle producing a major left to right shunt. The right coronary artery was ligatured at its point of entry into the right ventricle and the shunt was thereby terminated. No complication.

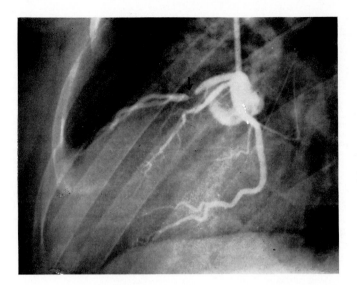

Fig. 105
Abnormal Left Coronary Arteriogram
Male aged 25 years

Left anterior oblique projection.
Judkins catheter.

Fig. 105. Localized severe narrowing (↓) of left anterior descending branch, possibly post-traumatic. (Courtesy of Dr. J. Fleming.)

Coronary Atheroma. Left Coronary Artery

Fig. 106. Left anterior oblique projection. Severe atheroma in first part (↑) of anterior descending branch of left coronary artery.

Note circumflex artery (→); obtuse marginal artery (⇉); left atrial branch (←).

Coronary Atheroma. Left Coronary Artery

Fig. 107. Right anterior oblique projection. Severe atheroma of circumflex branch (→). Note obtuse marginal branch (⇉).

Anterior descending branch (↑) is not well seen in this view and is severely narrowed.
Dominant left coronary artery supplying posterior interventricular branch (↑ ↑).

Coronary Atheroma. Retrograde Flow into Right Coronary Artery

Fig. 108A and B. (A) Left coronary arteriogram. Right anterior oblique projection. Note circumflex artery (→): anterior descending branch (↑).

(B) Two or three seconds later during the same injection. The posterior interventricular branch (↑↑) of the right coronary artery is now filling retrogradely, being supplied by branches of both the circumflex and the anterior descending branches of the left coronary artery. This retrograde flow is a reliable sign of obstruction of the proximal part of the right coronary artery.

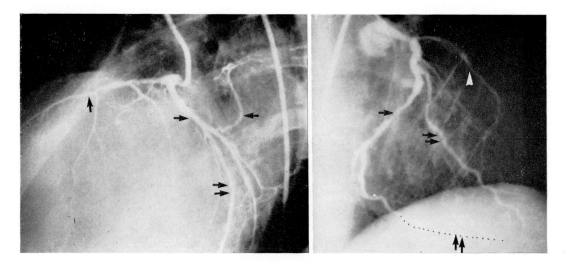

Fig. 106   Fig. 107

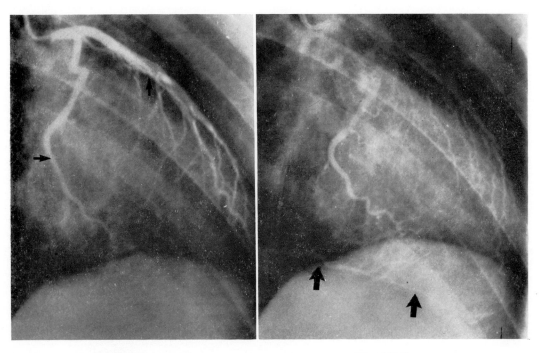

Fig. 108 A   Fig. 108 B

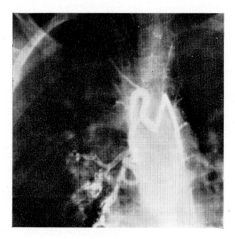

Fig. 109
Enlarged Bronchial Artery

Fig. 109. The child had pulmonary stenosis and transposition of the great vessels. The catheter is passed into the much enlarged right bronchial artery which enters the right hilum before ramifying in the lung. This enlarged bronchial artery is the principal blood supply of the right lung.

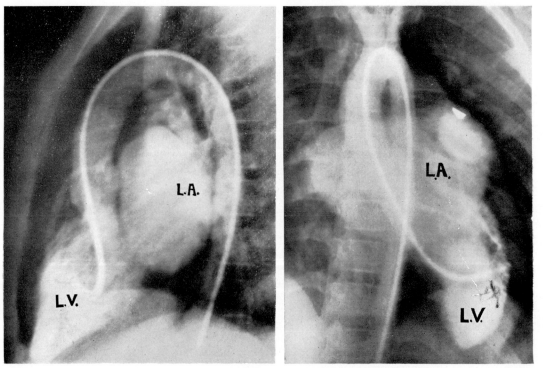

Fig. 110 A   **Fig. 110 B**

Congenital Mitral Incompetence (Boy aged 8 years)

Fig. 110 A and B. Left ventricular injection (L.V.) opacifies large left atrium (L.A.) by reflux through incompetent mitral valve.

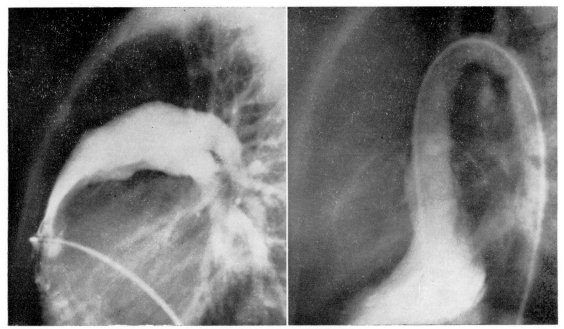

Fig. 111 A   Fig. 111 B

Hypertrophic Obstructive Cardiomyopathy
(4 years old boy)

Fig. 111 A. Injection into right ventricular outflow demonstrates a large curved indentation from behind
to compress posterior aspect of R.V. and main pulmonary artery.

Fig. 111 B. Retrograde left ventriculogram demonstrates indentation from in front, to compress anterior
aspect of left ventricle. Fig. A and B indicate mass in upper part of the interventricular septum.

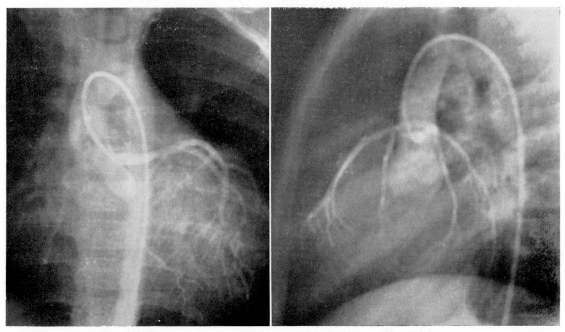

Fig. 111 C   Fig. 111 D

Fig. 111 C and D. Selective left coronary arteriogram demonstrates a dilated coronary arterial tree which
is stretched, basket-like (D) around a very vascular mass (C). This mass corresponds to the
lesion demonstrated in A and B, and is due to hypertrophied muscle in the upper part of the interventricular septum.

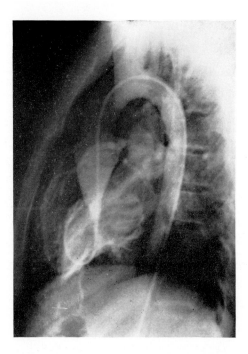

Fig. 112
Hypertrophic Obstructive Cardiomyopathy

Fig. 112. 'Carrot' sign in hypertrophic obstructive cardiomyopathy. Note the large coronary arteries and the great thickness of the ventricular wall. The aortic root is well shown and below it the ventricle has formed a triangular cavity resembling a carrot due to the gross hypertrophy of the muscle in the outflow of the left ventricle.

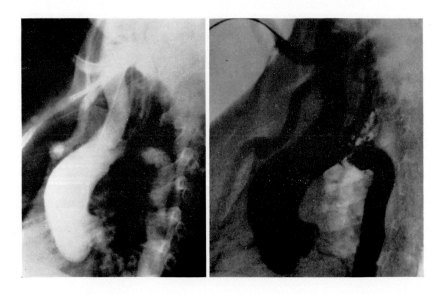

Fig. 113 A   **Fig. 113 B**

Photographic Subtraction

Fig. 113 A and B. Coarctation of aorta. Note much improved detail in region of coarctation on the subtraction film (B) compared to original radiograph (A).

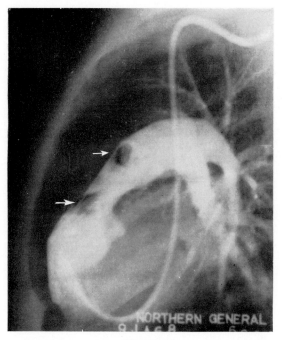

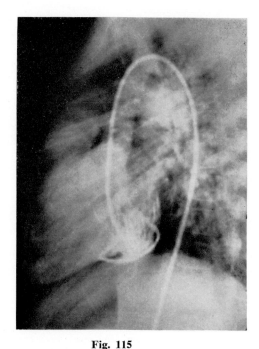

Fig. 114   **Fig. 115**

Air Embolism

Fig. 114.   Note two bubbles of air in main pulmonary artery due to faulty loading of Talley syringe. No adverse reaction. (Patient supine.)

Sub-endocardial Injection (Ventricular Septal Defect)

Fig. 115.   Retrograde left ventriculography with grey Kifa catheter. Striated appearance at posterior inferior angle of heart is due to deposition of contrast medium into myocardium. No adverse reaction.

Ventricular septal defect demonstrated by opacification of both ventricles, followed by both aorta and pulmonary artery. There is no suggestion on the lateral film of the interventricular septum, which lies too obliquely to be visualized in this projection. The left anterior oblique projection demonstrated the septum.

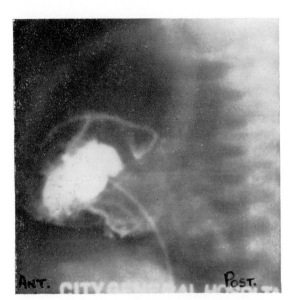 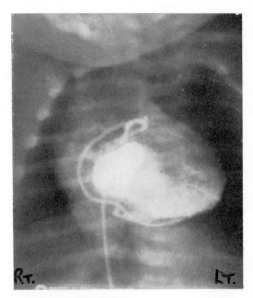

Fig. 116 A   Fig. 116 B

Extensive Sub-endocardial Injection

Fig. 116 A and B. Three week old infant with cyanotic congenital heart disease. It was impossible to find a catheter position in the right ventricle where the intra-cardiac E.C.G. was normal. Despite elevated S.T. segments, the angiographic injection was delivered and unfortunately resulted in a large intramural injection (the dense white blob). Note draining coronary veins which opacify within a second. No clinical adverse reaction. (Tricuspid atresia with tiny right ventricle.)

Index

Index

Filmset by Typesetting Services Ltd., Glasgow